ADVANCES
IN
IMMUNOPHARMACOLOGY 4

Previous Volumes in the Series

Volume 1 First International Conference, Brighton, 1980

Volume 2 Second International Conference, Washington, 1982

Volume 3 Third International Conference, Florence, 1985

Titles of Related Interest

ALEXANDER *et al.*	Bioreduction in the activation of drugs
MASIHI AND LANGE	Immunomodulators and non-specific host defence mechanisms against microbial infections
MITCHELL	The modulation of immunity
SIEST	Drug metabolism: molecular approaches and pharmacological implications
TIPPER	Antibiotic inhibition of bacterial cell wall biosynthesis

Journals of Related Interest *(sample copy gladly sent on request)*

Developmental and Comparative Immunology

Comparative Immunology, Microbiology and Infectious Diseases

Current Advances in Immunology

International Journal of Immunopharmacology

Molecular Immunology

ADVANCES
IN
IMMUNOPHARMACOLOGY 4

Proceedings of the Fourth International Conference
on Immunopharmacology,
Osaka, Japan, 16–19 May 1988

Editors

J. W. HADDEN
University of South Florida, Tampa, USA

F. SPREAFICO
Istituto di Ricerche Farmacologiche, Milan, Italy

Y. YAMAMURA
Osaka University Medical School, Osaka, Japan

K. F. AUSTEN
Harvard Medical School, Boston, USA

P. DUKOR
Sandoz Research Institute, Vienna, Austria

and

K. MASEK
Institute of Pharmacology, Prague, Czechoslovakia

PERGAMON PRESS

OXFORD · NEW YORK · BEIJING · FRANKFURT
SÃO PAULO · SYDNEY · TOKYO · TORONTO

U.K.	Pergamon Press plc, Headington Hill Hall, Oxford OX3 0BW, England
U.S.A.	Pergamon Press, Inc., Maxwell House, Fairview Park, Elmsford, New York 10523, U.S.A.
PEOPLE'S REPUBLIC OF CHINA	Pergamon Press, Room 4037, Qianmen Hotel, Beijing, People's Republic of China
FEDERAL REPUBLIC OF GERMANY	Pergamon Press GmbH, Hammerweg 6, D-6242 Kronberg, Federal Republic of Germany
BRAZIL	Pergamon Editora Ltda, Rua Eça de Queiros, 346, CEP 04011, Paraiso, São Paulo, Brazil
AUSTRALIA	Pergamon Press Australia Pty Ltd., P.O. Box 544, Potts Point, N.S.W. 2011, Australia
JAPAN	Pergamon Press, 5th Floor, Matsuoka Central Building, 1-7-1 Nishishinjuku, Shinjuku-ku, Tokyo 160, Japan
CANADA	Pergamon Press Canada Ltd., Suite No. 271, 253 College Street, Toronto, Ontario, Canada M5T 1R5

First edition 1989

Library of Congress Cataloging in Publication Data

Advances in Immunopharmacology.
Serial publication.
Serial catalog record and catalog card number
to be prepared.

British Library Cataloguing in Publication Data

International Conference on Immunopharmacology.—
4th. (1988)
Japan, Osaka
Advances in Immunopharmacology. 4
1. Immunopharmacology
I. Hadden, J. W. (John W.)
615'.7

ISBN 0-08-036149-8

Printed in Great Britain by BPCC Wheatons Ltd, Exeter

Contents

Secondary Immunodeficiency and its Therapy

Introduction and Overview on AIDS

JOHN L. FAHEY and BO HOFMANN

Center for Interdisciplinary Research in Immunology and Disease, Department of Microbiology and Immunology, UCLA School of Medicine, Los Angeles, CA 90024

Epidemiologic studies have defined the course of HIV infection and illness. Much experience has been gained in a study of the Natural History of AIDS being conducted as a multi-center AIDS cohort study (MACS) involving Los Angeles, Chicago, Pittsburgh and Baltimore where several thousand homosexual men at risk for AIDS have been seen every six months since 1984. An evaluation of the CD4 T cell changes revealed that CD4 T cell reduction is relatively rapid in the first year after infection for the group of those who seroconverted and that the rate of decrease for the mean of the group tended to reduce after one year (Fig.1) (Fahey, Giorgi, Martinez-Maza, Detels, Mitsuyusu, Taylor, 1987). The individuals within the larger population, however, show differences in the level of CD4 T cells and these relate to the onset of AIDS (Taylor, Fahey, Detels, Giorgi, 1988). When a large number of individuals who had been seropositive for several years were evaluated serially, many were found to have little or no reduction in CD4 T cell level over a several-year period. This plateau in the CD4 T cell level can occur at any level of CD4 T cells from 1,000 down to 200/mm^3 (Fahey, et al., unpublished). This suggests that the virus reaches a state of latency or low activity with which the host can cope, or that there are resistance factors which help to check the destructive activity of the HIV virus.

Several resistance factors have been postulated as contributing to the control of the virus. Neutralizing antibodies for the virus have been identified but not shown to relate to disease progression. Antibodies which produce antibody dependent cellular cytotoxicity (ADCC) have been identified (Ojo-Amaize, Nishanian, Keith, Houghton, Heitjan, Fahey, Giorgi, 1987) but additional studies so far have failed to reveal evidence that the level of ADCC antibodies correlated with the rate of CD4 T cell reduction or whether patients developed AIDS or remained AIDS free. Further studies of specific antibodies mediating ADCC activity, however, are underway.

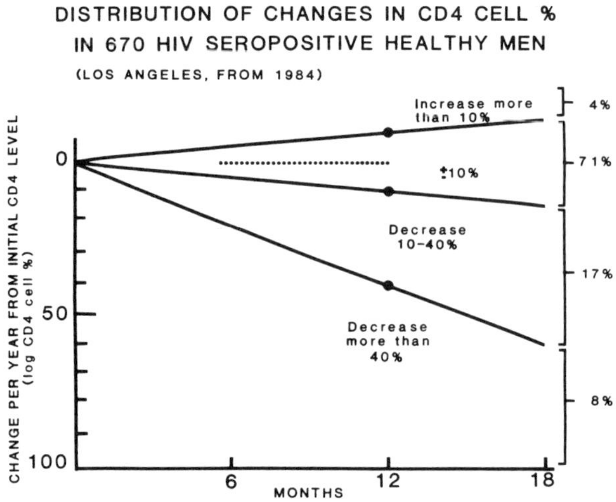

Fig. 1. Patterns of CD4 change in HIV-seropositive men. Homosexually active men (670) were followed serially at 6-month intervals. Seronegative homosexually active men varied only ± 10% in the slope of % CD4 cell measurements per year. The distributions of individuals within the persistently seropositive population with various slopes per year are presented.

There are many immunologic changes after HIV infection. Those seen at the time of diagnosis of AIDS are listed in Table 1.

TABLE 1

IMMUNE CHANGES IN AIDS

DEPRESSION	STIMULATION
Skin test anergy	Lymphadenopathy
WBC, Total lymphocytes	CD8 T cells
Total T cells	Immunoglobulins
CD4 T cells	Ig-secreting B cells
CD4:CD8 ratio	Soluble IL-2 receptor
T cell proliferative response	beta-2 microglobulin
mitogens, antigens	Neopterin
IL-2 receptor expression	IL-6
Lymphokine production	IL-1
IL-2, IFN gamma	
NK cell cytotoxicity	
Monocyte function	
chemotaxis	
antigen presentation	

In an effort to determine the relationship to prognosis, the tests that related to the occurrence of AIDS were found to be primarily the CD4 T cell levels, and related measurements, e.g., CD4:CD8 T cell ratio (Taylor, Afrasiabi, Fahey, Korns, Weaver, Mitsuyasu, 1986). Some but not all parameters reflecting immune stimulation also related to prognosis. Not related to AIDS prognosis were total numbers of B cells, total numbers of NK cells, NK cytotoxicity, serum IgG or IgM levels or delayed-type skin test anergy.

Immunopathogenesis is central to AIDS. Although several mechanisms have been shown to be able to decrease in CD4 T cell numbers in HIV infected cultures in vitro, the exact nature of the mechanism in vivo is still obscure (Table 2).

TABLE 2

POTENTIAL MECHANISMS OF CD4 REDUCTION

1. DIRECT CYTOPATHIC EFFECT VIA T4 RECEPTOR
2. SELECTIVE DEPLETION OF SUBSET OF T4 CELLS CRITICAL TO T CELL DEVELOPMENT FROM STEM CELLS
3. SOLUBLE FACTOR(S) WITH TOXIC EFFECT ON LYMPHOCYTE
   A. VIRAL PROTEIN
   B. CD4 CELL PRODUCT
4. AUTOIMMUNE REACTIONS

Cytopathogenic infection with HIV cannot entirely explain the destruction of CD4 cells since HIV expression in CD4 cells is very infrequent as demonstrated by in situ hybridization (Harper, Marselle, Gallo, Wong-Staal, 1986). Further, besides a decrease in CD4 numbers due to destruction, an impairment of the progenitor cells responsible for generation of new CD4 cells must be present since there is no evidence for CD4 T cell reconstituion of the type seen after bone marrow transplantation. A number of explanations have been offered for the CD4 reduction in vitro: binding of free or bound gp120 to the CD4 receptors of the CD4 cells resulting in syncytia formation (Sodroski, Goh, Rosen, Campbell, and Haseltine, 1986; Lifson, Feinberg and Reyes, 1986) and subsequent destruction of the cells. Binding of free gp120 on the surface of uninfected cells may also result in recognition of the cell as foreign and thus leading to destruction by the immune system (Klatzmann and Gluckman, 1986). Autoantibodies to CD4 cells and other lymphocyte subsets have also been demonstrated but are not expected to have in vivo importance, since they can be found in other diseases, e.g., after major surgery, which are not accompanied by immunodeficiency.

After exposure to HIV, the immune system responds to the infection by induction of antibodies to the individual proteins of the HIV virus. However, the existance of cell mediated immunity manifesting specific cytotoxic cells against HIV infected cells has been questioned since it may be difficult to distinguish between specific cytotoxic reactions and antibody dependent cytotoxicity. However, cytotoxicity against cells infected with genetic engineered vaccinia containing HIV gp120 genes indicates that such cells exist (Walker, Chakrabarti,

Moss, Paradis, Flynn, Durno, Blumberg, Kaplan, Hirsch and Schooley, 1987) although their role in the course of the infection is unknown.

Patients with HIV infection are often immunosuppressed at a time when they apparently have a substantial number of CD4 T lymphocytes left. Further, the low number of HIV antigen expressing cells in the peripheral blood indicates that other mechanisms than CD4 T cell depletion are involved in the developed immunosuppression. Several investigations of the function of the CD4 (Lane, Depper, Greene, Whalen, Waldmann, Fauci, 1985) and also the CD8 T lymphocyte subsets (Hofmann, Odum, Platz, Ryder, Svejgaard and Nielsen, 1985) indicate a defective proliferative response in these cells.

The monocytes/macrophages have also been demonstrated to be a target for HIV induced changes. A small subset of monocytes express CD4 receptors and may be infected via these receptors, other monocytes may become infected by direct internalization of the virus. HIV has no lysing effect on macrophages and HIV replication within macrophages is low. However, macrophages may transfer HIV to CD4 cells during antigen presentation.

Monocyte function is altered by HIV infection in some individuals with reduction of the helper component for T cell activation and proliferation and also for other macrophage functions (Prince, Moody, Shubin, Fahey, 1985) including the dendritic cells which are responsible for the stimulation of allogeneic cells as well as for presentation of microbial antigens for de novo responses (Hofmann, Odum, Jakobsen, Platz, Ryder, Gerstoft and Svejgaard, 1986).

Neopterin is produced in macrophages and serum levels are increased by HIV infection (Hutterer, Fuchs, Eder, Hausen, Knapp, Koller, Reibnegger, Werner, Wacher, Stingl, Wolff, 1987). Studies at UCLA (Melmed, et al., unpublished) have shown that HIV seroconversion is accompanied by a prompt rise in serum neopterin levels indicating that this change is an early response to HIV infection. Furthermore, the elevation of neopterin correlates well with the development of AIDS (almost as well as CD4 T cell levels). It appears that the macrophage functions may reflect several aspects of HIV infection. One is a direct stimulation of the monocytes and another is being the loss of normal regulatory processes because of reduced CD4 T cell levels. Further investigations of these mechanisms are in progress.

Multiple immunological abnormalities are characteristically associated with the immunodeficiency caused by HIV infection. It still has to be determined which of these abnormalities are primary and which are secondary to other defects, e.g., lack of induction from CD4 cells, lack of cytokine production, etc. Lysates of different HIV strains (Pahwa, Pahwa, Saxinger, Gallo and Good, 1985; Hofmann, Langhoff, Lindhardt, Platz, Ryder, Hyldig-Nielsen, Odum, Morling, Ulrich and Svejgaard, 1986) as well as purified gp120 (Mann, Lasane, Popovic, Arthur, Robey, Blattner and Newman, 1987) and peptides from gp41 (Chanh, Kennedy and Kanda, 1988) have been demonstrated to have suppressive properties in T cell proliferative assays. However, a suppressive factor produced in response to the HIV infection also remains a distinct possiblility. Further, sera from some asymptomatic subjects with antibodies to HIV seem to have a neutralizing effect on the suppressive effect of HIV lysate but whether this has any clinical importance remains to be investigated.

T cells are usually stimulated via the T cell receptor complex (T3-Ti) and/or the alternative pathway (CD2). Some investigations have pointed out that lymphocyte responses to PMW (Hofmann, Lindhardt, Gerstoft, Petersen, Platz, Ryder, Odum, Dickmeiss, Nielsen, Ullman and Svejgaard, 1987), which stimulates principally via the T3-Ti receptor, are more severely decreased than the response to PHA which stimulates via both the T3-Ti and T11 receptors. Direct stimulation of the CD2 pathway shows that this response seem to be largely preserved through the infection and even severely immunosuppressed AIDS patients seem to have a clear cut response (Hofmann, et al, unpublished). Stimulation of the membrane receptors usually result in an increase in the mobilization of intracellular calcium via an inositol trisphosphate dependent pathway and activation of protein kinase C via a diacyl glycerol dependent pathway. In normal T lymphocytes increased concentrations of intracellular calcium together with an activation of protein kinase C results in expression of receptors for interleukin-2, production of IL-2, and finally in DNA synthesis and proliferation. Our investigations have shown that PHA stimulation of lymphocytes from immunodeficient AIDS patients result in a normal increase in intracellular calcium. Furthermore, when both stimulatory pathways, the inositol trisphosphate pathway and the diacyl glycerol pathway, were stimulated directly with an ionophore and a phorbol ester, the expression of IL-2 receptors were normal in AIDS lymphocytes, while there was a severely decreased production of IL-2 (Hofmann, et al., unpublished). Thus, the HIV-induced changes in T lymphocytes appear to exist in mechanisms regulating functional gene expression.

The duality of HIV effects of the immune system is striking but the full significance is not well understood. HIV stimulation to the CD8 T cell system is evident in the increased number of CD8 cells that occurs within the first months after onset of HIV infection and is maintained until the terminal stages of illness in many individuals. Furthermore, the CD8 T cells exhibit evidence of activation in their phenotype and also immaturity (Salazar-Gonzalez, Moody, Giorgi, Martinez-Maza, Mitsuyasu, Fahey, 1985). They may, also, be functionally impaired.

B cell increases are not characteristically seen in the circulating blood but evidence of B cell stimulation is seen in the increased IgA and (frequently) IgG levels in individuals with HIV infection. The B cell activation can also be seen in terms of increased immunoglobulin secreting cells in the circulation. Also, phenotypic studies applying two-color flow cytometry have revealed evidence of activation and probably immaturity within the T cells during HIV infection (Martinez-Maza, Crabb, Mitsuyasu, Fahey, Giorgi, 1987). Evidence of increased number of B cells and CD8 T cells is also seen in the lymphadenopathy occurring in some individuals with HIV infection where both B cells and CD8 T cells are increased.

The immune system response to HIV infection is, indeed, complex. In addition to specific immunity as manifested by antibodies formed against many of the antigenic components of the HIV virus, the possibility of specific immunity in the cellular immune sytem has been described. Stimulation of the CD8 T cells and the B cells is clearly evident. The macrophages are altered with the HIV stimulation resulting in production of neopterin, IL-6, (Martinez-Maza, unpublished) and tumor necrosis factor. Finally, there is the damage occurring to the CD4 T cells with reduction in the CD4 T cell number. The diversity of immunologic responses to HIV infection has been delineated because of the interest of many investigators and the detailed knowledge of the immune system, its components and their function. Immunological research on AIDS is a part of the worldwide effort to develop improved means of therapy and prevention for AIDS as well as to learn from HIV infection about the mechanisms operating within the immune system in health and disease.

ACKNOWLEDGEMENTS

Bo Hofmann was supported by grants from the Danish Cancer Society and the Danish Medical Counsil.

The research of John L. Fahey is supported by NIH awards AI-15332, AI-23606, and AI-72631.

REFERENCES

Chanh, T.C., Kennedy, R.C. & Kanda, P. (1988). Synthetic peptides homologous to HIV transmembrane glycoprotein suppress normal human lymphocyte blastogenic response. Cellular Immunol., **111**, 77-86.

Fahey, J.L., Giorgi, J., Martinez-Maza, O., Detels, R., Mitsuyasu, R. & Taylor, J. (1987). Immune pathogenesis of AIDS and related syndromes. Ann. Inst. Pasteur/Immunol., **138**, 245-252.

Fauci, A.S. (1987). AIDS: Immunopathogenic mechanisms and research strategies. Clin. Res., **47**, 503-510.

Harper, M.E., Marselle, L.M., Gallo, R.C. & Wong-Staal, F. (1986). Detection of lymphocytes expressing human T-lymphotropic virus type III in lymphnodes and peripheral blood from infected individuals by in situ hybridization. PNAS, **83**, 772-776.

Hofmann, B., Odum, N., Platz, P., Ryder, L.P., Svejgaard, A. & Nielsen, J.O. (1985). Immunological studies in acquired immunodeficiency syndrome: Functional studies of lymphocyte subpopulations. Scan. J. Immunol., **21**, 235-243.

Hofmann, B., Odum, N., Jakobsen, B.K., Platz, P., Ryder, L.P., Nielsen, J.O., Gerstoft, J. & Svejgaard, A. (1986). Immunological studies in the acquired immunodeficiency syndrome: II active suppression or intrinsic defect-investigated by mixing AIDS cells with HLA-DR identical normal cells. Scand. J. Immunol., **23**, 669-678.

Hofmann, B., Langhoff, E., Lindhardt, B.O., Platz, P., Ryder, L.P., Hyldig-Nielsen, J.J., Odum, N., Morling, N., Ulrich, K. & Svejgaard, A. (1986). Patient antibodies against a potent suppressive factor associated with HTLV-III and possible therapeutic consequences. AIFO, **11**, 619621.

Hofmann, B., Lindhardt, B.O., Gerstoft, J., Petersen, C.S., Platz, P., Ryder, L.P., Odum, N., Dickmeiss, E., Nielsen, P.B., Ullman, S. & Svejgaard, A. (1987). Lymphocyte transformation to PWM as a predictive marker for development of AIDS and AIDS-related symptoms in homosexual men with HIV antibodies. Brit. Med. J., **295**, 293-296.

Hutterer, J., Fuchs, D., Eder, G., Hausen, A., Knapp, W., Koller, V., Reibnegger, G., Werner, E.R., Wacher, H., Stingl, H., Wolff, K. (1987). Neopterin as discriminating & prognostic parameter in healthy homosexuals, ARC, and AIDS patients. Wiener Klinische Wochenschrift, **15**, 531-535.

Klatzmann, D. & Gluckmann, J.C. (1986). HIV infection: Facts and hypotheses. Immunol. Today, **7**, 291-296.

Lane, H.C., Depper, J.M., Greene, W.C., Whalen, G., Waldmann, T.A. & Fauci, A. (1985). Quantitative analysis of immune function in patients with AIDS. N. Engl. Med., **313**, 79-80.

Lifson, J.D., Feinberg, M.B. & Reyes, G.R. (1986). Introduction of CD4-dependent cell fusion of the HTLV-III/LAV envelope glycoprotein. Nature, **323**, 725-728.

Mann, D.L., Lansane, F., Popovic, M., Arthur, L.O., Robery, W.G., Blattner, W.A. & Newman, M.J. (1987). HTLV-III large envelope protein (gp120) suppresses PHA-induced lymphocyte blastogenesis. J. Immunol., **138**, 2640-2644.

Mann, J.M. (1988). For a global challenge. World Health, 4-8.

Martinez-Maza, O., Crabb, E., Mitsuyasu, R.T., Fahey, J.L. & Giorgi, J.V. (1987). Infection with the human immunodeficiency virus (HIV) is associated with an in vitro increase in B lymphocyte activation and immaturity. J. Immunol., **138**, 3720-3724.

Ojo-Amaize, E., Nishanian, P., Keith, D.E., Houghton, R.L., Heitjan, D.F., Fahey, J.L. & Giorgi, J. (1987) Antibodies to human immunodeficiency virus in human sera induce cell-mediated lysis of human immunodeficiency virus-infected cells. J. Immunol., **139(7)**, 2458-2463.

Pahwa, S., Pahwa, R., Saxinger, C., Gallo, R.C. & Good, R. (1985). Influence of the human T-lymphotropic virus/lymphadenopathy-associated virus on function of human lymphocytes: Evidence for immunosuppressive effects and polyclonal B cell activation by banded viral preparations. Proc. Natl. Acad. Sci., **82**, 8198-8202.

Prince, H.E., Moody, D.J., Shubin, B.I. & Fahey, J.L. (1985). Defective monocyte function in acquired immune deficiency syndrome (AIDS): Evidence from a monocyte-dependent T cell proliferation system. J. Clin. Immunol., **5**, 21-25.

Sodroski, J., Goh, W.C., Rosen, C., Campbell, K. & Haseltine, W.A. (1986). Role of the HTLV-III/LAV envelope in syncytium formation and cytopathicity. Nature, **322**, 470-474.

Taylor, J., Fahey, J.L., Detels, R. & Giorgi, J. (1988). CD4 percentage, CD4 number, and CD4:CD8 ratio in HIV infection: Which to choose and how to use. (Submitted)

Walker, B.O., Chakrabarti, S., Moss, B., Paradis, T., Flynn, T. Durno, A.G., Blumberg, R.S., Kaplan, J.C., Hirsh, M.S. & Schooley, R.T. (1987). HIV-specific cytotoxic T lymphocytes in seropositive individuals. Nature, **328**, 345-348.

Taylor, J., Afrasiabi, R., Fahey, J.L., Korns, E., Weaver, M. & Mitsuyasu, R. (1986). Prognostically significant classification of immune changes in AIDS with Kaposi's Sarcoma. Blood, **67(3)**, 666-671.

AIDS Vaccine Development—1988

ROBERT B. COUCH

Department of Microbiology and Immunology, Baylor College of Medicine, Houston, Texas, USA

ABSTRACT

Effective control of AIDS will probably require development of an effective vaccine. Successes of the past in vaccine development have provided a framework for approaching the problem and a number of gene products have been described that could serve as vaccine immunogens. At present, all approaches to developing human immunodeficiency virus vaccines are being utilized. Acceptable virus vectors containing the human immunodeficiency gene segments for the envelope glycoprotein and recombinant DNA-produced envelope glycoproteins are receiving the most emphasis. In initial human trials, some products have been shown to be immunogenic. However, sufficient information on pathogenesis of HIV infection or vaccine effectiveness in animal models to ensure success in development of a vaccine is not available. A successful program will require cooperative efforts of scientists, government, and industry.

KEYWORDS

Human immunodeficiency virus vaccines; AIDS vaccines-1988.

INTRODUCTION

The prospect for a global medical crisis posed by the acquired immunodeficiency syndrome (AIDS) has prompted a scientific and governmental response to the problem of unprecedented magnitude. A part of this response has involved a program directed toward prevention of the development and progression of the disease in human populations. Since AIDS is the consequence of infection with the human immunodeficiency virus (HIV), traditional approaches to the control of infectious diseases are being evaluated for a possible contribution to the control of AIDS.

The three fundamental approaches to prevention of an infection are: 1) prevention of exposure, 2) chemoprophylaxis, and 3) immunization.

Efforts directed toward insuring a safe supply of blood and plasma products has significantly reduced transmission through their use. Efforts to alter behavior and thereby prevent transmission through intravenous drug abuse and sexual promiscuity are underway. The development of safe and effective antivirals that can be used for long-term prophylaxis of HIV infection is not likely in the near future. However, efforts are underway to determine the effectiveness of short-term post-exposure prophylaxis with Zidovudine among medical care personnel; in addition, trials of suppressive regimens among infected asymptomatic individuals are underway to determine if long-term prophylaxis can be given safely and be effective for prevention of the emergence of AIDS. Efforts toward developing vaccines for control of HIV infection have also been underway since the virus was isolated, a substrate for its cultivation was described, and the ability to measure immune responses was developed. This is appropriate since vaccines are probably the most highly effective and cost-beneficial means for disease control ever developed by the scientific establishment. Although knowledge is insufficient for projecting success in development, it is likely that effective control of HIV infection and AIDS will require development of an effective vaccine.

The Approach to Development of a Vaccine

The successes of vaccine development in the past have provided a framework for approaches to development of vaccines. This framework includes an understanding of antigens and of immune responses that have successfully conveyed immunity to other infections through vaccination. For virus infections, the major requirement has been development of neutralizing antibody to a level that correlates with protection against reinfection. Thus, determining whether immunity to reinfection with HIV exists and identifying its correlates must be considered a high priority for a vaccine development program.

Preclinical evaluation of vaccine candidates must indicate that the vaccine is immunogenic and potentially safe before proceeding to the clinical level. Providing this preclinical data involves immunogenicity and toxicology studies in conventional laboratory animals, toxicology evaluations *in vitro*, a precise definition of the components contained in the vaccine, and an indication that the manufacturing process leads to reproducible, stable preparations. At present, all preclinical studies should also include vaccination and subsequent challenge of chimpanzees with HIV.

Development at the clinical level involves establishing safety and immunogenicity in escalating numbers as an optimal vaccination dose, immunization route and schedule is developed. This information is then used for design of studies to establish efficacy in target populations. It should be stressed that features of an optimal clinical study are: a double-blind, placebo-controlled design; selection of a stable, compliant population; inclusion of adequate numbers for valid conclusions; objective endpoint criteria that are unambiguous; and obtaining of supporting data for understanding results.

Candidate Immunogens

The rapid and extensive elucidation of the molecular biology of HIV has identified a number of gene products that could serve as immunogens for vaccines. Potential immunogens are shown in Table 1.

TABLE 1 Viral Gene Products as Potential Immunogens for HIV Vaccines

Envelope proteins	-	gp 160, (gp 120, gp 41)
Gag (core) proteins	-	p 55, (p 18, p 24, p 15)
Polymerase proteins	-	p 66/51, p 31
Other proteins	-	p 27, p 23, p 20, p 14

HIV posseses a single envelope glycoprotein - gp 160; it consists of a gp 41 protein that provides a transmembrane anchor and gp 120, the attachment protein. The envelope glycoproteins have received the primary focus for vaccine development because of their traditional role as the protective antigen for viral vaccines and because successful subunit vaccines for retroviral disease in animals have contained envelope glycoproteins (Hunsmann, 1985). In this regard, it is of interest that a complex of gp 70 (external glycoprotein) and gp 15 (transmembrane anchor) was superior to gp 70 alone for prevention of friend leukemia in mice (Kleiser, 1986).

Gag proteins also serve as immunogens during natural infections. In order for protection to be mediated via a gag protein, one would presume that it must be expressed on the viral surface or on the surface of infected cells. The p 18 gag protein may be expressed on the surface since antibody to a related protein, α thymosin, can reportedly neutralize virus (Sarin, 1986) and p 12, a gag protein of friend leukemia virus is reportedly expressed on the surface of infected cells (Hunsmann, 1976). A possible expression of polymerase and other viral proteins at sites of exposure to antibody or sensitized lymphocytes dictates a need to evaluate all defined gene products as sites of potential immune attack.

Candidate Vaccines

All of the traditional and newer approaches to vaccine development are being explored with HIV and preliminary information on each one of them is available. Some have more or less promise than others.

Live attenuated vaccines. Live attenuated vaccines have generally been more effective than inactive preparations for prevention of virus infection. It is possible that a fundamental understanding of the role of each viral gene segment in the integrative and replicative process might make it feasible to develop a safe attenuated vaccine in the future. However, because of the potential for genetic integration with lifelong persistence, for tumor induction, and for reversion to virulence, any effort in the development of live attenuated vaccine requires more than we currently know about the virus and availability of an acceptable animal model for evaluating vaccine candidates before beginning what would still be a very laborious and lengthy process. Such an approach cannot receive serious attention at the present time.

Inactive vaccines. The majority of active effort toward vaccine development for HIV at present involves various approaches to developing specific antigens. A summary of the approaches being evaluated is in Table 2.

TABLE 2 Human Immunodeficiency Virus Vaccines Under Development

Inactivated whole virus
Purified proteins
Recombinant DNA-derived proteins
Bacterial systems
Yeast systems
Insect virus - cell systems
Mammalian cell systems
Infectious agents as gene vectors
Synthetic peptides
Anti-idiotypes

Whole virus inactivated vaccines have been made and used in man as part of a strategy of suppressive immunization of asymptomatic antibody-positive persons (Salk, 1986). The theory for this approach is that hyperimmunization with inactive antigen will maintain immune surveillance at a high level so that virus remains in the latent state. Potential problems for this approach include: 1) failure of "immune persons" to respond to the vaccine, 2) the development of immunopathology as a result of immunization, and 3) the fact that virus is already in the central nervous system, a relatively protected site from immune surveillance. Using whole virus vaccines before virus exposure carries the potential problem of a residual ability of nucleic acid to integrate into the cell genome with the consequent risks cited above for live virus vaccine. Moreover, among some of the oncoviruses, whole virus vaccines have exhibited low immunogenicity (Olsen, 1987). Thus, this type of preparation will also require a prolonged and intensive effort regarding safety before such vaccines can be considered as candidates for trials to prevent infection.

The remaining approaches in Table 2 constitute the major vaccine development effort at the present time. Purified envelope glycoprotein vaccines have been produced, given to animals, and shown to be immunogenic (Arthur, 1987). Chimpanzees have been challenged; however, no protection has been demonstrated. A problem with purified proteins is the low yield obtained from currently available viral growth methods. For this reason and because of the ease of indefinitely and reproducibly producing large quantities of proteins, the newer recombinant DNA procedures are most popular; these have included well described E. coli bacterial systems as well as yeast, mammalian cell and insect virus-cell systems. Bacterial and yeast systems have the advantage of high yield, relative simplicity, and consistency of the system and relative freedom from contamination with undesireable proteins and DNA. Mammalian systems are less acceptable in each of these categories. Mammalian cells and, to a lesser extent, yeast cell systems, can secrete a glycoprotein that undergoes appropriate proteolytic processing; such proteins may be identical to native glycoprotein. The yeast system has been used for preparing Hepatitis B vaccine, an effective, commercially-available vaccine preparation (Stevens, 1987). The insect cell system consists of baculovirus as a vector for infection and sensitive insect tissue cultures (Summers, 1987). The system has been used for producing a number of proteins because of a high efficiency that may yield large quantities of the desired protein. Candidate vaccines from each of these categories have been produced and evaluated for immunogenicity in animal systems; each has been shown to be immunogenic.

The second most popular approach for developing products currently is to use recombinant DNA technology for introducing gene segments for specific proteins into the genome of an infectious agent and then using that infectious agent as a vector for transmitting the information to the vaccinated animal for synthesis of the desired protein, usually an envelope glycoprotein. Many potential vectors are being evaluated for this purpose; they include vaccinia virus, adenovirus, herpes simplex virus, cytomegalovirus, and the BCG mycobacterium that is used for prevention of tuberculosis in the undeveloped world. The first vaccine used in man employed a vaccinia recombinant vector (Zagury, 1987). A similar preparation is under trial in the USA at present among vaccinia antibody-positive individuals who are homosexuals practicing low risk behavior. Potential problems of the vaccinia approach are the occurrence of the complications known to accompany vaccination, such as vaccinia necrosum and post-vaccinial encephalitis, and insufficient gene expression among vaccinia-immune persons at initial vaccination or at future reimmunizations for inducing an effective immune response. Essentially all adults in the world today have received prior vaccination with vaccinia virus.

Synthetic peptides and anti-idiotype vaccines represent two approaches to vaccine development that emerged from modern molecular biology. Among the potential problems of peptides are the absence of conformational epitopes, the difficulty in identifying acceptable carrier proteins, and the paucity of adjuvants currently acceptable for use in humans. A considerable research effort in adjuvants is underway and will contribute to development of protein and peptide vaccines for many infectious agents. Development of anti-idiotype vaccines is also a modern, potentially useful vaccine approach. Among the numerous difficulties to be overcome, however, are concerns of sensitization, identification of an acceptable production system, and concerns about induction of immunosuppression when the vaccine antigen mimics the viral antigen binding to CD-4 receptor.

Passive immunization with high titered antiserum is an alternative approach for immunization in limited situations, such as postexposure prophylaxis. Trials of passive immunization of chimpanzees with pooled human sera containing high titers of neutralizing antibody were not effective for prevention of infection of chimpanzees against intravenous challenge with infectious HIV (Prince, unpublished data). However, passive immunization of AIDS patients with similar high titered sera was followed by a decrease in the level of infection and detection of clinical improvement (Jackson, 1988). Thus, it may be possible to develop sera effective for passive immunization.

Current Clinical Trials

In a preliminary report of his experience with a vaccinia-HIV recombinant virus containing the envelope gene, Zagury and coworkers (1987) claimed a primary type vaccinia response with no effect on CD-4 or CD-8 cell counts in peripheral blood, or on lymphocyte proliferation and IL-2 production. A high titer of vaccinia antibody developed at 30 days (1:2430) and the HIV neutralization antibody titer rose to 1:40. This result was said to have been repeated in a few Zairians, again with no evidence of immunosuppression from vaccination and with the development of antibody in some. In order to enhance development of a CMI response, the investigators used autologous recombinant infected and inactivated lymphocytes as boosters. The latter approach to boosting is unique but not practical for large scale use. Theoretically, however, an inactive antigen could be equally effective for boosting provided it contains T-cell epitopes.

Preliminary results of a trial involving a gp 160 vaccine prepared in insect cell culture using a baculovirus vector are available. This protein is being given by Kovacs and coworkers (1988) in an escalating two dose schedule to homosexuals practicing low risk behavior and by the NIH multicenter trial group in a three dose schedule to a low risk, mostly heterosexual population. Doses of up to 80 ug has been given and antibody has been detected in Western blot tests and Elisa in some. No evidence of immunosuppression from the vaccination has been noted.

These early reports will be useful for comparison to animal immunization data and to provide valuable experience in recruiting and identifying problems in conducting human trials.

Remaining Problems and Challenges

Despite the initial clinical trial experience that has produced considerable insight into implementation and evaluation of HIV vaccines, many problems and challenges remain. Designing and implementing high quality clinical trials is a complex process; it is not too early to begin considerations for efficacy trials. Developing populations, ensuring comparability, assessing sample size and developing end point criteria and surveillance methods are equally as important as identifying a candidate vaccine and developing the dose, route, and schedule for a trial. An efficacy trial in a high-risk population carries with it an obligation to counsel on behavior control, an intervention that may require alterations in population size and surveillance methods. Implementation of an efficacy trial must, however, await the availability of a vaccine candidate and of sufficient knowledge to project with confidence that the vaccine will be effective and that it will be safe. Thus, the major needs regarding HIV vaccine development are still scientific.

Fundamental information on the infectious process is needed to support the vaccine effort. Determining the manner of acquisition of infection, whether infection is typically initiated with free or cell-associated virus, the initial route of spread, and whether immunity at the mucosal level is required would serve to focus vaccine development. But, more importantly, we must know whether protective immunity develops after infection or vaccination; if it exists, then the correlates of this immunity can serve as guidelines for the immune response required of a vaccine. Alternatively, a suitable animal model might serve as a surrogate for obtaining this information. In this regard, the chimpanzee, a primate phylogenetically close to man, can be infected with HIV; but, so far, these animals have not developed either immunosuppression or the organ system disease seen in AIDS (Derosiers, 1987). There is hope that simian immunodeficiency virus or feline immunodeficiency virus infections will be helpful in assessing vaccine principles, but these efforts are just beginning. Thus, development of an analogous animal model for AIDS in man carries a high priority.

Because of the deficiencies in knowledge of HIV infection, the major basis for believing a successful vaccine can be developed comes from the precedent of success in retroviral diseases in animals, particularly the oncoviruses (Hunsmann, 1985). There are, however, no clear vaccine successes for other lentivirus infections.

The other major problem that vaccine develoment for HIV faces is the genomic diversity exhibited by naturally-occurring isolates of HIV (Hahn, 1986). The antigenic variation described is reminiscent of the antigenic drift exhibited by type A and B influenza viruses. That diversity, however, is a sequential variation; HIV variation may not exhibit such a defineable pattern. Cross-reactive immunity, its potency and the mediators must be understood so as to include solutions in the design of vaccines. This is particularly important for assessing safety as this macrophage-trophic virus exhibits enhanced uptake in the presence of non-neutralizing antibody via Fc receptor attachment as described for the dengue viruses, a phenomenon believed to account for dengue shock syndrome (Halstead, 1988). A high degree of confidence regarding safety is needed before entering into expanded vaccine trials in risk groups.

Final Comment

The HIV vaccine development effort at all levels in the industrialized countries is unprecedented in its magnitude. However, despite the commitment of science and industry to the problem, considerable skepticism exists whether an effective vaccine can be made. Moreover, many insist that the risk of an adverse reaction is so great that even initial studies involving man should be postponed until a success is ensured and occurrence of an adverse effect is not a risk. On the other hand, there are those who believe the crisis is so great that the preparation eliciting the highest and broadest immune response must be identified rapidly and an efficacy trial initiated. Surely the best approach is to proceed with dispatch at all levels, but to do so with thoughtfulness, caution, and with appreciation that there are risks, but there are also benefits to be gained by the rapid identification of an effective vaccine. The high degree of expectation held by the public and the extreme degree of scrutiny the AIDS problem is receiving by the press dictate a need for cooperation by scientists, government, and industry to hasten the developmental process.

ACKNOWLEDGEMENT

Supported in part by contract N01 AI72629, NIAID, NIH.

REFERENCES

Arthur, L.O., Pyle, S.W., Nara, P.L., and others. (1987). Serological responses in chimpanzees inoculated with human immunodeficiency virus glycoprotein (gp120) subunit vaccine. Proc. Natl. Acad. Sci. USA, 84, 8583-8587.

Desrosiers, R.C., and Letvin, N.L. (1987). Animal models for acquired immunodeficiency syndrome. Reviews of Infect. Dis., 9, 438-446.

Hahn, B.H., Shaw, G.M., Taylor, M.E., and others. (1986). Genetic variation in HTLV-III/LAV over time in patients with AIDS or at risk for AIDS. Science, 232, 476-481.

Halstead, S.B. (1988). Pathogenesis of dengue: challenges to molecular biology. Science, 239, 476-481.

Hunsmann, G., Claviez, M., Moennig, V., and others. (1976). Properties of mouse leukemia viruses. X. Occurrence of viral structural antigens on the cell surface as revealed by a cytotoxicity test. Virology, 69, 157-168.

Hunsmann, G. (1985). Subunit vaccines against exogenous retroviruses: overview and perspectives. Cancer Research, 45, 4691s-4693s.

Jackson, G.G., Rubenis, M., Knigge, M., and others. (1988). Passive immunoneutralization of human immunodeficiency virus in patients with advanced AIDS. The Lancet, September 17, 647-651.

Kleiser, C., Schneider, J., Bayer, H., and others. (1986). Immunoprevention of friend leukaemia virus-induced erythroleukaemia by vaccination with aggregated gp70. J. Gen. Virol., 67, 1901-1907.

Kovacs, J.A., Megil, M.E., Deyton, L., and others. (1988). Phase I trial of a recombinant gp 160 candidate AIDS vaccine. Abstract, IV International Conference on AIDS, Stockholm, Sweden.

Olsen, R.G., Lewis, M.G., Lafrado, L.J., and others. (1987). Feline leukemia virus: current status of the feline induced immune depression and immunoprevention. Cancer and Metastasis Reviews, 6, 243-260.

Salk, J. (1987). Prospects for the control of AIDS by immunizing seropositive individuals. Nature, 327, 473-476.

Sarin, P.S., Sun, D.K., Thornton, A.H., and others. (1986). Neutralization of HTLV-III/LAV replication by antiserum to thymosin α_1. Science, 232, 1135-1137.

Stevens, C.E., Taylor, P.E., Tong, M.J., and others. (1987). Yeast recombinant hepatitis B vaccine: efficacy with hepatitis B immune globulin in prevention of perinatal hepatitis B virus transmission. J. Am. Med. Assoc., 257, 2612.

Summers, M.D., and Smith, G.E. (1987). A manual of methods for baculovirus vectors and insect cell culture procedures. Texas Agriculture Experimental Station Bulletin No. 1555.

Zagury, D., Leonard, R., Fouchard, M., and others. (1987). Immunization against AIDS in humans. Nature, 326, 249-250.

Current Immunotherapeutic Efforts and Future Prospects in Human HIV Disease

JOHN W. HADDEN

Program of Immunopharmacology, University of South Florida Medical College, 12901 Bruce B. Downs Blvd., Tampa, Florida 33612, USA

ABSTRACT

Therapy trials have demonstrated efficacy of α interferon in AIDS with Kaposi Sarcoma; have strongly suggested efficacy of DTC and isoprinosine in ARC; and are suggestive for efficacy of imreg, ampligen, thymopentin, and thymostimulin in ARC. Many other substances are under evaluation. No immunotherapeutic agent has been useful in AIDS with opportunistic infections, although many combined trials with AZT are beginning. The preclinical and clinical data indicate that without the presence of a functioning thymus, new T cells cannot be produced thus immunorestorative treatments with thymomimetic biologicals (thymic hormones and IL2) or drugs (DTC and isoprinosine) in HIV disease should be administered prior to the thymic destruction characteristic of AIDS. Combinations of agents may be useful. New agents and strategies may derive from recent data indicating that interleukins and pituitary-derived hormones and factors play a critical role in T cell and thymus development.

KEY WORDS

AIDS/ARC; HIV infection; immunotherapy; thymic hormones; interleukins I & II; and thymomimetic drugs.

The worldwide epidemic involving the human immunodeficiency virus (HIV) has offered a unique challenge to immunopharmacologists and immunotherapists. With incomplete knowledge about the pathogenesis of acquired immune deficiency syndrome (AIDS) and the AIDS-related complex (ARC), a large number of immunotherapy trials were initiated in an effort to stall or reverse the immunodeficiency of these diseases. It is the purpose of this chapter to summarize the current status of these efforts and to comment on our prospects for the future. The reader is referred to two prior reviews for more complete details and referencing concerning earlier trials (Hadden, 1984; Hadden, 1987).

Table I provides a summary of the agents involved in the immunotherapeutic efforts.

Table I Immunotherapeutic Agents Used to Treat HIV Infection in Humans

Adoptive Therapy		Drugs
Gammaglobulin*		Ampligen*
Marrow/thymus transplant		AS-101
Interferons α*		Bropirimine (ABPP)
β		Carrisyn
γ		CL 246738
Interleukin II		D-penicillamine
Thymic hormones	thymosin fraction V	Dextran
	thymostimulin TP-1*	Diethyldithiocarbamate (DTC)*
	thymulin	DNCB
	thymopentin*	Isoprinosine*
	thymosin α1	MTP-PE
	thymic humoral factor	
Imreg/transfer factor*		

* in widespread use or trials

Adoptive Therapy

Gammaglobulin - In the adult form of these diseases, memory β lymphocyte function is relatively intact although dysregulation and inability to respond to new antigens occurs. As a result, antibodies to high grade pyrogenic pathogens are preserved and infection resulting from breaches in antibody-mediated defenses are not common. In pediatric patients in whom primary exposures have not yet occurred, gammaglobulin therapy has proven useful to prevent or alleviate infection, particularly bacterial infections (Cavelli & Rubenstein 1986). Therapy with virus-inactivated plasma from HIV positive donors is under evaluation in a few selected AIDS patients by one group in England. Neutralizing mouse or human monoclonal antibodies would seem a reasonable trial when available (Fung et al 1987).

Cellular engineering - prior efforts with transfer of lymphocytes or transplantation of bone marrow or thymic fragments have been generally unsuccessful (see Hadden 1987); however, renewed attempts are under consideration with concommitant antiviral therapy with azidothymidine (AZT) (see Abrams et al 1987).

Biological Therapy

Interferons (IFN) - A number of trials with α interferon in the treatment of Kaposi sarcoma (KS) in AIDS have been published. Complete and partial response rates have varied from 20-50% (see Abrams et al 1987). The side effects involve a "flu-like" syndrome; however, immunosuppression characteristic of antimetabolite therapy of KS was not observed. These studies have not demonstrated immune restorative effects of α IFN in AIDS; however, a lower frequency of opportunistic infections (OI) were often noted and clinical tumor response tended to correlate with better immune function (see Hadden 1987). Beta and gamma IFN's and tumor necrosis factor (TNF) are currently under evaluation. Interestingly, one therapeutic approach to AIDS under evaluation is the use of sheep anti-alpha interferon globulin to neutralize the acid labile IFN observed in the serum of AIDS patients (Bellanti et al 1987).

Interleukin II (IL2) - Based upon reports that IL2 reversed in vitro a number of the defects associated with AIDS (see Hadden 1987), IL2 in purified (Jurkat) and recombinant (rIL2) form was administered in several studies to 68 patients with AIDS and ARC without obvious benefit. In a group of 24 AIDS patients given recombinant IL2 in high dose by continuous infusion (Fauci & Lane 1986,

Clifford Lane personal communication) increased lymphocyte counts and other T cell functions were observed. Side effects of IL2 are similar to those of IFN. Interestingly, in patients whose cells were cultured for HIV, viral expression was diminished not enhanced as one might fear. The AMFAR Directory (Abrams et al 1987) reports no current trials with IL2 alone; however, a trial with IL2 and AZT is reportedly in progress at Stanford University.

Thymic Hormones - The earlier studies clearly showed no benefit of the various thymic hormones in AIDS itself. Thymosin fraction V, thymopentin, thymostimulin (TP-1), and thymic humoral factor (THF) showed effects to modify T cell number and/or function in half of 40 patients with ARC. Based upon these preliminary studies in which clinical responses were not examined, Serono Laboratories embarked on multicenter AIDS and ARC trials with TP-1 in 8 centers in the USA as well as a number of centers in Europe (company source). In 60 AIDS patients, no significant effects were observed. In 103 ARC patients the preliminary data show no significant effect on conversion from ARC to AIDS; however, the immunologic data are still under evaluation. A combined protocol with AZT is under consideration. Similarly, Ortho Immunobiology Research Institute is in the process of recruiting patients for a controlled study of 160 ARC patients with thymopentin by injection (company source). Thymic humoral factor is under evaluation in a trial but details are not available. No ongoing trials are reportedly occurring with thymosin, thymosin alpha 1 or thymulin.

Leukocyte Extracts - Imreg 1 is derived from dialyzed leukocyte extracts and contains both an active dipeptide and tripeptide. A recent trial with 90 ARC and 50 control patients reportedly shows decreased conversion from ARC to AIDS without toxicity (company source). The lack of published data makes it difficult to comment on the immunopharmacology of this preparation and further details are awaited. Transfer factor prepared by conventional means (see Carey and Lederman 1987) is under evaluation in several AIDS and ARC patients in Denver. Prior attempts with transfer factor were unsuccessful (Dwyer 1984).

Drug Therapy

Sulphur-containing thymomimetic drugs (see Hadden 1985) - Imuthiol (diethyldithiocarbamate, DTC) was entered into a multicenter double blinded study of 92 ARC patients in France following reports of activity in several open trials (see Lang and Aleksile 1987). Treatment with DTC (400 mg/M^2/week) was associated with decreased conversion of ARC to AIDS (0 vs 4), increased CD4+ cells in 42%, weight stabilization, and loss of splenomegaly in those affected. Studies by Brewton et al (1987) and Hersh et al (1987) in AIDS and ARC patients showed less pronounced effects. Toxicity (skin rash, vomiting, fever, and chest pain) was noted at 800 mg/M^2/week while the lower doses were well tolerated. Merieux Laboratoire has in excess of 200 AIDS and ARC patients enrolled in carefully controlled trials designed to confirm the earlier study by Lang and Aleksile (1987). Combined treatment of DTC with AZT has occurred in a number of patients and while no results are available at this time, no incompatability of these agents has been observed.

D-Penicillamine has a structure and immunopharmacology similar to DTC. Like DTC, it has an anti-HIV effect in vitro. As a result of this latter action, it was introduced into trials in ARC and lymphadenopathy syndrome (LAS) patients (Schuloff et al 1986; Sarin et al 1987; Parenti et al 1987). A dose-dependent decrease in HIV expression or replication was observed; however at the more effective doses, decreased CD4+ cells or lymphoproliferative responses were observed. A large scale clinical trial is planned in Germany to follow up on these initial trials.

Thymomimetic Purines - Isoprinosine showed activity in a 28 day treatment study of 63 ARC patients to decrease symptom scores, increase CD4+ and CD11+

lymphocytes and NK cell activity, and to decrease conversion from ARC to AIDS over 3 months without toxicity (Wallace et al 1986; Bekesi et al 1987). An interim report (Hoehler and Robbins 1988) involving 200 ARC patients treated for 28 days showed no conversion from ARC to AIDS during treatment with isoprinosine in contrast to control (4% - $p > .05$) and significant increases in CD4+ cells and NK cell activity. The difference in conversion persisted to 1 year. Multicenter controlled trials have been initiated with continuous treatment in HIV+ and ARC patients in the US (700 patients), Scandinavia (1,000 patients), Italy (2,000 patients) and Australia (700 patients).

NPT 15392 is an analog of isoprinosine with very similar immunopharmacology (Hadden 1985). Based upon immunorestorative effects of this drug in T cell-deficient neonatal mice, a trial with this agent in ARC patients is being planned in Italy.

Other Compounds - Trials have been completed and abandoned with Azimexon and glucan (see Hadden 1987).

AS101 (ammonium salt of tellurium) is a T cell immunomodulator in Phase I trials in Israel.

DNCB (dinitrochlorobenzene) is a chemical sensitizer for delayed type hypersensitivity (DTH) and has some activity to nonspecifically increase T cell number and/or function. Mills (1986) reported preliminary findings to confirm these effects in AIDS and open trials are under discussion.

MTP-PE (muramyl tripeptide-phosphatidyl ethanolamine) in liposomes acts to stimulate the reticuloendothelial system (RES) and activate tumoricidal macrophages. Phase I toxicity trials have been initiated in AIDS-KS at the National Institutes of Health (NIH).

Interferon Inducers - Trials have been initiated with several compounds which can be classified immunopharmacologically as immunomodulators/interferon inducers.

Ampligen (a mismatched polymer of poly(1)-poly(c)) has been introduced into preliminary trials in patients with AIDS and ARC with and without AZT (Brodsky 1985, Carter et al 1987; Mitchell et al 1987). The initial findings include: decreased symptoms, increased T cell responses, and decreased virus expression in some patients without limiting toxicity. Large scale trials in ARC patients have been initiated to confirm these findings.

Bropirimine (ABPP) is an orally active immunomodulator under development by Upjohn (Abrams et al 1987). It was introduced in 20 AIDS patients with Kaposi sarcoma without significant clinical benefit nor significant toxicity although interferon induction occurred and lymphoproliferative responses were affected (company source). A trial in AIDS with opportunistic infections with and without AZT is in formulation.

CL 246,731 is an NK/interferon inducer in trials for AIDS-KS.

Carrisyn is an acetylated mannan preparation which has increased T cell responses and decreased viral expression in preliminary studies in ARC patients (McDaniel and McAnailey 1987) and further trials are reportedly under consideration.

Dextran sulphate is an immunomodulating glycan which additionally shows some anti HIV activity in vitro and is in toxicological evaluation in California.

Trends and Strategies

It is clear that α interferons have clinical efficacy as anti-tumor agents and α and β IFN and several interferon inducers are under evaluation in AIDS-KS. No other immunotherapeutic agent has been found to be useful in AIDS. In ARC, the thymic hormones have shown modest immunorestorative effects and two are undergoing widespread controlled testing for licensing (thymostimulin and thymopentin). Two thymomimetic drugs (DTC and isoprinosine) have shown immunorestorative effects and decreased conversion of ARC to AIDS and are in extended trials for licensing. A smattering of new agents (imreg, bropirimine, ampligen, and carrisyn) look interesting; however, the predicted limitations of monotherapy with immunorestorative biologicals and drugs have been reached and recognized. Palliation in AIDS-KS and in ARC would appear to be the best achievements possible.

The combination of existing immunotherapeutic agents (Hadden 1984) seems like a rational strategy; further combinations of immunotherapeutic agents and effective antiviral agents are an obvious next step. Trials (see AmFar Directory - Abrams et al 1987) are planned or underway in AIDS and ARC with azidothymidine (AZT) plus α interferon, isoprinosine, DTC, imreg, rIL2, colony stimulating factor (CSF), or bone marrow transplantation and with ribavirin plus isoprinosine or thymopentin. It remains to be determined whether the immunotoxicologies of these two antiviral agents will permit successful combination therapy with immunorestorative agents; the clinical efforts are warranted and their results anxiously awaited. Finally, it is increasingly evident that vaccine approaches (HIV-immunogen, HIV-iscom, HIV-specific active immunotherapy etc. (see Abrams et al 1987)) will be employed not only in immunoprophylaxis but also in immunotherapy to prevent asymptomatic HIV-positive individuals from progressing to ARC and ARC from progressing to AIDS. The use of these agents in combination with traditional and new synthetic adjuvants will be critical in enhancing the development of protective neutralizing antibodies. The role of delayed type hypersensitivity (DTH) to HIV is not clear; however, I strongly suspect DTH is critical in preventing disease progression. The use of vaccine-type approaches to induce and augment DTH to HIV will be important and the joint use of immunotherapeutic, particularly thymomimetic drugs (DTC and isoprinosine) and biologicals (thymic hormones and IL2) will be important to maximize the protection gained. While the pace is slow, significant progress through the combined use of antivirals, HIV antigens, and immunotherapeutic agents is envisioned.

Prospects for the Future with Immunotherapeutic Agents To Reverse T Cell Immunodeficiency

The lack of clearcut evidence on the mechanisms by which HIV cripples and destroys T lymphocytes and the role played by these T lymphocytes in resistance to HIV make it difficult to plan specific strategies for immunotherapy. The therapies in the past have thus been notably empirical. The observations that thymomimetic biologicals and drugs are only effective in ARC, i.e., in the stage of disease where T cells are present (although declining) yet dysfunctional implies a degree of reversibility of the virus-derived immunosuppressive influences manifest in this disease. Most of our prior experience with the immunotherapeutic agents has been under circumstances of normal or near normal immunity in animals or mild to moderately severe immunosuppression in humans (Hadden 1985). Under these circumstances the clearcut immunotherapeutic effects of these agents have been documented. The effects of the agents under these circumstances can be most clearly viewed as deriving from actions on preexisting functional T cells. The fact that similar effects are being achieved in ARC patients is not then surprising. Their lack of effect in AIDS, i.e., late stage disease with profound T lymphopenia implies they may be relegated to the modulation of a preexisting, peripheralized cellular immune system.

A fundamental question is whether the development of uninfected, new T cells from bone marrow precursors can be achieved in HIV disease. The extremely slow rate of viral transmission in this disease, the presence of antiviral chemotherapeutic agents and the known co-immunosuppressive influences produced by companion viruses (EBV, CMV, etc.) all suggest that, if individuals can be protected from new exposures to companion viruses and the HIV held in check, a significant clinical window exists for reconstituting the T cell system. The most dramatic efforts to restore the system historically have been provided by cellular engineering efforts using bone marrow and thymus transplantation. Their use tells us that months are required before T cell numbers and function appear and normality is reached (Touraine et al 1977). Their use in AIDS and ARC would be markedly limited since, in the presence of residual immunity, non syngeneic tissues would be rejected. With twin pairs in HIV disease being limited, other approaches need be explored.

There is a popular conception that thymus atrophy in the young adult is profound once the T cell system becomes established in the periphery and that persistent endocrine function extends into midlife and provides little more than a hormonal influence via the thymic hormones to maintain integrity of the peripheralized system. It is well known, but little appreciated, that the T cell system in the adult can be completely, although slowly, reconstituted from T cell precursors following irradiation or chemotherapy-induced destruction of the immune system (e.g., adult leukemia treated with bone marrow transplantation, post Chernobyl recovery, etc.). The question then is whether this type of reconstitution can be achieved in HIV disease using molecular rather than cellular means.

In order to approach this question experimentally, we decided to test the notion that T cells can be induced by in vivo drugs and biologicals. It is known that athymic nude mice develop functional T cells as they mature (Ikehara et al 1984), although it is not clear whether they evolve extrathymically or are processed by the residual cords of thymic epithelial cells apparent in these mice (Ikehara et al 1987). Successful therapeutic efforts to induce T cells in these mice have been reported with thymosin fraction V (Ikehara et al 1975), IL2 (Stötter et al 1980), isoprinosine and DTC (Renoux et al 1979). The most comprehensive of these studies was performed with thymosin fraction V in which the treatment required three months before functional T cells were evident. Marker profiles for T cells were not performed.

We designed our experiments essentially as described by Ikehara et al (1975). We employed thymosin fraction V provided by Allan Goldstein at a 5 mg/kg dose. Control animals were injected with sterile saline or given a syngeneic thymus transplant. Adult non-nude Balb/c mice were also used as control. Additional groups of animals were treated with:

- Buffy coat interleukins (2500 units IL2/kg) D. Dumonde & R. Wolstencroft, London
- Recombinant interleukin IL2 (rIL2)(2500 units/kg) Hoescht Pharmaceuticals
- Isoprinosine (50 mg/kg) - Newport Pharmaceuticals
- DTC (25 mg/kg) - Merieux Laboratoires

The animals were treated with a single daily injection 5 days/week for periods of 3, 6, and 12 weeks after which they were sacrificed. Spleens were weighed and spleen cells obtained for T cell marker analysis (Thy 1.2) and proliferative responses to stimulation with rIL2, concanavalin A (Con A), Con A + rIL2, and phytohemagglutinin (PHA). The proliferative responses were averaged and expressed as a proliferative index. The experiments were performed in two different laboratories, University of South Florida, Tampa (Hadden and Zheng) and Hoechst Pharmaceutical, Frankfurt (Caspritz). The results are expressed in Table II.

Table II Treatment of Athymic Nude Mice*

	3 Week		6 Week		12 Week	
	Thy 1.2	P.I.**	Thy 1.2	P.I.	Thy 1.2	P.I.
Thymus graft	1x	1x	2x+	3x	9x+	5x
Thymosin	1x	2x	1x	1x	1x	1x
Lymphokines	1x	3x	1x	>1x <2x	2x	2x
rIL2	ND	2x	1x	1x	2x	1x
DTC	1x	3x	1x	1x	3x	2x
Isoprinosine	1x	2x	1x	1x	2x	1x

* Data are expressed as multiples of control; 1x = no change

** Proliferative index - average response of spleen cells to rIL2, ConA, ConA + IL2, and PHA

ND = not done

\+ = high density; the remainder are low density Thy 1.2

During the twelve weeks of study the nude controls did not display significant numbers of T cells (Thy 1.2 - 10% or less - low density cells versus 39% high density cells for the adult control). The cells present showed a proliferation index less than 10% of adult control. Thymus transplant induced splenic T cells having the adult, high density phenotype progressively at 6 and 12 weeks and functional responses followed. None of the treatments affected T cell marker Thy 1.2 expression. All of the treatments produced a transient increase in proliferative index at 3 weeks; however, the effects were not enduring. We conclude that these therapeutic effects would be clinically insignificant. The differences between our data and those of Ikehara et al (1975) concerning thymosin fraction V may reside in difference in the dose and nature of the thymosin fraction V; the genetics of the mice (and thus perhaps in the degree of residual thymic epithelial cords); or in background issues relevant to endemic infection, a known inducer of Thy 1.2 cells in nude mice (Scheid et al 1975). In any case, we conclude that under the circumstances of our experiment, extra-thymic maturation of T cells was not induced in the absence of a thymus by the thymomimetic biologicals, thymic hormones and rIL2, or the thymomimetic drugs, DTC or isoprinosine.

These experiments confirm the more conventional dogma, i.e., that the thymus is essential for T cell development.

The application of this information to HIV disease is relevant in that, as ARC progresses to AIDS, there is a progressive destruction of the thymus (Savino et al 1986) and its secretory potential (Dardenne et al 1983). If therapy designed to promote T cell evolution is to be effective, it must be administered before this destructive process. The time at which that occurs is not known. Clarification of precisely when bioactive thymic hormone levels decline will be important information for predicting when this may occur.

It remains to be determined whether the treatments employed will be effective in the presence of a functioning thymus. To examine this we have employed neonatal mice of approximately 4 days of age. These mice have a sizeable thymus yet lack Thy 1.2 positive spleen cells having proliferative responses to IL2 or T cell mitogens. Treatment of these mice for 1 week (5X) with the mixed lymphokines results in a doubling of the Thy 1.2+ cells (5-10% moderate density) and a two fold increase of the Con A proliferative response (± IL2) (preliminary results). Recombinant IL2 alone at the same dose and IL1 were inactive; the experiments with the other agents are in progress. We also plan experiments to examine the effects of these agents in adult mice who have been rendered T cell-free through the use of lytic monoclonal antibodies. The results of these experiments should give us a better idea about whether and to what extent these thymomimetic biologicals and drugs will be useful to hasten the development of T cells in the presence of a functional thymus. Their compatibility with anti retroviral agents can then be tested and the best combined therapeutic strategies for ARC can be devised.

Speculation

In asking the question as to how to treat a patient or animal by immunopharmacological means to promote T cell development, it becomes apparent that we immunologists do not fully understand what are the normal signals which guide T cell evolution. If we were to know better how the thymus recognizes the need for replacing T cells in the periphery, we might be able to reconstruct these signals and magnify them to enhance the flow of new T cells into the periphery. It appears that signals would appropriately derive from two sources, lymphokines derived from lymphocytes and macrophages in the periphery and the central nervous system via autonomic innervation of the thymus or by hormonal influences from the pituitary/hypothalamus. I would like to summarize briefly recent experiments which give insight into both these types of signals because they may suggest new approaches for molecular strategies for reconstructing the T cell system.

A large amount of data indicates the thymic hormones (thymosin α1, thymopoietin, and thymulin) are products of thymic epithelial cells, circulate in the blood, and act on both prothymocytes and mature T cells. We (Chen et al 1983) and others (Andrews et al 1985) were unable to show that these hormones or other thymic epithelial cell products will induce intrathymic maturation of immature T cells. We found that IL2 would induce intrathymic maturation by both marker and functional criteria (Chen et al 1982, 1983; Hadden et al 1986) and suggested that IL2 might represent a signal from the periphery for T cell maturation. Others confirmed these observations (Conlon et al 1983) and showed IL2 receptors on immature intrathymic precursor cells (Raulet 1985). We (Hadden et al 1986; Wiranowska et al 1987) went on to show that prothymocytes from bone marrow precursors are regulated by IL2 in terms of both T cell marker expression (Thy 1.2 induction) and proliferation and that this regulation is markedly potentiated by coculture with thymic epithelial cells.

A role for IL1 in these processes has recently emerged. We have observed that IL1 shows a marked synergy with IL2 on the proliferation of immature cortical thymocytes (Hadden et al. 1988). Falk et al (1987) previously showed that the intrathymic precursor is similarly stimulated in a synergistic manner by IL1 and IL2. We (Hadden et al 1988) report at this meeting that the splenic prothymocyte (the bone marrow level) is also so stimulated. At the precursor level where no mitogen responsiveness exists, none is induced; however, at the cortical thymic levels when few mitogen responsive cells are present the synergy of IL1 and IL2 on proliferation of these cells is associated with marked induction of a mitogen response. IL1 has recently been shown to be produced by thymic epithelial cells (Le et al 1987) as well as thymic dendritic cells. We (Galy et al 1988) show at this meeting that IL1 stimulates the proliferation and the secretion of thymic epithelial cells. Thus IL1 may not only be an endocrine signal from the periphery but also an intrathymic autocrine/paracrine pathway regulating thymic epithelial cell function. IL1 may derive from either or both of these sources to act in synergy with IL2 in regulating T cell development. Other lymphokines may participate in these processes (e.g., IL3 and IL4); however, so far, in our experience, the effect of a natural mixed lymphokine preparation is mostly accounted for by its content of IL1 and IL2. These observations suggest that mixed lymphokine treatment would enhance T cell ontogeny and our preliminary data in neonatal mice cited supports this conclusion.

Evidence for a role of pituitary hormones/factors in thymic function and T cell development has also recently emerged. An intimate relationship between the thymus and pituitary has long been suggested (Pierpaoli et al 1969). Recent evidence indicates that thymic hormones participate in communication with the hypothalamus/pituitary to regulate hormone output (Spangelo et al 1987). IL1 has also been recently shown to regulate pituitary ACTH and prolactin production (Besedofsky et al 1987; Sapolsky et al 1987). Pituitary-derived prolactin and perhaps growth hormone regulate T cell function in the periphery (Russel et al 1985; Davila et al 1987; Kelley et al 1987). We present at this meeting (Hadden et al 1988) evidence that the pituitary makes a factor(s) which stimulates thymic epithelial cell growth. Others have presented evidence to indicate that pituitary hormones or hormone-producing implants can reverse the thymic involution and T cell functional deficiencies associated with dwarfism (Pierpaoli et al 1969) and with aging (Kelley et al 1987). These experiments suggest that treatment with pituitary thymotrophic hormone(s) and/or prolactin may be useful in fostering T cell development and function in ARC and HIV+ individuals. We have experiments in progress to test which of these strategies or a combination may be most useful and we plan to test their compatibility with AZT.

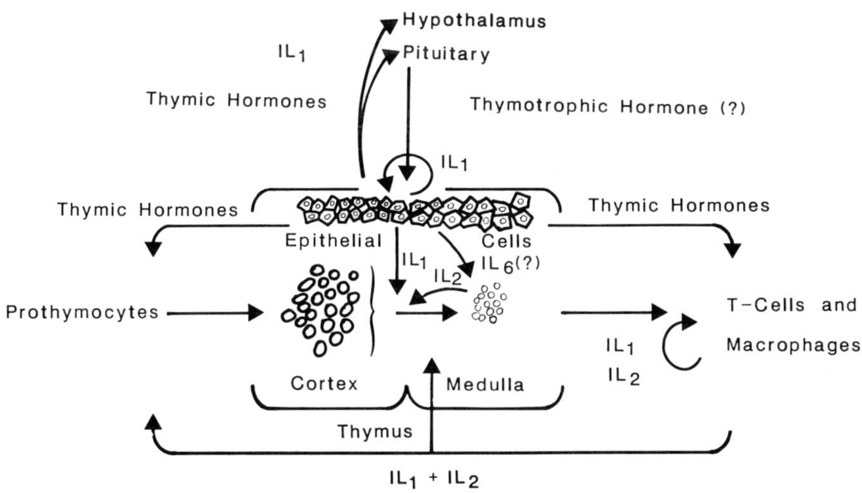

Figure 1 summarizes the developmental scenario as we currently view it. It suggests that therapeutic efforts may derive from interleukin products, and both pituitary and thymic epithelial cell products. Better understanding of how they act alone and in concert will aid us in determining how they may be administered exogenously or stimulated endogenously to foster T cell development.

REFERENCES

Abrams, D. et al., eds. (1987). AmFAR Directory of Experimental Treatments for AIDS and ARC. Vol. 1, Mary Ann Liebert, Inc.

Andrews, P., et al. (1985). Cell Immunol. 91, 455.

Bekesi, J.G. et al. (1987). J. Clin Lab Immunol. 24, 155.

Bellanti, J. et al. (1987). Abstract, III Int'l Conference on AIDS, Washington, DC, p. 18.

Besedovsky, H. et al. (1986). Science, 233, 652.

Brewton, G.W. et al. (1987). Abstract, III Int'l Conference on AIDS, Washington, DC, p. 225.
Brodsky, I. (1985). J. Interferon Res. 4, 669.
Carey, J.T. and Lederman, M.M. (1987). JAMA 257, 651
Carter, W. et al. (1987). Lancet 1, 1286.
Cavelli, T.A. and Rubenstein, A. (1986). Clin. Exp. Immunol. 65, 683.
Chen, S.S. et al. (1982). Int. J. Immunopharm. 4, 382.
Chen, S.S. et al. (1983). Proc. Nat'l Acad. Sci. 80, 5980.
Conlon, P.J. et al. (1983). J. Immunol. 128, 797.
Dardenne, M. and Bach, J.F. (1983). N. Eng. J. Med. 309, 48.
Davila, D.R. et al. (1987). J. Neurosci. Res. 18, 108.
Dwyer, J.M. et al. (1984). Clin. Immunol. Rev. 3, 25.
Falk, W. et al (1987). Lymph. Rep. 6, 75.
Fauci, A. and Lane, H.C. (1986). Int. Conf. on Acquired Immunodeficiency Syndrome (AIDS), Paris, France.
Fung, M.S.C. et al. (1987). Biotechnology 5, 15.
Galy, A. et al (1988). Int. J. Immunopharm. 10, (in press).
Hadden, E.M. et al (1988). Int. J. Immunopharm. 10, (in press).
Hadden, J.W. (1984). NYAS 437, 76.
Hadden, J.W. (1985). In: Symposium on Immunopharmacology (P.A. Miescher, et al., eds.). Vol. 23, Raven Press, p. 183.
Hadden, J.W. et al. (1986). In: Advances in Immunopharmacology 3 (L. Chedid, et al., eds.). Pergamon Press, p. 487.
Hadden, J.W. (1987). In: AIDS-Acquired Immunodeficiency Syndrome-And Other Manifestations of HIV Infections (G. Wormser, et al., eds.). Noyes Publishers, p. 992.
Hadden, J.W. et al. (1986). Lymph. Rep. 5, 49.
Hadden, J.W. et al. (1988). Int. J. Immunopharm. 10, (in press).
Hersh, E.M. et al. (1987). Abstract, III Int'l Conf. on AIDS, Washington, DC, p. 225.
Hoehler, F.K. and Robins, D.S. (1988). Current Ther. Res. 43,
Ikehara, S. et al. (1975). Nature 258, 335.
Ikehara, S. et al. (1984). Proc. Nat'l Acad. Sci. 81, 886.
Ihehara, S. et al. (1987). Thymus 10, 93.
Kelley, K.W. et al. (1987). In: Neuroimmune Interactions (B. Jankovic, et al., eds.). Vol. 496, p. 91.
Lang, J.M. and Aleksile, A. (1985). Lancet 11, 1066.
Le, P.T. et al. (1987). J. Immunol. 138, 2520.
McDaniel, H.R. and McAnailey, B.H. (1987). Clin. Res. 35, 483.
Mills, L.B. (1986). J. Acad. Dermatol. 14, 6.
Mitchell, W.M. et al. (1987). Lancet 1, 890.
Parenti, D.M. et al. (1987). Abstract, III Int'l Conf. on AIDS, Washington, DC, p. 220.
Pierpaoli, R. et al (1969). Immunol. 16, 217.
Raulet, D.H. (1985). Nature 314, 101.
Renoux, G. et al. (1979). J. Immunopharma. 1, 415.
Russell, D.H. et al. (1985). J. Immunol. 134, 3027.
Sapolsky, R. et al. (1987). Science 238, 522.
Sarin, P. et al. (1987). Abstract, III Int'l Conf. on AIDS, Washington, DC, p. 24.
Savino, W., et al (1986). Am. J. Pathol. 122, 98.
Scheid, M. et al (1975). Science 190, 1211.
Schulof, R.S. et al. (1986). Drug Res. October, 10
Simon, L.N. et al. (1984). In: Immune Modulation Agents and Their Mechanisms (R.L. Fenichel and M.A. Chirigos, eds.). Marcel Dekker, p. 426.
Stötter, H. et al. (1980). Eur. J. Immunol. 10, 719.
Touraine, J-L. et al. (1977). Proc. Nat'l Acad. Sci. 74, 3414.
Wallace, J.I. et al. (1986). Clin. Immunol. Immunopath. 39, 179.

Experience in the Immunotoxicity Testing of Recombinant Cytokines

YOSHIO HARADA, M.D., Ph.D.

Division of Drug Safety Research, Shionogi Research Laboratories, 3–1–1, Futaba-cho, Toyonaka, Osaka 561, Japan

KEY WORDS

Immunotoxicity: recombinant cytokines: interferons: interleukin-2: hepatotoxicity: selection of animal species.

INTRODUCTION

Cytokines have been reported as immunomodulating agents released from macrophages, lymphocytes or a variety of cell types when they were stimulated by antigens. The effects of a cytokine display a wide range of differentiating functions and growth regulations for immunocompetent cells. With rapid development of genetic engineering, highly purified diverse human cytokines manufactured by recombinant DNA technology became available in a large quantity for preclinical and clinical research or product marketing.

Recently, systemic exposure of these cytokines to humans under the greater than normal physiological concentration is promissingly expected for therapeutic purposes against cancer, some types of hepatitis and rheumatic arthritis. However, patients encounter various adverse effects such as flu-like symptoms (pyrexia, rigors or myalgia), leucopenia, eosinophilia, thrombocytopenia, anemia, immunoreaction in lymphoid tissue, neurobehavioral irregularities and abnormal hepatic functions (elevation of GOT and GPT values in serum) during the course of treatment (Bocci, 1982; Lotze, 1985). These undesirable effects following systemic administration of cytokines were not related to their pharmacological properties which were produced in small concentration on local exposure, but to their systemic response referred as "exaggerated pharmacology" (Galbraith, 1987). Therefore, in developing new cytokine products, to conduct a preclinical toxicity study using animals is particularly important not only to predict the untoward effects occurred as a consequence of activity of cytokines when exaggerated doses are used, but also to extrapolate the data obtained in experimental models to humans. In addition, pathophysiological mechanisms on the immunotoxicity must be considered to elucidate the potential consequences resulting from pharmacodynamic properties induced by the administration of cytokines.

Since we had some experiences in testing the safety of biotechnology products such as interferons and interleukin-2, the data obtained from the animal toxicity studies on these recombinant cytokines will be presented in this report.

TOXICITY OF INTERFERONS

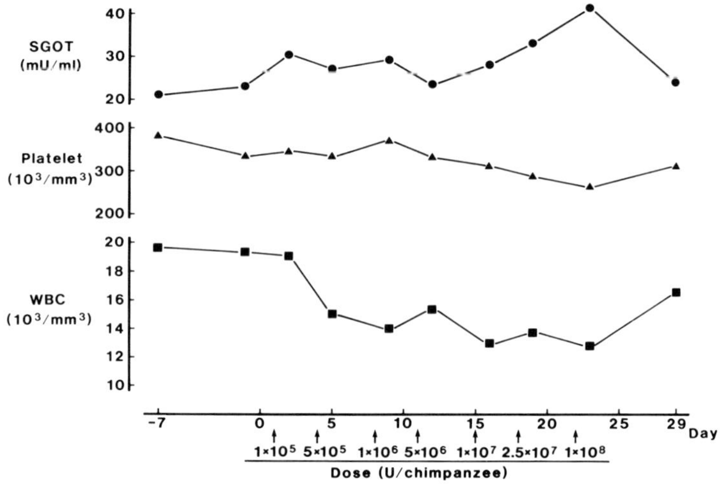

Fig. 1. Effect of r-γ-interferon administration on SGOT, platelet and WBC in chimpanzees

The effects of a single administration of recombinant DNA-derived human interferons alpha, beta and gamma were examined in both sexes of mice, rats and monkeys. All are inactive in these animals at doses of 5×10^6 - 1.6×10^8 U/kg of body weight which are about 50 - 1000 times higher than the intended human dosage (Kobayashi et al, 1986; Watson et al, 1986; Schellekens et al, 1986).

The subacute toxicity studies via the intravenous route which was proposed for human application have been performed using animals, in which rats were given γ-interferon at a dosage of 10^5 or 10^6 U/kg per day for 4 weeks and monkeys received a dosage of 10^6 or 10^7 U/kg per day for 4 weeks, respectively. Drug-related changes were not at all found in rats, because the interferon have minimal cross-species activity, and the neutralizing antibody against γ-interferon was detected in all the rats during the study. However, in cynomolgus monkeys, many diverse but similar side effects to those seen in human patients as described in the INTRODUCTION were observed, although the neutralizing antibody was detectable in half of the monkeys at the end of experiment. As these changes were dose-dependent and reversible after cessation of the treatment, these effects were interpreted as those induced by γ-interferon (Kobayashi et al, 1986; Kobayashi et al, 1986). In the study using chimpanzees that were thought phylogenetically most closest species to man in terms of difference of DNA sequence in a gene, the animals were administered 7 rising doses intravenously over a 22 day period and observed for 29 days for signs of toxicity. In addition to fever and sedation, decreased platelet and WBC counts and an elevation of SGOT levels occurred, as the higher doses of γ-interferon were dosed. These parameters were reversible and returned to the predose levels in a week after the last injection (Fig. 1) (Schellekens et al, 1986).

Furthermore, we have conducted a simulation test of γ-interferon in mouse in which recombinant DNA-derived mouse γ-interferon newly manufactured was dosed intravenously to C57Black mice for 30 days in order to infer the result of human interferon administered to humans. Sedation, slight anemia, leucopenia and increase of spleen weight were observed in this study. Histological examination revealed the activation of reticuloendothelial system in liver parenchyma and pulmonary alveoli. From the toxicological point of view, these findings seen in the mouse simulation study were similar to those obtained from the studies using

Table 1. Results of 4-Week and 13-Week Toxicity Tests of iv r-IL-2 in Sprague-Dawley Rats

Test	Results of toxicity tests
Survival:	Treatment-related death with 500 μg/kg
Observations:	Yellow discoloration (jaundice) in 500 μg/kg group
Haematology:	Slight anemia and thrombocytopenia in 50 and 500 μg/kg groups Leucocytosis with lymphocytosis and eosinophilia in all treated groups Eosinophilia in bone marrow in 50 and 500 μg/kg groups
Clinical chemistry:	Increased GOT, GPT, AP and bilirubin (50 and 500 μg/kg) Decreased α_1-, α_2-globulin and increased γ-globulin in the dose groups higher than 50 μg/kg
Organ weights:	Increased liver, spleen and lymph node weight in the dose groups higher than 25 μg/kg
Pathology:	The following histology seen in the dose groups higher than 5 μg/kg; Capsular fibrosis and hypertrophy of white pulp in spleen Portal and sinusoidal infiltration of macrophages, eosinophils and fibroblasts; and pseudolobular formation in liver Eosinophilia and fibrosis in subcutis Bile duct proliferation in 500 μg/kg group
Antigenicity:	Detectable in 4 weeks and dose dependent

monkeys including chimpanzees that were given human γ-interferon in large doses and over a long period of time. Therefore, for the safety evaluation of an interferon, it is concluded that selection of a test species that responds to the known activity of interferon is desirable to detect an unanticipated effects in human. However, as even primate forms the neutralizing antibody against human γ-interferon during a prolonged study, duration of toxicity study will be limited until the time that the neutralizing antibodies are formed, because their appearance will modify the kinetics of interferons and make the interpretation of toxic findings confounded due to immune complex disorders, hypersensitivity or anaphylaxis.

TOXICITY OF INTERLEUKIN-2

In acute toxicity of single intravenous administration of the recombinant DNA-derived human interleukin-2 (r-IL-2) at doses up to 0.5 - 5 mg/kg, which are about 500 - 5000 times higher than the clinical dose in humans, no changes were observed in any of the clinical, haematological or biochemical parameters in mice, rats and monkeys.

Prolonged toxicity test were conducted with male and female rats given r-IL-2 intravenously at a dosage of 5, 50 or 500 μg/kg per day for 4 weeks and at a dosage of 1, 5 or 25 μg/kg per day for 13 weeks (Table 1). In the control group given vehicle which contained human serum albumin (HSA), no abnormality was found at all throughout both studies, although formation of antibody against HSA was confirmed. However, mortality of rats was found in the 500 μg/kg group during the course of the 4 week study and was accompanied by the appearance of jaundice. All the rats receiving the lower doses survived through the experimental period. Leucocytosis, lymphocytosis and eosinophilia in peripheral blood were noted in all treated groups. Abnormal hepatic functions (increase of GOT, GPT, alkaline

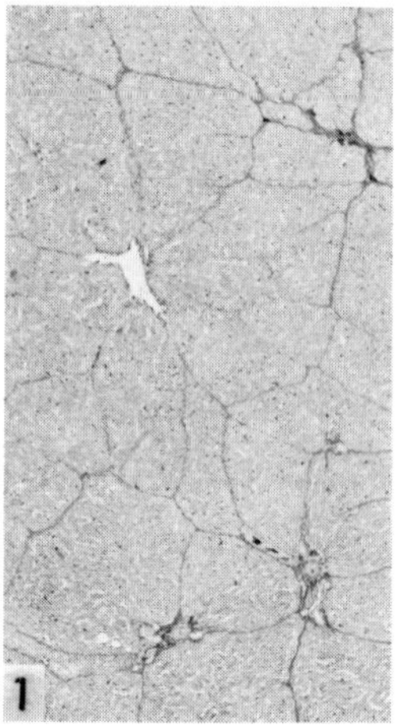

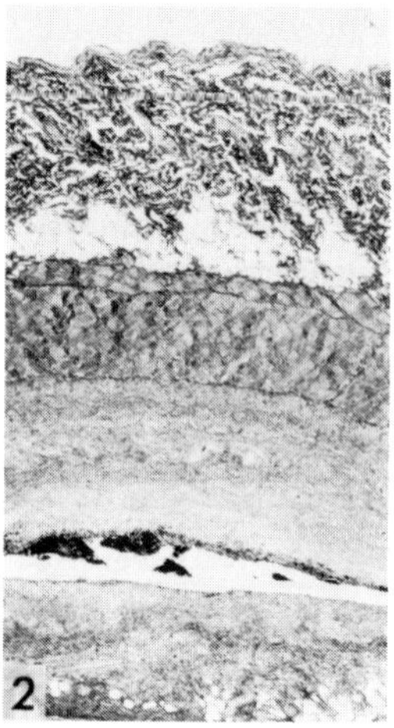

Photo. 1.

Liver of a rat received 25 μg/kg/day of r-IL-2 for 13 weeks shows pseudolobules in parenchyma with fibrosis and disruption of normal architecture.

Photo. 2.

Subcutis of the same rat reveals marked fibrosis extended to deep layer.

phosphatase and bilirubin levels) were found in association with slight anemia and thrombocytopenia in peripheral blood, eosinophilia in bone marrow as well as decreased α_1-, α_2-globulin and increased γ-globulin in the 50 and 500 μg/kg/day groups. Weight increase in liver, spleen and lymph node was observed in the groups higher than 25 μg/kg/day. Histological examination revealed marked infiltration of macrophages, eosinophils and fibroblasts at portal and sinusoidal regions as well as pseudolobular formation with increase of connective tissue in liver, capusular fibrosis and hypertrophy of white pulp in spleen, and fibrosis with eosinophilia in subcutis in rats receiving higher than 5 μg/kg/day (Photo. 1 & 2). In addition, bile duct proliferation at portal area was observed in the 500 μg/kg/day group.

After 5 weeks of withdrawal, all the changes subsided or returned to normal, but fibrotic proliferation remained in liver, spleen and subcutis. Regarding formation of neutralizing antibody against r-IL-2, it was detectable in a dose-dependent manner in the rats receiving higher than 5 μg/kg/day in 4 weeks after the start of the treatment, while it was not found in the 1 μg/kg/day group by the end of treatment for 13 weeks.

Interleukin-2 has been demonstrated to support the growth and enhance the functional capabilities of activated T lymphocytes as well as others such as macrophage and B cell mediated by IL-2 receptors on them. However, repeated administration of exogenous r-IL-2 in large quantities to rats developed various toxic changes in many tissues, as described in this report. One could therefore speculate that r-IL-2 may induce multipotential consequences resulting from a certain combination of other cytokines and lead to develop a variety of immunotoxicity. Then, in order to investigate whether recombinant human IL-2 exhibits its pharmacodynamic activity in animals, the immunomodulating effect of the r-IL-2 was monitored during the course of the rat 13-week test by procedures of flow cytofluorography and immunohistochemical analysis (Harada, 1987).

At first, peripheral blood cells in rats were analysed at specified intervals during the treatment period of the test. Although there were no changes in total WBC in the vehicle control, rats receiving 5 or 25 μg/kg/day of r-IL-2 showed dose-dependent leucocytosis in the middle of the administration period. Despite daily treatment, however, these changes returned to the predose level by the 12th week. While there was no change in neutrophils among the WBC differential, lymphocytosis was noted 2 - 4 weeks following the start of dosing and then

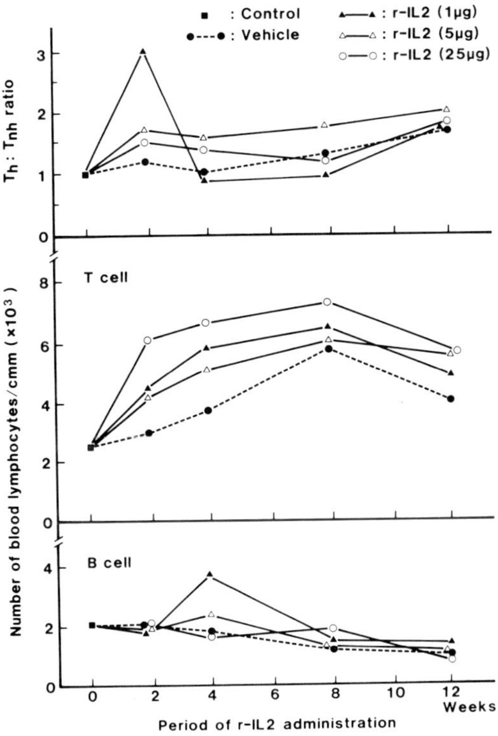

Fig. 2.

Effect of r-IL-2 administration on lymphocyte subsets in rat peripheral blood

declined to the predose level by the end of the study. In addition, considerable eosinophilia was particularly observed at the end of the study and monocytosis was found at a dose of 25 μg/kg/day during the dosing period.

Analysis of lymphocyte subsets in peripheral blood was conducted by a flow cytofluorography using EPICS-V after labeling lymphocyte subsets with the corresponding monoclonal antibodies. As shown in Fig. 2, no remarkable changes in the number of the B cell population identified by using anti-B cell monoclonal antibody (OX 6) was seen throughout the study. On the other hand, an increase of the T cell population identified by using anti-T cell monoclonal antibody (W3/13) was observed depending on the increased frequency of dosing of r-IL-2. Regarding the ratio of helper to non-helper T cells, which were recognized by using monoclonal antibodies against the corresponding cells (W3/25, OX 8), the helper T cells became dominant from 2 weeks following the commencement of the administration. These findings were interpreted that a large part of the lymphocytosis in peripheral blood in response to r-IL-2 treatment was due to an increase in helper T cells. However, in spite of the consecutive administration of r-IL-2, both lymphocytosis and increase of helper T cells tended to subside following the middle of the experimental period. These trends suggest that the effect of r-IL-2 was diminished in some degree by the neutralizing antibody against r-IL-2 elicited in animals during the study.

At specified intervals during the study, the rats were bled for analysis of peripheral blood and killed, and then the spleen and liver were removed and frozen to prepare for histological sections. Sections of spleen and liver were stained immunohistochemically by an indirect immuno-alkaline phosphatase

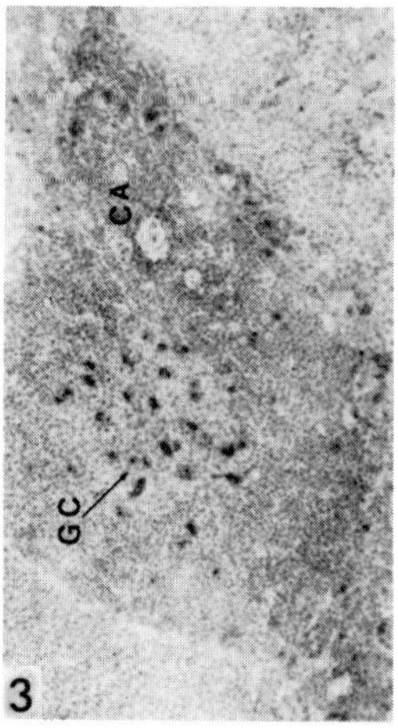

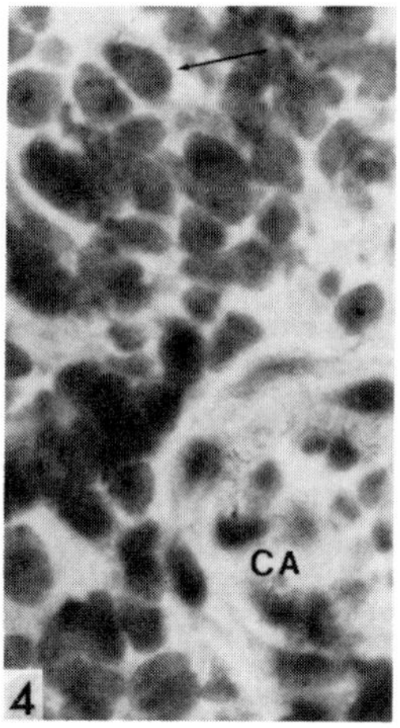

Photo. 3.

Spleen of a rat received 25 μg/kg/day of r-IL-2 shows MΦ aggregated at germinal center and transitional zone between white and red pulps.

Photo. 4.

White pulp of the above spleen shows $Ia^{+}M\Phi$ (arrow) infiltrated around a central artery (CA) and contacted with T cells.

technique using monoclonal antibodies against the corresponding cells (Cordell et al, 1984; Erber et al, 1984). Then, after taking the colored micro-photographs on each section, the distribution and frequency in number of various types of cells were quantitatively analysed by an image analyzer (VIDEO PLAN).

A section of the spleen obtained from rats receiving r-IL-2 administration was treated by anti-T cell monoclonal antibody. Enlarged white pulps were found which consisted of thymus dependent areas (TDA) stained a red-purple color and unstained thymus independent areas (TIDA). Compared with the vehicle control, a marked increase was observed not only in the TDA but also in TIDA (which is also called the B cell area) for the groups given 5 or 25 μg/kg/day of r-IL-2 four weeks after the start of the treatment. But, after that, the areas of TDA and TIDA tended to decrease their size.

Macrophages in a spleen section were identified by using anti-macrophage monoclonal antibody (M 53). They were demonstrated to be aggregated at germinal centers of white pulp and the transitional zone between white and red pulps in rats receiving 25 μg/kg/day of r-IL-2 (Photo. 3). When the number of macrophages in white pulp was scrutinized by an image analyzer at intervals during the toxicity study, a prominent increase of macrophages in the TDA and the follicle per unit area of spleen section was observed, depending on the increased frequency of administration of r-IL-2. On the contrary, neither increase nor decrease of macrophage numbers was found in the vehicle control. Among macrophages in spleen, Ia positive macrophages were identified by using anti-Ia positive antigen monoclonal antibody (OX 4). Many Ia positive macrophages aggregated around a central artery and intermingled with T cells in white pulp of the r-IL-2 treated rats (Photo. 4). This reaction may suggest that a synergism between Ia positive macrophages and T cells is produced by the r-IL-2 treatment.

These results obtained from the repeated intravenous administration of r-IL-2 to rats are summarized as follows. Observations in the peripheral blood reveal a moderate leucocytosis derived mainly from the increase of helper T cells within two weeks after the start of r-IL-2 administration. This fact indicates that r-IL-2 not only facilitates the rate of cell proliferation in the immunocompetent organs, i.e. thymus, lymph node, spleen and bone marrow which take a role as a source for supplying lymphocytes, but also stimulates the mobilization of these cells toward the peripheral blood. Simultaneously, the following changes were observed in the spleens of animals receiving r-IL-2. 1) Increased weight in

Table 2. Histopathological Findings in Liver of the Rats Dosed r-IL-2 (25 μg/kg/day) and Killed at Specified Intervals

Duration of administration (Weeks)		0	2	4	8	12	After 5-week withdrawal
Histopathological changes* in parenchymal tissue	Vacuole in hepatocyte	-	±	±	±	±	±
	Fatty degeneration	-	-	-	-	-	-
	Amyloid deposition	-	-	-	-	-	-
	Pseudo-lobule	-	-	-	±	+	+
Cell-infiltration* in portal region	T ($W3/13^+$)	-	-	-	-	±	± (Lymphocyte)
	B ($OX\ 6^+$)	-	-	±	±	±	
	Mφ ($M53^+$)	-	+	+	++	++	±
	$Ia^+M\phi$ ($OX\ 4^+$)	-	+	+	++	++	
	N ($P67^+$)	-	-	-	-	+	±
	M	-	±	±	+	±	±

* Arbitrary grade: -; absent, ±; very weak, +; weak, ++; extensive.
T; T cell, B; B cell, Mφ; macrophage, $Ia^+M\phi$; Ia positive macrophage, N; neutrophil, M; mast cell.

spleen where the hypertrophy of both TDA and TIDA were evident in white pulp, and 2) Increased number of macrophages including Ia positive macrophages contacted with T cells. As a result, it is suggested that exogenous r-IL-2 activates lymphoid tissues, establishes an immunologically effective micromilieu in the tissue for the synergism between the macrophage and the T cell, and promotes the effect of immunomodulation in the whole body.

Regarding a section of the liver obtained from the same rats employed for the immunohistochemical study of spleen, the following changes were observed in animals receiving 25 μg/kg/day of r-IL-2 (Table 2). 1) Vacuolar degeneration in hepatocytes appeared from 2 weeks following the start of dosing and throughout the period of treatment and remained for 5 weeks after withdrawal. However, no fatty degeneration or amyloid deposition was confirmed in the vacuoles by specific staining respectively. 2) Pseudolobules in parenchyma were formed in association with fibrosis and disruption of normal architecture from 8 weeks after the commencement of treatment. These fibrotic changes were still left after the cessation of administration of r-IL-2. 3) Portal mononuclear cell infiltration which extended into hepatic parenchyma were observed from 2 weeks after the start of treatment. These infiltrates were identified immunohistochemically by using the monoclonal antibodies against the correspond-

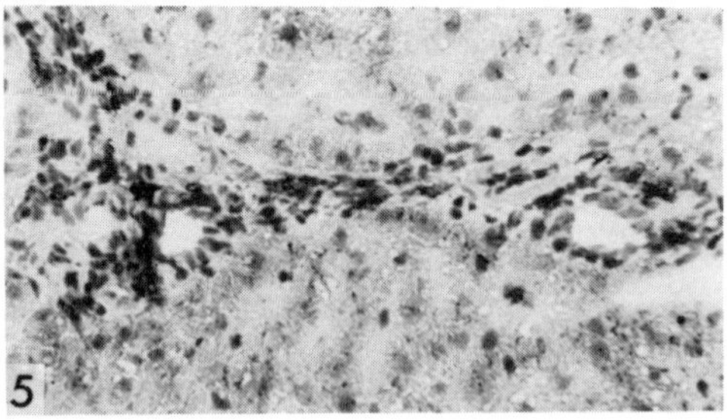

Photo. 5.

Liver of a rat received 25 μg/kg/day of r-IL-2 shows perivascular infiltration of MΦ and Ia^{+}MΦ.

ing cells described previously in the sections of spleen. Depending on the increased frequency of dosing of r-IL-2, macrophages and Ia positive macrophages which infiltrated at first became noticeable (Photo. 5), followed by infiltrates of mast cells and B lymphocytes, and finally by neutrophils and T lymphocytes at the end of treatment. After 5 weeks of withdrawal, these infiltrates remained at perivascular area. These findings may suggest that although the etiology of hepatotoxicity is unclear, prolonged administration of r-IL-2 could stimulate the extravasation of mononuclear cells into hepatic parenchyma and the release of other cytokines through unpredictable mechanism within the immune system. Then, in combination with other cytokines, r-IL-2 would harm hepatocytes and facilitate fibrosis which might cause genesis of liver cirrhosis.

Using cynomolgus monkeys of both sexes, repeated toxicity studies of r-IL-2 were also conducted by intravenous route at a dosage of 5, 50 or 500 μg/kg per day for 4 weeks and at dosage of 1, 5 or 25 μg/kg per day for 40 weeks. The results of the studies are summarized in Table 3. All monkeys receiving 500 μg/kg/day were sacrificed in extremis during the course of the 4-week study. Except for these decedents, all the monkeys in the other groups survived through the experimental period. Throughout the study, loose faeces, lethargy and subdued behavior were observed in animals given higher than 50 μg/kg/day. Flaky dry skins were noted in monkeys receiving 25 μg/kg/day for 40 weeks, despite the remaining of good appetite. Haematological changes, such as anemia, thrombocytopenia, neutropenia and eosinophilia were found in the groups dosed at higher than 25 μg/kg/day. In clinical chemistry, increased GOT, LAP and bilirubin levels which were suggestive of hepatotoxicity were found in the higher dose groups. Histologically, for the monkeys receiving higher than 50 μg/kg/day of r-IL-2, conspicuous mononuclear cell infiltration was observed around the perivascular area in parenchymal tissues of liver and lungs which were very similar to those seen when large doses of r-IL-2 were given to rats. Increased weight of spleen and hypertrophy of white pulp were demonstrated in the animals given higher than 25 μg/kg/day. Interesting findings on antibody formation were as follows; despite daily consecutive administration of r-IL-2 up to 40 weeks, no neutralizing antibody against r-IL-2 was detected by means of radioimmunoassay in sera of any monkeys, but positive antibody against HSA in vehicle was detected in all the treated monkeys including the vehicle control.

In addition to the above studies, the continuous infusion of r-IL-2 using a mini-osmotic pump (model 2001) implanted subcutaneously in mice was performed at doses of 10,000, 30,000 and 100,000 U/kg/h. All the mice survived up to the time of killing at 8 days. Slight anemia, leucocytosis with lymphocytosis and eosinophilia in peripheral blood were noted in the highest dose group. In the same group, increased GOT, GPT, LDH and bilirubin levels were observed in serum chemistries. Enlargement of liver and spleen and atrophy of thymus were seen in the mice receiving higher than 30,000 U/kg/h. Histological examination revealed dose-dependent infiltrations of lymphoblastoid or macrophage -like cells, which contained a few eosinophilic large granules in cytoplasma in liver, spleen, lymph

Table 3. Results of 4-Week and 40-Week Toxicity Tests of iv r-IL-2 in Cynomolgus Monkeys

Test	Results of toxicity tests
Survival:	Treatment-related death with 500 μg/kg
Clinical symptoms:	Loose faeces, lethargy, subdued behavior, coughing and vomiting in 50 and 500 μg/kg groups Flaky dry skin in 25 μg/kg group
Haematology:	Slight anemia, thrombocytopenia, neutropenia and eosinophilia in the groups dosed at higher than 25 μg/kg
Clinical chemistry:	Increased GOT, LAP and bilirubin in 500 μg/kg group
Organ weights:	Increased spleen weight in the groups dosed at higher than 25 μg/kg
Pathology:	Mononuclear cell infiltration in lungs, liver, spleen, thymus and parenchymal tissues of many other organs in 50 and 500 μg/kg groups Capsular fibrosis on spleen in 25 μg/kg group
Antigenicity:	No detectable antibody formation until 40 weeks of dosing

nodes and subcutaneous infusion sites. These toxic findings in mice demonstrated a striking similarity to those obtained in our rat and monkey studies or others (Matory et al, 1985).

CONCLUSIONS

It has long been a principle for safety evaluation of a compound that animal tests should be conducted in a species that responds to the test material in a manner similar to humans. From the studies described in this report, rodents did not show any biological response to the recombinant human γ-interferon due to minimal cross-species activity of the protein, but primates demonstrated similar toxic effects to those seen in human patients given therapeutic doses of the interferon. On the other hand, since interleukin-2 was known active across the barrier of animal species-specificity, the immunomodulating effect of recombinant human IL-2 was confirmed in rats by means of flow cytofluorography and immunohistochemical analysis during the toxicity study. In addition, a variety of immunotoxicity represented by a hepatotoxicity were acknowledged not only in rodents but also in primates, and these toxicities had similarity to those seen in human patients following intravenous administration of r-IL-2. Therefore, unlike the preclinical safety evaluation of xenobiotics, selection of species which respond to the intended pharmacological effect of cytokines is the most serious issue (Hobson et al, 1987). Additionally, our study indicated that both quantity and duration of dosing should be carefully monitored during systematic administration of r-IL-2 to patients, because of occurrence of hepatotoxicity which might lead to liver cirrhosis following the prolonged period of the treatment.

Because of the high degree of species specificity in molecular structure of cytokines, their capacity to elicit neutralizing antibody should be carefully delineated during toxicity study with various species of animals. Furthermore, many researchers expected animals to make antibody quite easily against human species-specific protein and pointed out the duration of a repeated toxicity study to be decided by the development of antibody, because the antibody might neutralize and remove the test protein and subsequently mask its toxicity or result in immune complex disorders (Dayan, 1987; Zbinden, 1987). However, it was surprizingly demonstrated in our monkey study that no neutralizing antibody against r-IL-2 has been detected in sera of monkeys, despite daily administration at a dose up to 25 μg/kg/day for more than 40 weeks. This outcome verified that primates turned out to be the most appropriate species for studies of biotechnological products, especially for chronic toxicity with r-IL-2.

With recent increasing desire to expand the clinical therapeutic indication of cytokines to the treatment for chronic non-life-threatening diseases, such as hepatitis B or rheumatic arthritis, regulatory authorities would like to require chronic toxicity study using a newly invented animal model for safety evaluation in human. To fulfil this requirement, a suitable model must be considered, but a transgenic mouse carrying a gene of cytokine may become a good model for this type of study, as reported by Dr. Metcalf et al, (1987).

ACKNOWLEDGEMENTS

Technical assistance for immunohistochemistry and helpful suggestions were received from Professor A. Yamashita of Hamamatsu Medical School.

REFERENCES

Bocci, V. (1982). Drugs Exptl. Clin. Res. 8, 683-689
Cordell, J.L., Falini, B., Erber, W.N., Ghosh, A.K., Abdulaziz, Z., MacDonald, S., Pulford, K.A.F., Stein, H. and Mason, D.Y. (1984). J. Histochem. Cytochem. 32, 219-229
Dayan, A.D. (1987). In: Preclinical Safety of Biotechnology Products Intended for Human Use: (ed C.E. Graham) Alan R. Liss, Inc. 89-106
Erber, W.N., Prinching, A.J. and Mason, D.Y. (1984). Lancet 1, 1042-1045
Galbraith, W.M. (1987). In: Preclinical Safety of Biotechnology Products Intended for Human Use: (ed C.E. Graham) Alan R. Liss, Inc. 3-14
Harada, Y. (1987). In: Preclinical Safety of Biotechnology Products Intended for Human Use: (ed C.E. Graham) Alan R. Liss, Inc. 127-142
Hobson, W.C. and Fuller, G.B. (1987). In: Preclinical Safety of Biotechnology Products Intended for Human Use: (ed C.E. Graham) Alan R. Liss, Inc. 55-71
Kobayashi, F., Furukawa, H., Torii, M., Nemoto, Y., Hirashiba, Y., Yoshizaki, T., Takano, K., Ikeuchi, J. and Nina, N. (1986). Kiso to Rinsho (in Japanese) 20, 4905-4105
Kobayashi, F., Matsuura, M., Ogawa, M., Maruyama, T., Yoshizaki, T., Hasegawa, N., Nishibe, Y., Teshima, K., Nakano, A., Hanafusa, T., Sato, K., Wada, T., Yamashita, T., Muto, M., Nakai, K. and Harada, Y. (1986). Kiso to Rinsho (in Japanese) 20, 4140-4173
Kobayashi, F., Torii, M., Furukawa, H., Hasegawa, N., Yoshizaki, T. and Ikeuchi, J. (1986). Kiso to Rinsho (in Japanese) 20, 4121-4137
Lang, R.A., Metcalf, D., Cuthbertson, R.A., Lyons, I., Stanley, E., Kelso, A., Kannourakis, G., Williamson, D.J., Klintworth, G.K., Gonda, T.J. and Dunn, A.R. (1987). Cell 51, 675-686
Lotze, M.T., Matory, Y.L., Ettinghausen, S.E., Rayner, A.A., Sharrow, S.O., Seipp, C.A.Y., Custer, M.C. and Rosenberg, S.A. (1985). J. Immunol. 135, 2865-2875
Matory, Y.L., Chang, A.E., Lipford III, E.H., Braziel, R., Hyatt, C.L., McDonald, H.D. and Rosenberg, S.A. (1985). J. Biol. Resp. Modif. 4, 377-390
Schellekens, H., de Reus, A., Wiersema, H.D., Hirschi, M., Nooter, K., van Es, A.A., Dawson, A. and Harada, Y. (1986). Kiso to Rinsho (in Japanese) 20, 4180-4190
Schellekens, H., van Eerd, P.M.C.A., de Reus, A., Hartevelt, N., Boekesteijn, A.J.J., Hoek, L.A., Struyck, A.J.J., Hirschi, M., van Es, A.A., Dawson, A. and Harada, Y. (1986). Kiso to Rinsho (in Japanese) 20, 4191-4208
Watson, M., Brett, D., Heywood, R., Gibson, W.A., Dawson, A. and Harada, Y. (1986). Kiso to Rinsho (in Japanese) 20, 4175-4179
Zbinden, G. (1987). In: Preclinical Safety of Biotechnology Products Intended for Human Use: (ed C.E. Graham) Alan R. Liss, Inc. 143-159

Immunopharmacology of Neuroendocrine Interaction

Overview on Neuroimmunomodulation and a Possible Role for Serotonergic System

K. MAŠEK

Institute of Pharmacology, Czechoslovak Academy of Sciences, Prague, Czechoslovakia

ABSTRACT

The recent advances in the field of neuroimmunomodulation have been remarkable. The list of neurotransmitters, immunotransmitters and hormones which are involved in the bidirectional communication between neuroendocrine and immune systems is steadily increasing. The possible role of serotonergic system in neuroimmunomodulation is discussed in more details.

KEYWORDS

Neuroimmunomodulation, neurotransmitters, immunnotransmitters, hormones, 5-HT, MDP, receptors

A growing body of data support the concept of the existence of a close bidirectional communication between the neuroendocrine and immune systems. Messages from the brain reach the immunocompetent cells through the autonomic nervous and endocrine systems and via a great number of hormones and neurotransmitters affect the function of the immune system. Evidence on the existence of a close communication between the brain and immune systems has been gathered quite recently and consists of data at anatomical, physiological as well as pharmacological levels. The autonomic nerve endings were found to be present in all major lymphatic organs and the electrolytic or chemical lesions at the central or peripheral sites always influenced the immune function. The neuroanatomical aspects of the interaction between the neural and immune systems has been recently reviewed (Livnat et al. 1985).

The list of hormones and neurotransmitters which can influence the immune response is steadily increasing and currently we have at least 30 well characterized transmitters or hormones which have been reported to influence the immune response. For a great number of these substances their receptors have been identified to be present on immunocompetent cells, but it has to be mentioned that most of the neurotransmitters or hormones can bind with more than just one receptor type. The list of substances that might influence the immune response is presented in Table 1.

TABLE 1 Modulators of Immune Response

Neurotransmitters	**Neuroactive peptides**
Acetylcholine	Substance P
Catecholamines	Neurotensin
Serotonin	VIP
(Benzodiazepines ?)	Cholecystokinin
	Enkephalins
Hypothalamic hormones	**Hormones**
Somatostatin	Corticosteroids
Corticotrophin Releasing hormone	Insulin
	Glucagon
Pituitary hormones	Gonadal hormones
Vasopressin	**Others**
Oxytocin	Prostaglandins
ACTH	Histamine
TSH	Bradykinin
Prolactin	Bombesin
Growth hormone	
Endorphins	
Products of immune cells	
Interleukins	TSH
Thymosins	VIP
Lymphokines (MIF, CSF)	Histamine
Interferons	Serotonin
ACTH	Prostaglandins
β-Endorphin	Others ?

Each of the neurotransmitters or hormones may act through a different kind of second messenger systems such as cAMP, cGMP or through phosphatidyl inositol pathway.

The brain, on the other hand, receives signals from resting or activated immune cells via afferent nerves or soluble products which are synthetized by immunocompetent cells such as interferons, interleukins, thymosins, endorphins, but also hormones which are classically associated with the neuroendocrine system such as corticotropin (ACTH), thyrotropin (TSH) and most probably others (Weigent and Blalock, 1987). More evidence however is needed to better understand the real role of these hormones and factors that trigger their synthesis by immune cells. We consider as crucial the findings that some of the receptors for neurotransmitters or hormones are common for cells of neuroendocrine and immune systems and furthermore, an important question on the role of such sets of common receptors and/or molecular mechanisms involved in the response of the organism to internal or external stimuli was thus opened. The possible ways of interactions between the neuroendocrine and immune system are summarized on Figure 1.

Since the other speakers of this Symposium will cover in more details the possible role of hormones shared by the neuroendocrine and immune systems as well as the role of immunotransmitters in neuroimmunomodulation I will review to a greater extent the anatomical, biochemical and pharmacological evidence which was accumulated by our group as well as by some others during the past several years with respect to the role of serotonergic system and serotonergic receptors in neuroimmunomodulation.

FIGURE 1

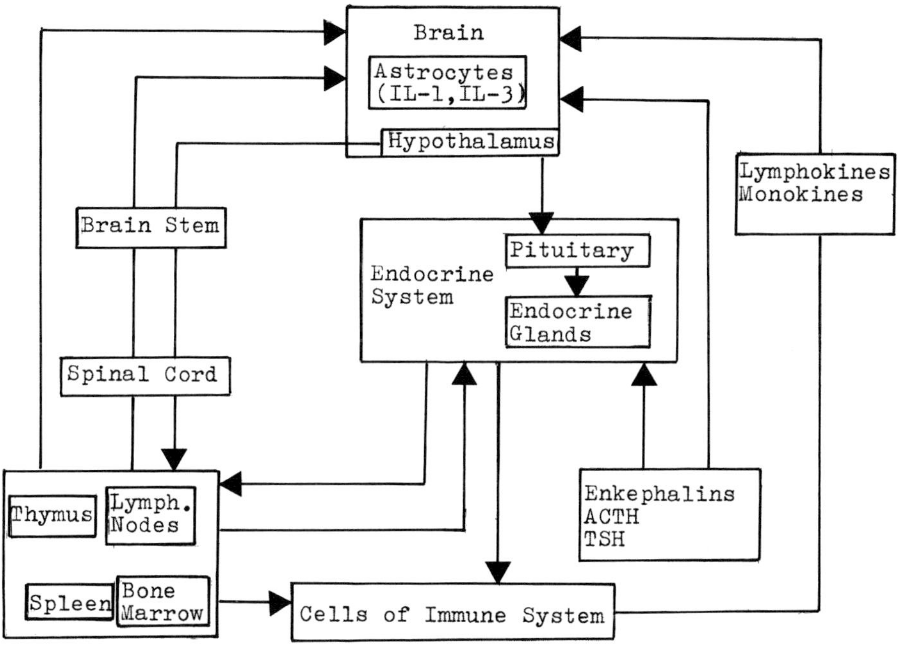

During the studies that investigated the mechanism of action of bacterial cell wall product muramyl peptides (MDP), our group has discovered years ago that these potent immunomodulatory compounds have also a number of other pharmacological activities and some of them were evidently linked to the central nervous system. These are particularly the effects on temperature, sleep and pain threshold control. With the biochemical approaches we have been able to show that MDP in doses which stimulate the immune response markedly increases the 5-HT turnover in several regions of the brain stem which suggests the activation of serotonergic structures. Simultaneously we have noted also the changes in temperature, sleep and pain threshold. The effect is evidently specific since we have not observed the effects on other neurotransmitter systems; and MDP-DD analoque, which is biologically inactive, had no comparable effect. The involvement of specific serotonergic structures, particularly B 6, B 7 and B 8 with the corresponding pathways to hypothalamus is suggested by the result of small electrolytic lesions which markedly potentiated the effect of MDP on delayed hypersensitivity response (Mašek et al., 1985).

The possible role of serotonergic system in the immune response induced by MDP as well as temperature, sleep and pain threshold changes caused by MDP has been confirmed by a number of experiments with different serotonergic agonists and antagonists and also in the experiments in which we have inhibited the serotonin synthesis by para-chlorphenylalanine (Mašek and Kadlecová, 1987). In vitro experiments with the brain tissue slices where we have measured release of ^{3}H-serotonin under the influence of MDP and the results of experiments with different isolated tissues such as guinea-pig ileum, rat stomach strip, rat colon ascendens and the guinea-pig and mouse vas deferens further support the hypothesis on the importance of interaction of MDP with serotonergic receptors in its mechanism of action on the immune as well as nervous systems. The results of experiments with different antagonists of 5-HT receptor subtypes as well as the results of binding studies strongly suggest possible involvement of 5-HT_1 receptors (Fillion et al., 1988).The results of our most recent experiments in vivo where MDP was administered in doses of 1 and 60 µg/hr for 7 and 14 days by Alzet osmotic minipumps are in good agreement with previously described effects in vitro when we have reported super- and sub-sensitivity, respectively, of serotonin receptor system (Kadlec et al., 1984). In these experiments where the higher dosage regimen was applied we have noticed in serum of tested animals the presence of a factor which blocked the serotonin receptor and which may have a character of antibodies.

The results of our experiments with model compound muramyl peptide, a compound which has both immunopharmacological and neuropharmacological properties thus bring further support for an important modulatory role of 5-HT system in the interaction between neuroendocrine and immune systems. At present, we cannot strictly rule out also the involvement of interleukins which are released by MDP; however, the incubation of MDP with peritoneal macrophages and the addition of such a mixture to the organ bath did not cause any effect different from the addition of MDP alone when tested on serotonergic contractions.

Our finding that muramyl peptide, a subunit of bacterial cell wall, which is naturally present in some tissues, may interact with the serotonergic receptor can of course have important consequences since such interaction may influence serotonergic transmission which is playing an important role in a number of physiological functions. However, it might have an important role also in the development of some diseases which involve the central nervous and immune systems.

REFERENCES

Fillion, G., M. Bonnet, M. P. Fillion, L. Morelet, N. Prudhomme, K. Mašek, M. Flegel, N. Corvala and J. M. Launay (1988). Hypothetical role of the serotonergic system in neuroimmunomodulation: Preliminary molecular studies. In: Interaction between the neuroendocrine and immune systems. Ed. J. Hadden, K. Mašek and G. Nistico, Pytagora Press, Milan, p. 00.

Kadlec, O., K. Mašek, O. Gulda, V. Růžička, M. Parant and L. Chedid (1984). Smooth muscle stimulation by an immunomodulatory compound muramyl dipeptide: does it involve serotoninergic system? Pharmacology, 29, 31-39.

Livnat, S., S. Y. Felten, S. L. Carlson, D. L. Bellinger and D. L. Felten (1985). Involvement of peripheral and central

catecholamine systems in neural-immune interactions. J. Neuro-immunol., 10, 5-30.
Mašek, K., O. Kadlecová and P. Petrovický (1985). The involvement of brain structures in the adjuvant effect of muramyl dipeptide. Brain Research Bull., 15, 443-466.
Mašek, K. and O. Kadlecová (1987). Muramyl peptides, serotonergic system and sleep. Ann. N. Y. Acad. Sci., 496, 517-521.
Weigent, D. A. and J. E. Blalock (1987). Interactions between the neuroendocrine and immune systems: common hormones and receptors. Immunol. Rev., 100, 80-108.

A Molecular Basis for Bidirectional Communication between the Neuroendocrine and Immune Systems

ERIC M. SMITH, Ph.D. and EVE W. JOHNSON

Departments of Psychiatry and Behavioral Sciences and Microbiology, The University of Texas Medical Branch, Galveston, Texas 77550

KEYWORDS

Hormones: lymphokines: proopiomelanocortin: ACTH: endorphins: hormone receptors: intracellular messengers.

COMMUNICATION BETWEEN THE NEUROENDOCRINE AND IMMUNE SYSTEMS

There is currently much interest in the relationship between the mind and the immune system. A great deal of anecdotal and recent scientific evidence supports a concept linking the seemingly disparate systems. This relationship has been difficult to directly establish since the mechanisms involved were not known. Recent studies have suggested a number of possible connections that might link the brain and the immune system. There are at least two general mechanisms for their interactions. The first involves direct modulation of the immune system by the sympathetic nervous system, as suggested by the innervation of immune organs such as the spleen, thymus, and bone marrow (Felton, et al., 1985). Evidence for this direct modulation is that sympathectomy and lesioning of specific regions of the brain can be shown to enhance and/or suppress immune responses (Miles, et al., 1985; Roszman, et al., 1985) and the firing rate of hypothalamic neurons is altered during an immune response (Besedovsky, et al., 1977). Furthermore, lymphocytes are known to possess beta-2 adrenergic receptors as well as other neurotransmitter receptors (Felten, et al., 1985).

A second means for interactions between mind and immune system involves hormonal influences on immune function. Hormonal influence on immune reactions has been known for some time, exemplified in particular by the immunosuppressive effects of glucocorticoids (for review see Cupps and Fauci, 1982). Recently, we and others found that neuroendocrine peptide hormones will modulate T and B lymphocyte functions as well as other immunocyte responses (Besedovsky, et al., 1977; Cupps and Fauci, 1982; Johnson, et al., 1982a, 1982b; Wybran, et al., 1979; Hazum, Chang, and Cuatrecasas, 1979; O'Dorisio, et al., 1981; Gilman, et al., 1982; McCain, et al., 1982; Johnson, et al., 1984). Furthermore, lymphocytes themselves can synthesize biologically active neuroendocrine hormones (Blalock and Smith, 1980; O'Dorisio, et al., 1980; Smith and Blalock, 1981; Smith, et al., 1983; Lolait, et al., 1984; Ruff and Pert, 1984) as well as possess specific hormone receptors (Blalock, et al., 1985; Johnson, et al., 1986; Wybran et al., 1979; Hazum et al., 1979; O'Dorisio et al., 1981; Lopker, et al., 1980; Payan, Breuster and Goetzl, 1984; Pert, et al., 1985). In addition thymic hormones (Healy, et al., 1983), and lymphokines (Lotze, et al., 1985; Woloski, et al., 1985; Besedovsky, del Ray, and Sorkin, 1981) have been shown to exert hormonal effects. Thus, we feel that one way in which bidirectional communication takes place between the immune and neuroendocrine systems is via signal molecules and receptors which are common to cells of both systems.

PRO-OPIOMELANOCORTIN (POMC) PRODUCTION BY LEUKOCYTES

Stimulated lymphocytes produce molecules that are very similar, if not identical, to the peptide hormones: corticotropin (ACTH), endorphin (END), thyrotropin (TSH), human chorionic gonadotropin (hCG), prolactin (PRL), and possibly others (Table 1). The immunoreactive (ir) hormone produced is variable depending upon

TABLE 1

LEUKOCYTE PRODUCTION OF NEUROENDOCRINE HORMONES

Hormone	Cell type	Stimulus	Reference
ACTH	Lymphocyte	Virus, mitogens, CRF[a]	Blalock and Smith, 1980 Smith, et al., 1982, 1986 Harbour-McMenamin, et al., 1985 Westly, et al., 1986
	Macrophage	None	Lolait, et al., 1984
Bombesin	Macrophage[b]	None	Ruff, et al., 1984
hCG	Lymphocyte	MLR[c]	Harbour-McMenamin, et al., 1986a
END	Lymphocyte	Virus, mitogen, CRF	Smith, et al., 1986
	Macrophage	None, LPS[d]	Lolait, et al., 1984
ENK[e]	Lymphocyte	T-lymphocyte mitogen	Zurawksi, et al., 1986
GH[f]	Lymphocytes	None, GHRH	Weigent, et al., 1987
Oxytocin	Thymus	None	Geenan, et al., 1986
PRL	Lymphocytes	Con A[g]	Hiestand, et al., 1986
TSH	Lymphocyte	T-lymphocyte mitogen	Smith, et al., 1983
VIP[h]	PMN	None	O'Dorisio, et al., 1980
	Mast cell	None	Cutz, et al., 1978

[a]Corticotropin Releasing Factor
[b]Oat cell carcinoma cell of macrophage origin
[c]Mixed lymphocyte reaction
[d]Lipopolysaccharide
[e]Enkephalin
[f]Growth Hormone
[g]Concanavalin A
[h]Vasoactive Intestinal Peptide

the stimulus (Table 1) and thus may represent a mechanism for affecting differential homeostatic host responses. The kinetics of ir hormone production also varies with the inducer and may be another differentiating factor. Virus induction of ir ACTH occurs early, peaking at 18-24 hours concomitant with interferon alpha (IFN-α) production (Smith and Blalock, 1981). Lipopolysaccharide (LPS) induction of ir-ACTH peaks later, 48 hours after stimulation, and parallels mitogenic activity (Harbour-McMenamin, et al., 1985). The antigenic relatedness of these molecules to pituitary-derived hormones has been determined by immunofluorescence studies of their production and by immunoaffinity purification of the ir hormones. Presumably both T and B lymphocytes can synthesize these proopiomelanocortin (POMC)-related products because when 100% of the cells are infected and synthesizing Newcastle disease virus (NDV) antigens, all of the cells stain positive for ACTH and endorphins (END). Lolait, et al., (1984) found ACTH and END are also produced constitutively by nonstimulated macrophages. When foreign cells, which stimulate B-cells but not T-cells to produce IFN (Weigent, et al., 1981), are used as inducers, only 20-30% of the cells stained positive with anti-ACTH antiserum (Smith and Blalock, 1981). The B cell mitogen LPS induces B-lymphocytes but not T-cells to produce ACTH and END (Harbour-McMenamin, et al., 1985 and 1986b). Thus, all leukocytes appear to be capable of synthesizing ACTH and endorphins so long as the proper stimulus is used. These molecules are synthesized _de novo_, as induction of ir hormones can be inhibited in the presence of actinomycin D and cycloheximide (Blalock and Smith, 1982). Further evidence of _de novo_ synthesis is that these peptides can be intrinsically labelled by inducing lymphocytes in the presence of radiolabelled amino acids (Blalock and Smith, 1985).

Structurally, lymphocyte-derived ACTH and endorphins are very similar if not identical to their pituitary prototypes. ir-ACTH and pituitary ACTH share the following properties: antigenicity, molecular weight, resistance to acid inactivation, and migration time on reverse-phase HPLC (Blalock and Smith, 1985). Sizing on SDS polyacrylamide gels indicates that the molecular weight of the ACTH-like molecule is 4.5 K, which is identical to that of the 39 amino acid pituitary ACTH molecule (Smith and Blalock, 1981). Lymphocyte END, like β-END, has an apparent molecular weight of 3.6 Kd (Smith, et al., 1986). To date the only structural differences between lymphocyte and pituitary ACTH and END have been noted when LPS is used as a stimulus: ACTH and END species in this system are processed to approximately 3 Kd and 2 Kd respectively, compared to pituitary ACTH (4.5 Kd) and END (3.6 Kd). These differences are apparently not structural but due to a novel enzymatic activity (Harbour, et al., 1987). In addition, two laboratories have been able to detect POMC mRNA in splenocytes (Westly, et al., 1986) and macrophages (Lolait, et al., 1986). It appears then, that the same POMC gene expressed in pituitary cells is also induced in leukocytes.

Functionally, lymphocyte-derived ACTH also closely resembles pituitary ACTH. Ir-ACTH induces both steroidogenisis and morphological change (rounding) by mouse adrenal tumor cells (Blalock and Smith, 1980; Blalock and Smith, 1981; Smith, et al., 1986). Lymphocyte END is also biologically active, binding to opiate receptors both _in vitro_ and _in vivo_ (Harbour-McMenamin, et al., 1985; Blalock and Smith, 1981). These effects could be immediately reversed or prevented by the opiate antagonist naloxone. Therefore during an infection lymphocytes may be able to affect pain sensation, temperature regulation, neurotransmitter activity, or other opiate-mediated functions, by secretion of END.

OTHER NEUROENDOCRINE HORMONES PRODUCED BY LEUKOCYTES

In contrast to virus infection, lymphocytes stimulated with the T cell mitogen staphylococcal enterotoxin A (SEA) synthesize a molecule related to thyrotropin (TSH) (Table 1; Smith, et al., 1983). This ir-TSH consists of two polypeptide chains identical in size to the α and β chains of TSH and, like the pituitary hormone, appears to glycosylated. Mixed lymphocyte cultures produce a molecule that is immunologically, structurally, and functionally related to hCG (Table 1,

Harbour-McMenamin, et al., 1986a). Recent studies have detected prolactin and growth hormone immunoreactivity and mRNA in leukocytes (Montgomery, et al., 1987; Hiestand, et al., 1986; Weigent, et al., 1987). Thus it seems that, depending on the particular lymphocyte stimulus, a variety of hormone-related molecules can be produced which in turn may influence homeostasis. Besides classic immune stimuli such as mitogens and viruses, lymphocyte hormone production can be induced by the same hypothalamic releasing hormones that control their production by pituitary cells (Smith, et al., 1986; Kruger, et al., 1987; Harbour, et al., 1988). Corticotropin releasing hormone (CRH) stimulates leukocyte ACTH production (Smith, et al., 1986) and mitogenisis (McGillis, et al., 1987). Recent findings have shown that thyrotropin-stimulating hormone (TRH) and leutinizing hormone releasing hormone (LHRH) stimulate leukocyte production of ir-TSH and ir-LH respectively (Kruger, et al., 1987; Harbour, et al., 1988; Ebaugh et al., 1988). Although it has not been examined rigorously, these releasing hormones would appear to act in a specific manner to induce lymphocyte hormone production, since multiple hormones are not detected simultaneously in these cultures. On a structural and functional basis the lymphocyte products appear identical to their pituitary prototypes. Harbour, et al., (manuscript in preparation) have found mRNA expression of both α and β chain genes of TSH. In the case of ir-LH the molecule seems, at the protein level, to be identical to the pituitary prototype and is definitely not hCG. Therefore, depending upon the stimulus used, different hormones are produced that conceivably would have a variety of effects on immune and neuroendocrine responses.

COMMON MOLECULAR MECHANISMS

An important question concerning specificity is raised by leukocyte production of multiple hormones when treated with various stimuli. It would seem that specificity of response could occur at several levels. The first would be at the level of the surface membrane. This could occur as either expression of a binding site on specific cell subtypes (i.e., B or T-lymphocytes) or in the specificity of the binding. The first example certainly applies in the ACTH system. Different inducers with known tropisms for different lymphocyte types cause varying percentages of lymphocytes to synthesize ACTH. NDV will induce ACTH in both B and T lymphocytes, if they are infected at a multiplicity of infection greater than one (Smith and Blalock, 1981). Bacterial LPS will induce ACTH only in B cells (Harbour-McMenamin, et al., 1986b), and CRF causes only 40% of peripheral blood monocytes to synthesize ACTH (Smith, et al., 1986). Thus, probably only 40% of these lymphocytes possess CRF receptors, which is supported by a study of CRF binding in cryostat sections of mouse spleen indicating that binding occurs only in certain regions of the organ (Webster and deSouza, 1987). In the latter study, the authors felt that macrophages were the primary population which bound CRF. Other cell types stimulated by CRF in our study to produce ACTH might have been indirectly induced by macrophage-synthesized cytokines. Alternatively, lymphocytes might have fewer CRF receptors which in an *in situ* binding assay may appear as background binding. Use of an antiserum to the ACTH receptor (Bost, et al., 1985) has demonstrated a differential distribution of cells bearing these receptors within lymphoid organs and among cell types, including B cells, T cells, and macrophages (Johnson, et al., manuscript in preparation). In addition, activation of lymphocytes upregulates expression of a number of surface antigens and receptors; concanavalin A stimulation of thymocytes raises the precentage of cells expressing ACTH receptors from $\leq$ 1% to 90% within 48 hours (Johnson, et al., manuscript in preparation).

The ability of different ligands to induce ACTH production by lymphocytes suggests that some features of the response may be common or nonspecific. For example, do CRF and LPS bind to the same B cell receptor or have common intracellular pathways? The same question holds for TRH and SEA induction of TSH. Binding studies with ^{3}H-TRH show that SEA will not interfere with TRH-specific binding (Harbour, et al., 1988). Thus, in this case SEA and TRH do not share binding sites, although it would seem likely for some mitogens to bind and activate hormone receptors.

Common intracellular pathways, i.e., induction of common intracellular messengers, may play a role in production of lymphocyte hormones. In the IFN system, it has been shown that activation of IFN receptors on endocrine cells stimulates the same activity that a hormone does and that the response is mediated by common intracellular mechanisms (Blalock and Stanton, 1980). In the case of lymphocyte ACTH production, we have hypothesized that cAMP may be a common intracellular mediator. CRF stimulates cAMP production and release in anterior pituitary cells upon activation of its receptor (Westlund, et al., 1985). The POMC gene contains a cAMP regulatory sequence, and thus cAMP is thought to be involved in stimulating pituitary cell expression of POMC (Roberts, 1986). Since CRF will induce lymphocytes to synthesize ACTH (Smith, et al., 1986) these findings suggest that CRF may also activate adenylate cyclase in lymphocytes, which may play a role in inducing lymphocyte ACTH production. Table 2 shows that CRF does induce an increase in splenocyte cAMP production at doses similar to those required for ACTH production. LPS is known to induce production of cAMP and this may be the intracellular mechanism for its induction of ACTH also. This evidence is still preliminary, and definitive proof of our hypothesis awaits more direct experiments, such as the use of dibutyryl cAMP to induce splenocyte ACTH production. However this experiment is intriguing and suggests that other adenylate cyclase activators may also induce ACTH production. Our results also argue that the CRF binding site on cells of the immune system may be a bona fide CRF receptor, similar to the pituitary prototype which is structurally and functionally linked to adenylate cyclase. Thus not only are receptor structures on lymphocytes similar to neuroendocrine receptors, but the intracellular mechanisms which they trigger when occupied by specific ligand appear to be the same. In a similar vein, glucocorticoids such as the synthetic compound dexamethasone turn off POMC expression in both pituitary (Eipper and Mains, 1980) and lymphoid cells (Smith, et al., 1982), both of which are known to have glucocorticoid receptors. It would be naive to think of cAMP as the only intracellular mediator for POMC expression. Many studies on IL-2 are finding that cAMP, phosphoinositol and Ca^{2+} pathways are equally important and co-involved with IL-2 action. This will probably also be the case with POMC.

TABLE 2

CRF INDUCTION OF cAMP IN MOUSE SPLEEN CELLS

Treatment	cAMP (pMole/10^6 cells/25 min.)
Mock	48.1 ± 2.2
forskolin (10^{-5} M)	173.6 ± 2.0
CRF (2.5 ug/ml)	67.3 ± 5.1
CRF (1 ug/ml)	92.5 ± 18.7
CRF (0.1 ug/ml)	55.4 ± 4.2

Cells were incubated with the indicated concentrations of forskolin or corticotropin releasing factor (CRF). The reaction was stopped by addition of trichloroacetic acid after 25 minutes, and cAMP levels measured in a conpetitive binding assay as described by Peterson, et al., 1982.

IMPLICATIONS

This discussion has centered on induction of neuroendocrine hormones in lymphoid cells, but it should not be forgotten that these hormones also modulate a variety of classical *in vitro* immune responses. These include regulatory effects on antibody production (Johnson, et al., 1982b), lymphokine production (Johnson, et al., 1984), and more (see Smith, et al., 1988 for review). Such lymphokine-like immunomodulatory activity can also occur through activation of common intracellular pathways via different surface membrane receptors. Similarity between endocrine and immune cell receptor structure and function raises a question on timing of lymphocyte exposure to hormones/lymphokines. Many hormones are released in a pulsatile fashion which may have major differences when compared to the bolus type of exposure typically done in in vitro culture systems.

Finally, it does not seem so strange that lymphocytes express so many proteins when it is considered that macrophages make and release hundreds of different products important for normal immune function, and that neurons are known to release several peptide and nonpeptide neurotransmitters simultaneously. Furthermore, many of the pituitary hormones are induced by multiple signals, such as CRF and vasopressin in the case of POMC expression. Thus, future research will probably find many more mechanisms and structures common to both the neuroendocrine and immune systems.

ACKNOWLEDGMENTS

We thank Karen E. Goodwin for typing the manuscript. This research was supported in part by the Office of Naval Research (N00014-84-K-04-86) and a James W. McLaughlin Predoctoral Fellowship to E.W.J.

REFERENCES

Besedovsky, H.O., Sorkin, E., Felix, D., and Hass, H. (1977). European Journal of Immunology, 7, 323-325.
Besedovsky, H.O., del Rey, A. and Sorkin, E. (1981). The Journal of Immunology, 126, 385-387.
Blalock, J.E. and Smith, E.M. (1981). Biochemical and Biophysical Research Communications, 101, 472-478.
Blalock, J.E, and Smith, E.M. (1980). Proceedings of the National Academy of Sciences of the United States of America, 77, 5972-5974.
Blalock, J.E. and Smith, E.M. (1985). Federation Proceedings, 44, 108-111.
Blalock, J.E. and Smith, E.M. (1982). In: Human Lymphokines: Academic Press.
Blalock, J.E., Bost, K.L. & Smith, E.M. (1985). The Journal of Neuroimmunology, 10, 31-40.
Blalock, J.E. and Stanton, J.D. (1980). Nature, 238, 406-408.
Bost, K.L., Smith, E.M. and Blalock, J.E. (1985). Proceedings of the National Academy of Sciences of the United States of America, 82, 813-817.
Cupps, T.R. and Fauci, A.S. (1982). Immunological Reviews, 65, 133-155.
Cutz, E.W., Chan, W., Track, N.S., Goth, A. and Said, S. (1978). Nature, 275, 661-662.
Ebaugh, M.J. and Smith, E.M. (1988). The FASEB Journal 2, A1642.
Eipper, B.A. and Mains, R.E. (1980). Endocrine Reviews, 1, 1-27.
Felten, D.L., Felten, S.Y. Carlson, S.L., Olschowka, J.A. and Livnat, S. (1985). The Journal of Immunology, 135, 755s-765s.
Geenen, V., Legros, J., Franchimont, P., Baudrihaye, M., Defresne, M. and Boniver, J. (1986). Science, 230, 508-511.
Gilman, S.C., Schwartz, J.M., Milner, R.J., Bloom, F.E., and Feldman, J.D. (1982). Proceedings of the National Academy of Science of the United States of America, 79, 4226-4230.
Harbour, D.V., Smith, E.M. and Blalock, J.E. (1987). J. Neuroscience Research, 18, 95-101.
Harbour, D.V., Smith, E.M. and Meyer, W.J. (1988). J. Biological Psychiatry, 23, 797-806.
Harbour-McMenamin, D., Smith, E.M. and Blalock, J.E. (1985). Infection and Immunity, 48, 813-817.
Harbour-McMenamin, D., Smith, E.M. and Blalock, J.E. (1986a). Proceedings of the National Academy of Science of the United States of America, 83, 6834-6838.

Harbour-McMenamin, D., Smith, E.M. and Blalock, J.E. (1986b). ICSU Short Reports, 4, 378-379.
Hazum, E., Chang, K., and Cuatrecasas, P. (1979). Science, 205, 1033-1035.
Healy, D.L., Hodgen, G.D., Schulte, H.M., Chrousos, G.P., Loriaux, D.L., Hall, N.R. and Goldstein, A.L. (1983). Science, 222, 1353-1355.
Hiestand, P.C., Meker, P., Nordmann, R., Alfons, G. and Permmongkol, C. (1986). Proceedings of the National Academy of Sciences U.S.A. 83, 2599-2603.
Johnson, H.M., Farrar, W.L. and Torres, B.A. (1982a). The Journal of Immunology, 129, 983-986.
Johnson, H.M., Smith, E.M., Torres, B.A., and Blalock, J.E. (1982b). Proceedings of the National Academy of Science of the United States of America, 79, 4171-4174.
Johnson, H.M., Torres, B.A., Smith, E.M., Dion, L.D., and Blalock, J.E. (1984). The Journal of Immunology, 132, 246-250.
Kruger, T.E., Smith, E.M. and Blalock, J.E. (1987). Federation Proceedings 46, 926.
Lolait, S.J., Lim, A.T.W., Toh, B.H. and Funder, J.W. (1984). Journal of Clinical Investigation, 73, 277-280.
Lolait, S.J., Clements, J.A., Markwick, A.J., Cheng, C., McNally, M., Smith, A.I. and Funder, J.W. (1986). Journal of Clinical Investigation, 77, 1776-1779.
Lopker, A., Abood, L.G., Hoss, W. and Lionetti, F.J. (1980). Biochemical Pharmacology, 29, 277.
Lotze, M.T., Frana, L.W., Sharrow, S.O., Robb, R.J. and Rosenberg, S.A. (1985). The Journal of Immunology 134, 156-166.
McCain, H.W., Lamster, I.B., Bozzone, J.M., and Grbic, J.T. (1982). Life Sciences, 31, 1619-1624.
McGillis, J.P., Park, A., Dallman, M. and Payan, D.G. (1987). Federation Proceedings, 46, 1062.
Miles, K., Chelmicka-Schorr, E., Atweh, S., Otten, G., and Arnason, B.G.W. (1985). Journal of Immunology, 135, 797s.
Montgomery, D.W., Zukoski, C.F., Shah, G.N., Buckley, A.R., Pacholczyk, T. and Russel, D.H. (1987). Biochemical and Biophysical Research Communications 145, 692-698.
O'Dorisio, M.S., Hermina, N.S., O'Dorisio, T.M., and Balcerzak, S.P. (1981). The Journal of Immunology, 127, 2551-2554.
O'Dorisio, M.S., O'Dorisio, T.M., Cataland, S. and Blacerzak, S.P. (1980). Journal of Laboratory Clincal Medicine, 96, 666-672.
Payan, D.G., Brewster, D.R. and Goetzl, E.J. (1984). The Journal of Immunology, 133, 3260-3265.
Pert, C.B., Ruff, M.R., Weber, R.J. and Herkenham, M. (1985) The Journal of Immunology, 135, 820s-826s.
Peterson, J.W., Molina, N.C., Houston, C.W. and Fader, R.C. (1983).
Plotnikoff, N.P., Murgo, A.J., Miller, G.C., Corder, C.N. and Faith, R.E. (1985). Federation Proceedings, 44, 118-122.
Roberts, J.L. (1986). In: Advances in Gene Technology: Molecular Biology of the Endocrine System: Cambridge University Press. 14-17.
Roszman, T.L., Jackson, J.C., Cross, R.J., Titus, M.J., Markesbery, W.R., and Brooks, W.H. (1985). The Journal of Immunology, 135, 769s-772s.
Ruff, M.R. and Pert, C.B. (1984). Science, 225, 1034-1036.
Smith, E.M., Phan, M., Coppenhaver, D., Kruger, T.E., and Blalock, J.E. (1983). Proceedings of the National Academy of Science, USA, 80, 6010-6013.
Smith, E.M. and Blalock, J.E. (1981). Proceedings of the National Academy of Science, USA, 78, 7530- 7534.
Smith, E.M., Meyer, W.J. and Blalock, J.E. (1982). Science, 218, 1311-1312.
Smith, E.M., Morrill, A.C., Meyer, W.J. and Blalock, J.E. (1986). Nature, 321, 881-882.
Smith, E.M. and Blalock, J.E. (1988). Int. J. Neurosci. 38, 455-464.
Webster, E.L. and DeSouza, E.B. (1987). Federation Proceedings, 46, 540.
Weigent, D.A., Wear, W.E., Bost, K.L. and Blalock, J.E. (1987). Federation Proceedings, 46, 926.

Weigent, D.A., Langford, M.P., Smith, E.M., Blalock, J.E. and Stanton, G.J. (1981). Infection and Immunity, 32, 508-512.
Westlund, K.N., Aguilera, G. and Childs, G.V. (1985). Endocrinology 116, 439-445.
Westly, H.J., Kleiss, A.J., Kelly, K.W., Wang, P.K.Y. and Yuen, P.H. (1986). Journal of Experimental Medicine, 163, 1589-1594.
Woloski, B.M.R.N.J., Smith, E.M., Meyer, W.J., Fuller, G.M. and Blalock, J.E. (1985). Science, 230, 1035-1037.
Wybran, J., Appelbroom, T., Famaey, J.P., and Govaerts, A. (1979). The Journal of Immunology, 123, 1068-1070.
Zurawski, G., Benedik, M., Kamb, B.J., Abrams, J.S., Zurawski, S.M. and Lee, F.D. (1986). Science, 232, 772-775.

Enhancement of Mammalian Sleep by Immune Modulators

J. M. KRUEGER, L. A. TOTH, L. JOHANNSEN, F. OBAL, M. OPP and A. B. CADY

Department of Physiology and Biophysics, University of Tennessee, Memphis, 894 Union Avenue, Memphis, Tennessee 38163, USA

ABSTRACT

The central nervous and immune systems are closely interwoven in host defense and share many regulatory substances. Yet, despite the common observation of sleepiness during infectious disease, it was only recently shown that sleep is altered during bacterial infection. Bacterial components that may, in part, induce this somnogenic effect include muramyl peptides (MPs) derived from cell wall peptidoglycan and endotoxin or its lipid A moiety; animals respond to certain MPs or lipid A's with excess SWS. Poly I:C, a synthetic dsRNA, also enhances SWS; thus, viral products may also alter sleep-wake cycles as well. These bacterial/viral products may exert their somnogenic actions, in part, via altered cytokine production and release. Interleukin-1β (IL1β), tumor necrosis factor (TNF), and interferon$_{\alpha 2}$ (INF) enhance SWS and are produced by brain cells. IL1β-mRNA is found in normal brain. This, plus data suggesting that MPs may be constituents of normal tissue that are produced during macrophage processing of bacterial cell walls, suggests these immune response modifiers may be important in regulating normal sleep, as well as being involved in the enhanced SWS observed during infectious disease. Cytokines are linked to neuroendocrine substances that may be involved in sleep regulation. For example, IL1β enhances growth hormone (GH) release; GH is tightly coupled to SWS in humans, and GH-releasing factor (GRF) enhances sleep. IL1β and IL1α cause corticotropin-releasing hormone (CRF) release; CRF induces adrenocorticotropin hormone (ACTH) release. ACTH and α-melanocyte-stimulating hormone (ACTH$_{1-13}$, αMSH), inhibit sleep, and αMSH antagonizes IL1β-enhanced SWS. Thus, several factors may work together as a multi-level network of biochemical pathways to regulate sleep-wake cycles.

KEYWORDS

Bacteria : sleep : fever : electroencephalogram : interleukin-1 : interferon : tumor necrosis factor : MDP : endotoxin : muramyl peptides : infection.

INTRODUCTION

Influences of the central nervous system (CNS) on manifestations of infectious disease, such as the development of fever, acute-phase responses, and stimulation of the immune system to invoke both specific and nonspecific host defenses against invading organisms, have been postulated (Ader, 1981). One behavioral manifestation of infectious disease that is undoubtedly centrally mediated is increased lassitude or sleepiness. Anecdotal observations suggest that many people experience such feelings during infectious disease, and bed rest is frequently prescribed by physicians as an aid in recuperation (Guilleminault and Mondini, 1986). To date, however, relatively little research has been applied to the study of sleep during disease.

Recent work in our laboratory has been directed toward elucidating endogenous and exogenous factors that mediate mammalian sleep, and has provided insights into possible relationships between immune function and sleep. We have demonstrated that certain bacterial products (i.e., muramyl peptides [MPs] and endotoxin [lipopolysaccharide, LPS]), as well as a number of endogenous immune response modifiers (i.e., interleukin-1 [IL1], interferon α_2 [INF], and tumor necrosis factor [TNF]), all potentiate slow-wave sleep (SWS). Many of these factors also induce fever, produce alterations in several acute-phase reactants, and are potent immune modifiers. Such observations, taken together, suggest that sleep alterations might occur during bacterial disease, when levels of both bacterial products and endogenous immunomodulators are probably high.

Bacterial infection and sleep. Recently we have begun a systematic investigation of the effects of infectious disease on sleep (Toth and Krueger, 1988). In these studies, rabbits were inoculated intravenously with *Staphylococcus aureus* or *Escherichia coli*. *S. aureus* is a gram-positive bacterium with a cell wall composed largely of peptidoglycan, the monomeric subunits of which are MPs. *E. coli*, on the other hand, is a gram-negative bacterium with a cell wall containing LPS but only a thin layer of peptidoglycan. Thus, these organisms differ substantially in the amount of MPs in the cell wall, as well as in the presence of LPS. Such differences could influence the types of substances derived from the organisms, as well as the nature of the immune response and sleep patterns they stimulate in the host.

Typical sleep patterns for individual rabbits inoculated with these organisms are shown in Fig. 1. Both infectious agents produced significant deviations from normal sleep in infected animals. After a delay of 4-6 h, *S. aureus* enhanced SWS for up to 18 h postinoculation; after this time, sleep was decreased relative to the control period. The enhanced and suppressed sleep were respectively accompanied by increases and decreases in the average electroencephalographic (EEG) slow wave amplitudes during SWS. The magnitude of EEG slow wave amplitudes is thought to reflect the depth of sleep, and similar changes have been reported during recovery sleep following total sleep deprivation (Borbely and Neuhaus, 1979; Pappenheimer *et al.*, 1975). Inoculation with *E. coli* also produced a marked elevation in SWS, with accompanying increases in EEG slow wave amplitudes; however, in contrast to the effects of *S. aureus*, these effects occurred during the first 4 h after inoculation. Both infectious agents induced significant reductions in rapid-eye-movement sleep (REMS).

In addition to the alterations in sleep, inoculation with these organisms also produced clinical changes indicative of infectious disease, including leukogram changes (neutrophilia and lymphocytopenia), increased plasma cortisol levels, and fever. However, all of these effects could be dissociated temporally from the somnogenic effects, thus suggesting that these phenomena are, in part, independently regulated.

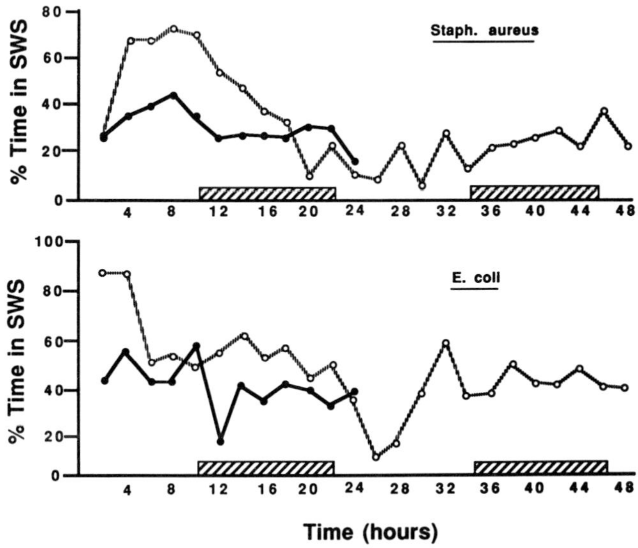

FIG. 1. Effects of bacterial inoculation on slow-wave sleep. Panels indicate the percentage of time in slow-wave sleep of individual rabbits for 24 h prior to (●——●) and 48 h after (o---o) the i.v. administration of 6 x 10^7 colony-forming units of S. aureus or E. coli. Shaded areas on the abscissa indicate the "lights-off" period.

The somnogenic effects of S. aureus were also evident, although attenuated, if the bacteria were killed prior to inoculation. In addition, administration of the bacteriocidal antibiotic cephalothin markedly attenuated both the somnogenic and the clinical effects of S. aureus inoculation. These observations, as well as the marked delay in the onset of enhanced sleep, suggest that the host's response to proliferation of the organism in vivo may also be involved in the production of somnogenic responses. The somnogenic effects of E. coli inoculation were not altered by the use of heat-killed bacteria. Several likely candidates for the mediation of increased SWS during the early stages of bacterial infection include MPs, endotoxin or LPS, and a number of endogenous immune mediators that are induced by these substances, including IL1, IFN, and TNF.

Macrophage processing of bacterial cell walls. Our findings that bacterial infections alter sleep raised the question: Can certain chemical structures of the infectious agent responsible for the effects on sleep be identified? MPs have been identified as sleep-promoting substances in brain and urine (Fig. 2) (Krueger et al., 1982a). Several analogs of these substances have subsequently been tested and are also somnogenic (see below). Although synthetic pathways for MPs have not been described in mammals, mammalian systems have the enzymatic machinery necessary for digesting bacterial cell walls and for the cleavage of MPs from these cell walls. For example, lysozyme is capable of cutting the sugar backbone of peptidoglycan. This enzyme occurs in several mammalian tissues and is in especially high concentrations in macrophages. Murine bone marrow-derived macrophages can digest the cell wall of intact S. aureus, depending on the specific chemical nature of the cell walls (Wecke et al., 1986). Further, macrophages which process cell walls of Bacillus subtilis release small MPs into the culture medium (Vermeulen and Grey, 1984).

Preliminary data suggest that the digestion of bacterial cell walls by macrophages can indeed be a step in the production of somnogenic MPs. S. aureus radiolabeled in their cell walls were incubated with murine bone marrow-derived macrophages. In response, these macrophages released radioactive substances of low molecular weight. These substances, which were not contaminated with substances of high molecular weight, such as lymphokines, or more lipophilic materials such as prostaglandins, enhanced SWS, depressed REMS, and were pyrogenic when injected intracerebroventricularly (icv) in rabbits (Johannsen et al., 1987). It is tempting to speculate that macrophage digestion products of cell walls of gram-positive bacteria are directly involved in the host response to infection, leading to enhancement of SWS and reduction of REMS, as well as other effects. In this regard, it has been proposed that MPs are similar to vitamins in that they are required by, but cannot be synthesized by, the host (Adam and Lederer, 1984).

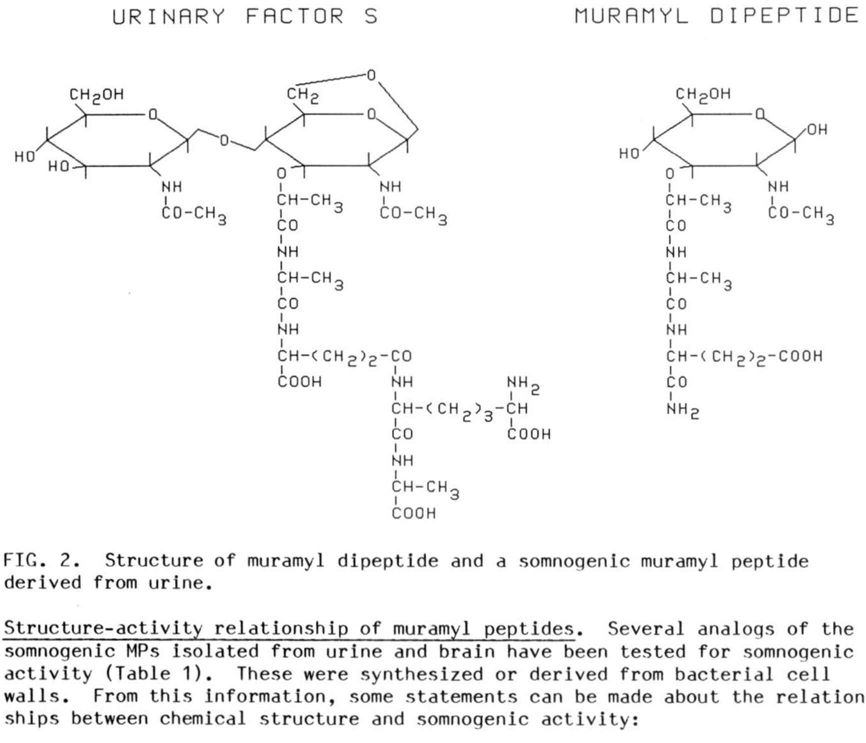

FIG. 2. Structure of muramyl dipeptide and a somnogenic muramyl peptide derived from urine.

Structure-activity relationship of muramyl peptides. Several analogs of the somnogenic MPs isolated from urine and brain have been tested for somnogenic activity (Table 1). These were synthesized or derived from bacterial cell walls. From this information, some statements can be made about the relationships between chemical structure and somnogenic activity:

1) The minimal structure of MPs necessary for somnogenic activity is muramyl dipeptide (MDP) (compound 1, Fig. 2), which is also the minimal structure necessary to replace mycobacteria in Freund's complete adjuvant (Ellouz et al., 1974).

2) Stereospecifity: MDP contains L-ala and D-isogln moieties and is somnogenic. When D-ala is substituted for L-ala (compound 2, Table 1), or when L-isogln is substituted for D-isogln (compound 3, Table 1), somnogenic activity is lost (Krueger et al., 1982b).

3) Amidation/deamidation: Somnogenic activity is lost by converting terminal carboxyl groups to unsubstituted amides, e.g., the gamma carboxyl of isogln (compound 4, Table 1) (Krueger et al., 1984b) and the ε carboxyl of dap (compound 5, Table 1) (Krueger et al., 1987b).

4) Changes in the sugar moiety: If muramic acid is destroyed by periodate oxidation (compound 6, Table 1) or if 3-O-(2-D-propionyl)-D-glucose (compound 7, Table 1) is substituted for it, somnogenic activity is lost (Krueger et al., 1984b). In contrast, if the muramic acid contains a 1,6-anhydro ring (compound 8, Table 1), somnogenic activity is enhanced (Krueger et al., 1987b).

TABLE 1. Somnogenic (S), Pyrogenic (P), and Immune (I) Activities of Various Muramyl Peptides.

Sugar | Peptide	ICV Dose (pmol)	S	P	I	Ref.
1) MurNAc-L-Ala-D-iGln (MDP)	10	-	-	+	*
	50	+	+		*
	75	+	+	+	**
2) MurNAc-D-Ala-D-iGln	100	-	-	-	**
	1000	-	-	-	**
3) MurNAc-L-Ala-L-iGln	200	-	-	-	**
4) MurNAc-L-Ala-D-Glu-$(NH_2)_2$	2000	-	-	+	*
5) MurNAc-Ala-gamma-Glu-epsilon-Dap(NH_2)	10	-	-		***
	100	-	-		***
	1000	-	-		***
6) MurNac-L-Ala-D-iGln periodate cleaved	200	-			*
7) D-Glucose-3-O-(D-2-propionyl)-	200	-	-		*
L-Ala-D-iGln	2000	-	-		*
8) (1,6-anhydro)MurNAc-	1	+	+		***
Ala-gamma-Glu-Dap-Ala	10	+	+		***
9) MurNAc-L-Ala-D-Gln	200	-	-	+	*
	2000	-	+	+	*

*Krueger et al., 1984b; **Krueger et al., 1982a; ***Krueger et al., 1987b.

The biological activities of MPs can, in part, be separated by using different analogs. Several analogs are immune modifiers without having pyrogenic or somnogenic effects (compound 4, Table 1) or are immunogenic and pyrogenic but not somnogenic (compound 9, Table 1). MPs that are somnogenic and not immunomodulatory have not been described, although such a differentiation could be dose-related. Although all somnogenic MPs tested in our rabbit bioassay model (Krueger et al., 1987b) were also pyrogenic, these two effects can be separated using antipyretics, which inhibit the pyrogenic but not the somnogenic effect (Krueger et al., 1982b).

Endotoxin/lipid-A. While MPs seem to mediate the somnogenic effects of gram-positive bacteria, sleep responses after injection of E. coli are much more rapid in onset, suggesting that LPS may also be important in eliciting sleep responses. MPs share many biological activities with LPS and their lipid-A moiety. These substances, like MPs, also are somnogenic (Krueger et al., 1986), stimulate the acute-phase response (Mashburn et al., 1984), potentiate nonspecific resistance to infection (Ribi et al., 1985), and induce fever (Tonamoto et al., 1984). Furthermore, as with MPs, there are certain specific structural features of lipid-A which are important for their biologic activities (Humme et al., 1986; Kanagasaki et al., 1986; Kotani et al., 1986). For example, conversion of diphosphoral lipid-A's to their monophosphoral analogs reduces their toxicity, although both diphosphoral and monophosphoral lipid-A are somnogenic (Krueger et al., 1986). Like MPs, lipid-A's and LPS have the capacity to enhance IL1, IFN, and TNF production and release.

Viral products/polyriboinosinic acid:polyribocytidylic acid. Sleep disturbances resulting from viral encephalitis have played an important historic role in sleep research. About 50 years ago, von Economo associated disturbances of sleep-wake cycles with specific virally induced CNS lesions (von Economo, 1930). These studies led him to postulate that sleep was an active process regulated by specific brain areas, including the hypothalamus and mesencephalon. More recently, viral infections have been linked to a number of syndromes, e.g., chronic fatigue syndrome, that have associated sleep disorders (reviewed, Krueger et al., 1988a). Despite these observations and the anecdotal reports of increased sleepiness during viral disease, as is the case with bacterial infections, there are no reports in the literature in which sleep was systematically monitored over the course of viral infection.

It has been postulated that double-stranded RNA (dsRNA) produced during the replication of RNA viruses is responsible for systemic symptoms associated with viral disease (Carter and DeClercq, 1974). Many systemic symptoms of viral disease, e.g., fever, can be elicited by a synthetic dsRNA, polyriboinosinic: polyribocytidylic acid (poly I:C). As an initial attempt to determine whether viral products may also be involved in altered sleep/wake cycles, we examined the somnogenic properties of poly I:C. This compound injected either i.v. or icv increased SWS, suppressed REMS, and induced fever (Krueger et al., submitted). Poly I:C-induced responses were distinct from those elicited by bacterial products in that LPS and MPs, but not poly I:C, induced changes in plasma copper, an acute-phase reactant. Further, the effective somnogenic dose of poly I:C given centrally did not produce significant changes when given i.v., suggesting a CNS site of action.

Cytokines. IL1, IFN, and TNF may mediate the somnogenic actions of the bacterial and possibly viral products discussed above. In rabbits, IL1β, whether derived from rabbit peritoneal exudate cells, human macrophages, or recombinant sources, enhanced rabbit SWS, suppressed REMS, and induced fever (Krueger et al., 1984a; Shoham et al., 1987b). Further, human IL1β was reported to enhance sleep in cats (Susic and Totic, 1987). IL1 also enhanced EEG slow-wave amplitudes in a manner similar to that observed after sleep deprivation (Krueger et al., 1984a; Tobler et al., 1984). The somnogenic actions of IL1 could be separated from its pyrogenic actions since antipyretics blocked IL1-induced fevers, but not IL1-enhanced SWS (Krueger et al., 1984a).

Another facet of temperature regulation, brain temperature changes coupled to states of vigilance, was not affected by IL1 (Walter et al., 1986). IFN and TNF had similar effects on rabbit sleep, although the time course of enhanced SWS induced by each substance was unique. Thus, after ICV injection, IL1 enhanced SWS during the first hour, then, depending on the dose, produced excessive SWS for 2-6 additional hours. In contrast, IFN-enhanced SWS was not observed until postinjection hour 2 (Krueger et al., 1987a), and TNF induced a biphasic enhancement of SWS with peaks observed in hours 1 and 3 postinjection (Shoham et al., 1987b).

In addition to sleep effects, these cytokines have other actions that are mediated via the CNS. The list includes fever (Dinarello, 1984), stimulation of hepatic synthesis of certain acute-phase proteins (Blatteis et al., 1984), and stimulation of pituitary and hypothalamic hormone/neuropeptide secretion (Sapolsky et al., 1987). Many of these CNS effects of cytokines may be mediated via their direct actions on neurons. For example, Hori et al. (1988) describe IL1-induced increases in firing rates of preoptic cold-sensitive neurons and decreases in firing rates of warm-sensitive neurons in vitro.

Further, Shibata et al. (1988) described differential sensitivities of hypothalamic neurons in brain slice preparations to IFN, IL1β, and TNF.

Challenges to the immune system are followed by changes of the blood levels of many pituitary hormones; some of these hormones may also be produced by lymphocytes (Weigen and Blalock, 1987). Increased secretion of pituitary hormones are also implicated in host defense (Nagy et al., 1983). Cytokines are involved in the stimulation of growth hormone (GH) (Atkins et al., 1986) and adrenocorticotropin hormone (ACTH) (Besedovsky et al., 1986) secretion. GH secretion is normally coupled to sleep (Sassin, 1977), and GRF has recently been shown to promote sleep in rats and rabbits (Obal et al., in press). It may be that cytokines have a direct effect on pituitary cells (Bernton et al., 1987), but stimulation of ACTH secretion is likely to be mediated primarily through the release of hypothalamic CRF (Sapolsky et al., 1987). IL1 induces α-MSH release in the CNS, and this effect may be mediated through corticotropin-releasing hormone (CRF) (Lipton and Clark, 1986). ACTH and α-MSH are two opiomelanocortin-derived peptides proposed as controlling the peripheral and central effects of IL1, respectively. Indeed, αMSH inhibits normal sleep and can block IL1β-enhanced sleep (Opp et al., submitted) and fevers (Lipton and Clark, 1986).

In vivo, the source of cytokines responsible for CNS actions remains unclear. IL1 , TNF, and IFN have all been described as CNS products. IL1β-mRNA, but not IL1α-mRNA, has a wide distribution throughout normal brain (Farrar et al., 1987). Further, neurons containing IL1β-immunoreactivity have been described in human hypothalamus (Breder et al., 1988). However it is not clear, especially during infections that are localized outside the CNS, whether CNS-derived cytokines are involved in their CNS actions. Attempts to determine if cytokines cross the blood-brain barrier have been inconclusive (reviewed, Blatteis, 1985). Regardless of whether the CNS actions of cytokines result from cytokines of central or peripheral origin, there are clear differences between the CNS actions of cytokines and those of substances that induce cytokine production. For example, injection of IL1β, but not IFN or TNF, into the preoptic area induces enhanced plasma Cu levels (Blatteis et al., 1987). Similarly, somnogenic doses of MDP that enhance plasma Cu when given icv are ineffective if given i.v. (Shoham et al., 1987a). In contrast, somnogenic doses of poly I:C, whether given icv or i.v. failed to alter plasma Cu (Krueger et al., submitted). These results indicate that perhaps MDP and poly I:C induce a different array of cytokines or have differential effects on neurons, thus leading to a different range of biological actions.

The brain regions responsible for the mediation of the various CNS effects of cytokines remain unknown. Receptors for IL1 have been demonstrated throughout the CNS (Farrar et al., 1987). IL1 (Blatteis, 1985) and IFN (Dafny et al., 1988) seem to interact with opiate receptors, providing a possible explanation for opiate-like effects of cytokines. Prostaglandins (PGs) have repeatedly been implicated in the mediation of the effects of cytokines on the CNS. PGE_2 has been the most intensively studied of the PGs and is associated with an upward shift of the thermoregulatory set point (reviewed, Hellon, 1975). Also, PGD_2 induces SWS in rats (Ueno et al., 1983) and rabbits. Thus, PGs may be mediators of fever and sleep regulation. However, PGs may not be essential for mediating all cytokine effects since blocking arachidonate metabolism often fails to interfere with cytokine actions (reviewed, Blatteis, 1985).

CONCLUSION

It is clear that infectious agents and several immune response modifiers and neuroendocrine hormones whose production and release are altered during infectious processes have the capacity to alter sleep. The somnogenic actions of these substances are undoubtedly related to each other (reviewed, Krueger et al., 1988b). Unlike other physiological systems, the function of sleep and the brain mechanism for sleep are almost completely unknown. The recent identification of these somnogenic substances and their interrelationships will likely be important tools in addressing these issues in sleep research. Indeed, our results could indicate a role for sleep in host defense. Perhaps more importantly, they raise the question of whether sleep regulation is a manifestation of the normal symbiotic relationship between microbes and their host.

ACKNOWLEDGMENTS

This work was supported by the National Institutes of Health (NS-25378), the Office of Naval Research (N00014-85-K-0773), and the U. S. Army Research and Development Command (DAMD-17-86-C-6194).

REFERENCES

Adam, A. and Lederer, E. (1984). Medicinal Res. Rev. 4, 111-152.
Ader, R. (1981). Psychoneuroimmunology. Academic Press.
Atkins, M., Gould, J., Allegretta, M., Li, J., Dempsey, R., Rudders, R., Parkinson, D., Reichlin, S. and Mier, J. (1986). J. Clin. Oncol. 4, 1380-1391.
Bernton, E., Beach, J., Holaday, J., Smallridge, R. and Fein, H. (1987). Science 238, 519-521.
Besedovsky, H., Del Rey, A., Sorkin, E., Dinarello, C. (1986). Science 233, 652-654.
Blatteis, C. (1985). In: The Physiologic, Metabolic, and Immunologic Actions of Interleukin-1: (eds M. Kluger, J. Oppenheim and M. Powanda). A.R. Liss. 107-120.
Blatteis, C.M., Ahokas, R.A., Dinarello, C.A. and Ungar, A.L. (1987). Fed. Proc. 46, 683.
Blatteis, C., Hunter, W., Llanos-Q., J., Ahokas, R. and Mashburn, T., Jr. (1984). Brain Res. Bull. 12, 689-695.
Borbely, A.A. and Neuhaus, H.U. (1979). J. Comp. Physiol. 133, 71-87.
Breder, C., Dinarello, C. and Saper, C. (1988). Science 240, 321-324.
Carter, W. and DeClercq, E. (1974). Science 186, 1172-1178.
Dafny, N., Lee, J. and Dougherty, P. (1988). J. Neurosci. Res. 19, 130-139.
Dinarello, C. (1984). Rev. Infect. Dis. 6, 51-95.
von Economo, C. (1930). J. Nerv. Mental Dis. 71, 249-259.
Ellouz, F., Adam, A., Ciorbaru, R. and Lederer, E. (1974). Biochem. Biophys. Res. Comm. 59, 1317-1325.
Farrar, W., Hill, J., Harel-Bellan, A. and Vinocour, M. (1987). Immunol. Rev. 100, 361-377.
Guilleminault, C. and Mondini, S. (1986). Arch. Int. Med. 146, 1333-1335.
Hellon, R. (1975). Pharmacol. Rev. 26, 289-321.
Hori, T., Shibata, M., Nakashima, T., Yamasaki, M., Asami, A., Asami, T. and Koza, H. (1988). Brain Res. Bull. 20, 75-82.
Humme, J., Matsuura, M., Kanagasaki, S., Kawakubo, Y., Kojima, Y., Shibukawa, N., Kumazawa, Y., Yamamoto, A., Tanamoto, K., Yesuda, T., Imoto, M., Yoshimura, H., Kusumoto, S. and Shiba, T. (1986). J. Biochem. 98, 395-406.
Johannsen, L., Wecke, J. and Krueger, J.M. (1987). Soc. Neurosci. Abstr. 13, 260.
Kanagasaki, S., Tanamoto, K., Yesuda, Y., Homma, J., Matsuura, M., Nakatsuka, M., Kumazawa, Y., Yamamoto, A., Shiba, T., Kusumoto, S., Imoto, M., Yoshimura, H. and Shimamoto, T. (1986). J. Biochem. 99, 1203-1210.
Kotani, S., Takada, H., Takahashi, I., Tsuijimoto, M., Ogawa, T., Ikeda, T., Harada, K., Okamura, H., Tamura, T., Tanaka, S., Shiba, T., Kusumoto, S., Imoto, M., Yoshimura, H. and Kasai, M. (1986). Infect. Immun. 52, 872-884.
Krueger, J.M., Pappenheimer, J.R. and Karnovsky, M.L. (1982a). J. Biol. Chem. 257, 1664-1669.
Krueger, J.M., Pappenheimer, J.R. and Karnovsky, M.L. (1982b). Proc. Natl. Acad. Sci. USA 79, 5102-5106.

Krueger, J., Walter, J., Dinarello, C., Wolff, S. and Chedid, L. (1984a). Am. J. Physiol. 246, R994-R999.
Krueger, J.M., Walter, J., Karnovsky, M.L., Chedid, L., Choay, J.P., Lefrancier, P. and Lederer, E. (1984b). J. Exp. Med. 159, 68-76.
Krueger, J., Kubillus, S., Shoham, S. and Davenne, D. (1986). Am. J. Physiol. 251, R591-R597.
Krueger, J., Dinarello, C., Shoham, S., Davenne, D., Walter, J. and Kubillus, S. (1987a). Int. J. Immunopharm. 9, 23-30.
Krueger, J.M., Rosenthal, R.S., Martin, S.A., Walter, J., Davenne, D., Shoham, S., Kubillus, S.L. and Biemann, K. (1987b). Brain Res. 403, 249-257.
Krueger, J., Obal, F., Jr., Opp, M., Cady, A., Johannsen, L. and Toth, L. (1988a). In: Sleep and Biological Rhythms: (eds J. Montplaisir, R. Godbout and Y. Lamarre). Oxford (in press).
Krueger, J.M., Toth, L.A., Cady, A.B., Johannsen, L. and Obal, F., Jr. (1988b). In: Sleep Peptides: Basic and Clinical Approaches: (eds S. Inoue and D. Schneider-Helmert) Springer-Verlag. 95-129.
Krueger, J., Majde, J., Blatteis, C., Endsley, J., Ahokas, R. and Cady, A. (submitted). Am. J. Physiol.
Lipton, J. and Clark, W. (1986). Ann. Rev. Physiol. 49, 613-623.
Mashburn, T., Llanos-Q., J., Hunter, W., Ahokas, R. and Blatteis, C. (1984). Pflugers Arch. 402, 157-161.
Nagy, E., Berczi, I. and Friesen, H. (1983). Acta Endocrinol. 102, 351-357.
Obal, F. Jr., Alföldi P., Cady, A.B., Johannsen, L., Sasy, G., and Krueger, J.M. (in press). Am. J. Physiol.
Opp, M., Obal, F., Jr. and Krueger, J. (submitted).
Pappenheimer, J.R., Koski, G., Fencl, V., Karnovsky, M.L. and Krueger, J.M. (1975). J. Neurophysiol. 38, 1299-1311.
Ribi, E., Cantrell, J. and Takayama, K. (1985). Clin. Immunol. News 6, 33-48.
Sapolsky, R., Rivier, C., Yamamoto, G., Plotsky, P. and Vale, W. (1987). Science 238, 522-524.
Sassin, J.R. (1977) In: Neurobiology of Sleep and Memory: (eds R. Drucker-Colin and J. McGaugh). Academic Press. 361-372.
Shibata, M., Blatteis, C., Krueger, J., Obal, F., Jr. and Opp, M. (in press). In: Thermoregulation Research and Clinical Applications: (eds P. Lomax and E. Schonbaum). Karger.
Shoham, S., Ahokas, A., Blatteis, C. and Krueger, J. (1987a). Brain Res. 419, 223-228.
Shoham, S., Davenne, D., Cady, A., Dinarello, C. and Krueger, J. (1987b). Am. J. Physiol. 253, R142-R149.
Susic, V. and Totic, S. (1987). Sleep Res. 16, 150.
Tanamoto, K., Zahringer, U., McKenzie, G., Galenos, C., Rietschel, E., Luderitz, O., Kusumoto, S. and Shiba, T. (1984). Infect. Immun. 44, 421-426.
Tobler, I., Borbely, A., Schwyzer, M. and Fontana, A. (1984). Eur. J. Pharmacol. 104, 191-192.
Toth, L.A. and Krueger, J.M. (1988). Infect. Immun., in press.
Ueno, R., Honda, K., Inou , S. and Hayaishi, O. (1983). Proc. Natl. Acad. Sci. USA 80, 1235-1237.
Vermeulen, M.W. and Grey, G.R. (1984). Infect. Immun. 46, 476-483.
Walter, J., Davenne, D., Shoham, S., Dinarello, C. and Krueger, J. (1986). Am. J. Physiol. 250, R96-R103.
Wecke, J., Kwa, E., Johannsen, L. and Giesbrecht, P. (1986). In: Biological Properties of Peptidoglycan: (eds P.H. Seidl and K.H. Schleifer) Walter de Gruyter. 197-202.
Weigen, T. and Blalock, J. (1987). Immunol. Rev. 100, 79-107.

Physiological Roles of Histamine H_3-Receptors

J-M. ARRANG*, M. GARBARG*, J-C. LANCELOT**, J-M. LECOMTE***, H. POLLARD*, M. ROBBA**, W. SCHUNACK**** and J-C. SCHWARTZ*

*Unité 109 de Neurobiologie et Pharmacologie, Centre Paul Broca de l'INSERM, 2ter rue d'Alésia, 75104 Paris, France
**Laboratoire de Pharmacie Chimique, U.E.R. des Sciences Pharmaceutiques, 1 rue Vaubénard, 14032 Caen, France
***Laboratoire Bioprojet, 30 rue des Francs Bourgeois, 75003 Paris, France
****Institut für Pharmazie, Freie Universität Berlin, Konigin-Luise-Straße 2 + 4, D 100 Berlin, FRG

ABSTRACT

The third histamine receptor was first identified on brain neurons and seems to be also present in other cells such as the lung mast-cells. Hence the novel and potent H_3-receptor agonist (R)α-methylhistamine might find therapeutic applications in allergic diseases.

KEYWORDS

Histamine H_3-receptors ; Release regulation ; Synthesis regulation ; Brain ; Lung ; Neurone ; Mast-cell.

INTRODUCTION

Two major breakthroughs have dominated the history of histamine (HA) receptors pharmacology : the discovery of "antihistamines" (now designated H_1-receptor antagonists) by Bovet and colleagues in France in 1937 and, in 1972, that of H_2-receptor antagonists by Black and colleagues at S.K. and F. in the U.K. These compounds together with more or less selective agonists have greatly helped to clarify and classify the actions of HA in various tissues and have provided extremely useful therapeutic agents.

More recently, it was observed that HA inhibited its own synthesis and release in brain slices via a negative feedback process operating at the level of histaminergic nerve-endings (Arrang et al., 1983, 1985, 1987b). We established that these actions of HA were mediated by a novel subclass of receptors (H_3) although no selective H_3-receptor agonist or antagonist was as yet available.

We now describe the actions of (R)α-methylhistamine (α-MeHA), a chiral agonist, and thioperamide, an antagonist derived from imidazolylpiperidine, which both display high selectivity and nanomolar potency in vitro. These drugs modify in opposite directions HA synthesis and/or release from not only brain slices but also cerebral and peripheral tissues in the living rat.

ALPHA METHYLHISTAMINE AND THIOPERAMIDE : TWO POTENT AND SELECTIVE LIGANDS

None of the selective H_1- or H_2-receptor agonists is able to mimic the actions of HA at H_3-receptors and some of them even behave as antagonists. In contrast, we have identified α MeHA as a compound fully meeting these requirements. In the H_3-receptor assay system in which depolarization-induced release of [^{3}H]HA from brain slices is evaluated (Arrang et al., 1983), the (R)isomer of α MeHA exerted its agonist effect at nanomolar concentrations, being approximately 100-times as potent as the (S)isomer and 15-times as potent as HA itself (Fig. 1). (R)α MeHA potencies relative to HA being only 0.5 % and 1 % at reference H_1- and H_2-receptor systems respectively (table 1), it can be regarded as a highly potent and selective H_3-receptor agonist.

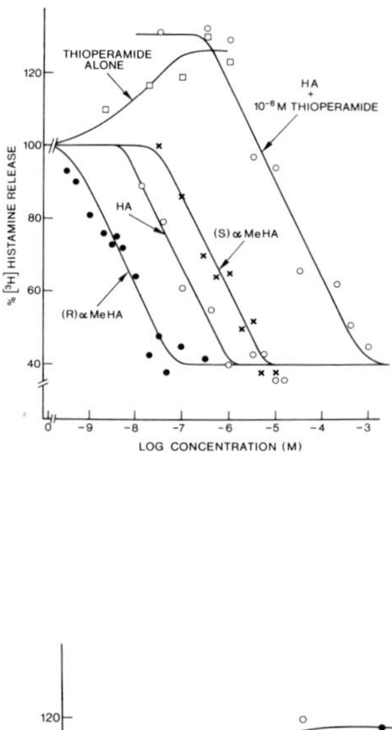

Fig. 1.

Effects of various histamine derivatives on the K^+-induced release of [^{3}H]histamine from slices of rat cerebral cortex. After preincubation with L-[^{3}H]histidine, slices were incubated for 2 min with 2 or 30 mM K^+. Drugs were added 5 min before the start of incubations, at the end of which [^{3}H]histamine was assayed in tissue and medium. The spontaneous efflux of [^{3}H]-HA (2 mM K^+) represented 5.0 ± 0.2 % of the total. In the absence of added agents, the [^{3}H]-HA release evoked by 30 mM K^+ (expressed as percent of total [^{3}H]-HA released over spontaneous efflux) represented 14.2 ± 0.6 %. Results are expressed as percent of this value (= 100 %). From Arrang et al, 1987a.

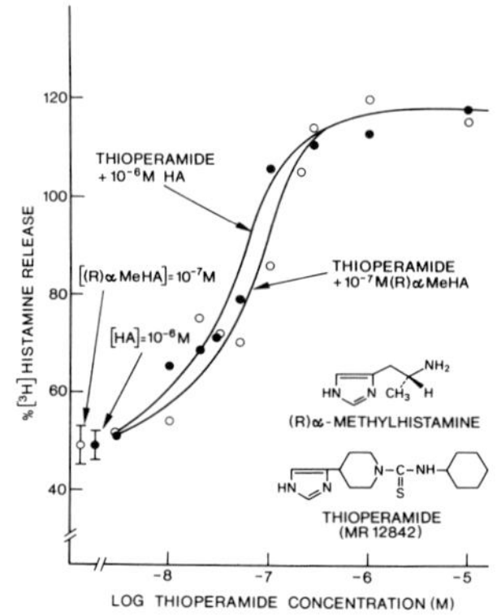

Fig. 2

Reversal by thioperamide of the HA or (R)α MeHA-induced inhibitions of [^{3}H]HA release from slices of rat cerebral cortex. The K^+-evoked release of [^{3}H]HA was performed and evaluated as described in Fig. 1. The IC_{50} values of thioperamide were 48 ± 9 nM and 74 ± 17 nM when opposed to HA and (R)α MeHA respectively. From Arrang et al., 1987a.

Thioperamide i.e. N-cyclohexyl-4-(imidazol-4-yl)-1-piperidinecarbothioamide competitively blocks H_3-autoreceptors regulating [^{3}H] HA release (Figs. 1 and 2) with a mean apparent Ki of 4 nM, calculated in disregard of the influence of endogenous HA (table 1).

TABLE 1 : Compared potencies of various imidazole derivatives at the three subclasses of HA receptors.

AGENTS	H_1-RECEPTOR	H_2-RECEPTOR	H_3-RECEPTOR
AGONISTS (relative potencies)			
HA	100	100	100
(R)α-MeHA	0.49 [a]	1.02 [c]	1,550
(S)α-MeHA	0.49 [a]	1.74 [c]	13
ANTAGONIST (Ki values)			
Thioperamide	> 100 μM [b]	> 10 μM [d]	4 nM

(a) Contraction of the isolated guinea-pig ileum.
(b) Competition with [^{3}H] mepyramine binding in membranes of guinea-pig cerebellum.
(c) Isolated guinea-pig right striatum.
(d) Cyclic AMP accumulation in slices from guinea-pig hippocampus.

The relative potencies were calculated as the ratio EC_{50} of HA/EC_{50} of agonist x 100.

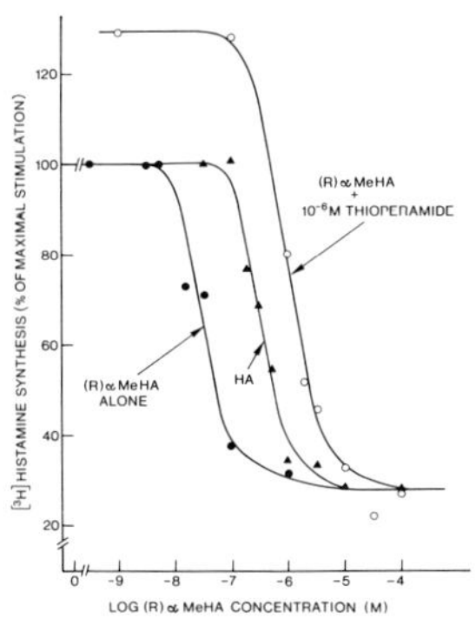

Fig. 3.

Effects of (R)α MeHA and thioperamide on the K^+-induced stimulation of [^{3}H]HA synthesis in slices of rat cerebral cortex. Slices were incubated for 30 min at 37°C in the presence of [^{3}H]histidine and 2 or 30 mM K^+. Drugs were added at the beginning of incubations. In the absence of any drug, [^{3}H]HA synthesis represented about 2,000 d.p.m/mg protein (2 mM K^+) and 4,000 d.p.m/mg protein (30 mM K^+). The difference was taken as the maximal stimulation. From Arrang et al., 1987a.

H_3-autoreceptors appear to control not only [^{3}H]HA release from but also [^{3}H]HA synthesis in depolarized cerebral histaminergic neurons (Arrang et al, 1987b). Consistently, (R)α-MeHA potently inhibited the K^+-induced stimulation of [^{3}H] histamine formation in slices of rat cerebral cortex and thioperamide antagonized in a surmountable manner the (R) α MeHA-induced inhibition of [^{3}H] HA synthesis with a nanomolar potency (Arrang et al., 1987a) (Fig. 3).

IN VIVO ACTION

The availability of potent agents acting selectively at H_3-receptors made it possible for the first time to assess the physiological rôle of these receptors in the control of HA synthesis and release in the brain and peripheral organs of living animals.

Opposite effects of the agonist and the antagonist were found when [^{3}H] HA formation in cerebral cortex was evaluated after administration of its [^{3}H] precursor. Hence (R)α-MeHA (10 mg/kg, i.v.) significantly decreased [^{3}H]HA formation by about 30 % and this was reversed by thioperamide (10 mg/kg, i.p.) which, alone or in combination with (R) α-MeHA, markedly enhanced the [^{3}H]amine formation (table 2).

A qualitatively similar effect occurred at the level of the hypothalamus, where HA perikarya (and also terminals) are located. Hence it seems that both α-MeHA and thioperamide cross the "blood-brain barrier" at reasonable dosages and that brain HA neurons activity can be modulated bi-directionally via H_3-receptors occupation. Thioperamide seems to be the first drug known to clearly increase this activity.

Most interestingly, [^{3}H]HA synthesis was modified in lung in the same manner as in brain (table 2), suggesting the presence of H_3-receptors therein, an hypothesis confirmed by radioligand binding studies (see below). Since a large part of lung HA is located within mast-cells found in abundance within the bronchial mucosa, in the alveolar septal connective tissue and in the pleura, it seems likely that these cells are endowed with H_3-receptors controlling the amine synthesis and, possibly, release.

The effects of the H_3-receptor antagonist on [^{3}H]HA formation were less clear-cut in other peripheral tissues. For instance in skin, where mast-cells of the connective tissue type are abundant, or spleen, (R)α-MeHA also decreased by about 30 % the [^{3}H]HA formation but the reversal by thioperamide was less clear and the H_3-receptor antagonist did not promote [^{3}H]HA formation over control levels. In these tissues, the presence of H_3-receptors remains to be confirmed by other approaches.

TABLE 2 : Effects of treatments with (R)α-Methylhistamine and thioperamide on [³H]histamine formation in various rat tissues

TISSUES	[³H]HISTAMINE LEVELS (dpm/g x 10^{-2})			
	CONTROLS	TREATED WITH		
		(R)α-MeHA	THIOPERAMIDE	(R)α-MeHA + THIOPERAMIDE
Cerebral cortex	32 ± 2	22 ± 2** (- 29 %)	75 ± 8** (+ 138 %)	63 ± 5** (+ 99 %)
Lung	51 ± 4	37 ± 3** (- 29 %)	96 ± 16** (+ 86 %)	73 ± 12* (+ 42 %)

Rats (13-38) received 250 µCi of [³H] L-histidine 10 min before sacrifice. (R) α-MeHA was administered (10 mg/kg, i.v.), together with the [³H] aminoacid whereas thioperamide (10 mg/kg, i.p.) was administered 1 h before. [³H]HA was isolated by ion-exchange chromatography. *$P < 0.04$; **$P < 0.005$ as compared with controls.

ASSAY AND VISUALIZATION OF H_3-RECEPTORS

The high apparent affinity of (R)α-MeHA in functional studies suggested that the drug might constitute, when radiolabelled, a suitable probe for H_3-receptors assay and visualization.

Indeed [³H](R)α-MeHA was found to bind in a reversible and saturable manner to cerebral cortex membranes. Sites labelled with [³H](R)α-MeHA were pharmacologically identified as H_3-receptors by competition studies with a variety of compounds (Fig. 4, left).

In membranes of guinea-pig lung specific binding sites could also be detected and unambiguously characterized as H_3-receptors in spite of their extremely low density which confirms the presence of H_3-receptors outside the brain (Arrang et al., 1987a) (Fig. 4, right).

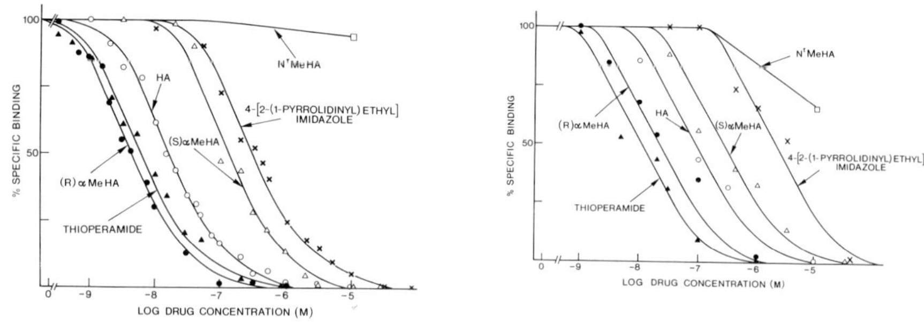

Fig. 4 : Inhibition of [^{3}H](R)α-MeHA binding to membranes of rat cerebral cortex (left) and guinea-pig lung parenchyma (right) by various imidazole derivatives. Membranes (0.4 - 0.5 mg protein) were incubated for 60 min at 25°C with 1-2 nM of [2.5 -^{3}H](R)α-MeHA and increasing concentrations of unlabelled substances. Specific binding was defined as that inhibited by 1 μM thioperamide. From Arrang et al., 1987a. Figs. 1-4 reprinted by permission from Nature, Vol. 327, n° 6118, pp. 117-123. Copyright (c) 1987 Macmillan Magazines Ltd.

CONCLUSIONS

The potent and selective agents that we have designed confirm the existence of a third subclass of HA receptors. In addition, they may be useful in trying to clarify the role of HA neurons in the CNS. The latter are thought to regulate states of vigilance, energy metabolism, cerebral circulation, pituitary secretions, etc.. and these hypothesis might be checked by the utilisation of H_3-antagonists, the first agents known to markedly enhance their activity. Hence, H_3-receptor ligands may find applications in neurology and psychiatry. The presence of H_3-receptors in HA-forming cells from peripheral tissues containing mast-cells e.g. in lung suggests that H_3-receptor agonists may find therapeutic applications in the field of allergy and inflammation, particularly if they control not only HA release but perhaps also other mast-cell functions.

REFERENCES

Arrang, J.M., Garbarg, M. and Schwartz, J.C. (1983). Nature, 302, 832-837.

Arrang, J.M., Garbarg, M. and Schwartz, J.C. (1985). Neuroscience, 15, 553-562.

Arrang, J.M., Garbarg, M., Lancelot, J.C., Lecomte, J.M., Pollard, H., Robba, M., Schunack, W. and Schwartz, J.C. (1987a). Nature, 327, 117-123.

Arrang, J.M., Garbarg, M. and Schwartz, J.C. (1987b). Neuroscience, 23, 149-157.

Black, J.W., Duncan, W.A.M., Durant, C.J., Ganellin, C.R. and Parsons, M.E. (1972). Nature, 236, 385-390.

Bovet, D. and Staub, A.M. (1937). C.R. Soc. Biol. (Paris) 124, 547-549.

Immunoregulatory Molecules, Receptors and their Immunopharmacological Implications

Cell-Cell Contact- and Cytokine-controlled B Lymphocyte Responses and their Potential Influences in Hematopoiesis

ANTONIUS ROLINK[1], MARTIN STREB[1], HAJIME KARASUYAMA[1,2] and FRITZ MELCHERS[1]

[1] *Basel Institute for Immunology, Basel, Switzerland*
[2]*Present address: Department of Immunology, Faculty of Medicine, University of Tokyo, Tokyo, Japan*

KEYWORDS

B cell responses: Cell-cell contacts: cytokines

INTRODUCTION

Cell-cell contacts and the production and reception of soluble cytokines control the development of the different lineages of blood cells from pluripotent stem cells. These stem cells give rise to progenitors committed either to the lymphoid or the myeloid series of cell lineages (Wu et al., 1968; Wu, 1967; Abramson, Miller and Phillips, 1977; Fleishmann, Custer and Mintz, 1982; Micklem et al., 1966; Keller et al., 1985; Dick et al., 1985). From the earliest myeloid progenitor, the colony-forming unit of spleen (CFU-S), proliferation and differentiation generate clones of megakaryocytes and platelets, erythroblasts and erythrocytes, basophils (mast cells), eosinophils, neutrophils (granulocytes), and monocytes and macrophages. With the possible exception of monocytes, all these cell lineages develop to terminally differentiated cells without falling into a resting state. This is different for cells of the lymphoid lineages. From (yet unidentified) progenitors for all lymphoid cells, progenitors develop which are committed to either the T or the B lymphocyte lineage. They become precursors when they begin to rearrange their T cell receptor (TcR), respectively immuno-globulin (Ig) genes (for references see Steinmetz, 1986). When precursors become mature, antigen-sensitive cells, they fall into a resting state. Lymphocytes will not develop into their terminally differentiated effector functions, but rather die, unless they are stimulated to do so. Stimulation in the immune system of lymphocytes is usually initiated by external influences, i.e. by foreign antigens.

The activation of B lymphocytes from their resting state to proliferation and to maturation into the effector function of Ig secretion is one example how antigen, T cells and accessory cells cooperate with B cells by cell-to-cell contacts and through the production and reception of soluble cytokines in this immune response. It also shows that this activation can spread to other lineages of blood cells, again through cell-to-cell contacts and by the actions of cytokines. The activation of primary, surface IgM-expressing murine B cells can be dissected into several steps.

CYTOKINE PRODUCTION BY THE ANTIGEN-SPECIFIC, MHC-RESTRICTED INTERACTION OF HELPER T CELLS WITH ACCESSORY CELLS.

When antigen enters the immune system, it is taken up by accessory (A) cells, such as macrophages or dendritic cells, is processed - in the case of proteins to peptides - and then presented in association with membrane molecules encoded by genes of the major histocompatibility complex (MHC) (Unanue and Cerottini, 1970; Chesnut and Grey, 1981; Lanzavecchia, 1985). In a second step, the complexes of processed antigen and MHC class II molecules on A cells are then recognized by the TcR and by CD4 molecules expressed on helper T cells. This recognition results in the production and secretion of cytokines by A cells and by helper T cells. The spectrum of cytokines produced by A cells includes interleukin (IL)-1, IL-6, complement C3-like α factors, and other growth factors such as Endo GF and FGF (Oppenheim et al., 1986; Bazin and Lemieux, 1987; Lernhardt et al., 1987). Two types of helper T cells appear to exist: T_{H1} produce IL-2, IL-3 and γ-interferon (γIFN); T_{H2} IL-3, IL-4, IL-5 and, maybe, IL-6 (Mosmann and Coffman, 1987). With the exception of the complement C3-like α factor, all the genes encoding these cytokines have been cloned, sequenced and expressed. We, ourselves, have introduced the cDNA genes for murine IL-2, IL-3, IL-4 and IL-5, and the cDNA gene for human IL-6, into a bovine papilloma virus-based vector, and have transfected eukaryotic cells with vectors containing single genes. In this way we have generated cell lines which produce and secrete constitutively tens of thousands of units of these cytokines into one milliliter of tissue culture medium (Karasuyama and Melchers, 1988).

THE ACTIONS OF CYTOKINES ON RESTING B CELLS

Resting B cells are refractory to the proliferation-inducing action of cytokines (Andersson et al., 1980; Melchers et al., 1980; Schreier et al., 1980). They, however, are inducible to maturation into Ig-secreting cells without proliferation with media conditioned by the interaction of cloned helper T cells with antigen-pulsed A cells, previously called T cell-replacing factors (TRF). IL-5, at 1-10 units/ml, and IL-2, at 100-1000 units/ml, but not human IL-1 (a gift of Dr. Lomedico, Research Laboratories, F. Hoffmann-La Roche, Nutley, N.J.), murine IL-3 and IL-4, nor human IL-6, all at concentrations up to 1000 units/ml, were found to induce maturation of resting B cells to Ig-secreting cells without proliferation. Limiting dilution analyses of resting B cells in the presence of IL-5 and inert rat thymus filler cells showed that 1-2% of all cells mature without division (Lernhardt et al., 1987; Karasuyama, Rolink and Melchers, 1988).

EXCITATION OF B CELLS FROM THE RESTING STATE

B cells can be excited from the resting state in T cell independent and T cell dependent ways by antigen. T cell independent antigens usually crosslink surface IgM molecules, possible even without uptake and processing of the antigen and, thereby, render the B cells susceptible to the proliferation-inducing and propagating actions of cytokines. T cell dependent antigens are often monovalent, bind to surface IgM, are taken up, processed and then presented in association with MHC class II molecules on the B cells. The TcR and CD4 molecules of helper T cells then recognize the complexes of antigen and MHC class II molecules. As a result B cells become excited, susceptible to cytokine action (for review and references see Melchers, 1988).

PROGRESSION THROUGH THE CELL CYCLE

Three restriction points control the cell cycle of activated B cells (Melchers and Lernhardt, 1985). The first, early in the G_1 phase, parallels much of the original activation from the resting state, i.e. is effected by interactions with surface Ig on B cells. Ig-specific monoclonal antibodies, immobilized on Sepharose beads, will suffice to control this point in the cell cycle in a polyclonal and MHC-unrestricted fashion, i.e. without antigen processing and MHC recognition by helper T cells. Entry into S phase is controlled by α factors. It is likely that these α factors are related to the complement component C3, and that they act through the C3d-specific complement receptor CR_2 (Erdei et al., 1985; Melchers et al., 1985). Entry into mitosis is controlled by β factors. We have recently shown that both IL-2 and IL-5 can act as β-type B cell growth factors. They both act at low concentrations, i.e. at 1-10 units/ml, and, therefore, at concentrations, where IL-5 (but not IL-2) also induces maturation without proliferation in resting B cells (Lernhardt et al., 1987; Karasuyama, Rolink and Melchers, 1988).

IL-2 receptor-specific monoclonal antibodies inhibit the β-type B cell growth factor activity of IL-2, but not of IL-5, indicating that IL-2 and IL-5 use separate receptors for signalling at the same restriction point in the B cell cycle (Karasuyama, Rolink and Melchers, 1988).

Human IL-1, murine IL-3 and IL-4, and human IL-6 have no effects at either restriction point in the B cell cycle. They cannot replace Ig-specific antibodies, nor α factors, nor β-type BCGF (such as IL-2 or IL-5) in their proliferation-propagating activities with B cells. In other assays, done in other laboratories, IL-1, IL-4 and IL-6 have, however, been shown to have activities with B cells.

The definition of the activity of a cytokine depends on the assay used. Clonal assays, as they are customary for cells of the myeloid lineages, are often not available for normal lymphocytes, since both the activation and the cell cycle progression phases are not only dependent on soluble cytokines, but also on cell-to-cell contacts. Furthermore, the efficiency of plating of normal lymphocytes drops to zero at cell concentration below 5×10^4 cells/ml in tissue culture. Cultures of normal lymphocytes, even when excessively enriched for a given type of cell by lysis of contaminating cells with appropriate monoclonal antibodies and complement, and by cell sorter purification with cell-specific monoclonal antibodies are never 100% pure, as single cells would be. Consequently, actions of cytokines on lymphocytes may be direct, or may be indirect via contaminating cells. In many instances, studies on lymphocyte activation do not really measure the completion of one or several cell cycles, but monitor early changes in surface marker expression, biochemical signalling reactions, thymidine uptake, cell size, RNA content, which all might occur without mitosis.

When we measure the effects on activated B cells, we monitor only proliferation, and do so by counting cells. We also monitor maturation, but only as the development of large numbers of Ig-secreting, plaque-forming cells, and only as induced in small, resting cells. We, therefore, restrict ourselves to polyclonal responses of large numbers of B cells, probably to the LPS-sensitive, primary, extrafollicular, surface IgM-positive B cell subpopulations. Responses of other, minor B cell subpopulations, and responses of B cells which do not lead to cell cycle progression, may go undetected in our assays.

The differences in assay conditions and the lack of an unambiguous assignment of the activity of a cytokine to a direct action on B cells may explain why we differ in our conclusions of the activities of IL-1, IL-4 and IL-6 from those of other laboratories (for a collection of literature see Melchers and Andersson, 1986; Lernhardt et al., 1987; Karasuyama, Rolink and Melchers, 1988).

RECEPTORS FOR IL-5

Since we had constructed a Ig-nonproducing X63Ag8.653 hybridoma cell line which produces and secretes constitutively large quantities (usually 5000-50,000 units/ml in 24 hours) of mIL-5 (Karasuyama and Melchers, 1988), and since a column containing mIL-5 specific monoclonal antibody had been kindly made available to us by Dr. K. Takatsu (Department of Biology, Institute of Medical Immunology, University of Kumamoto, Kumamoto, Japan) (Harada et al., 1987) we

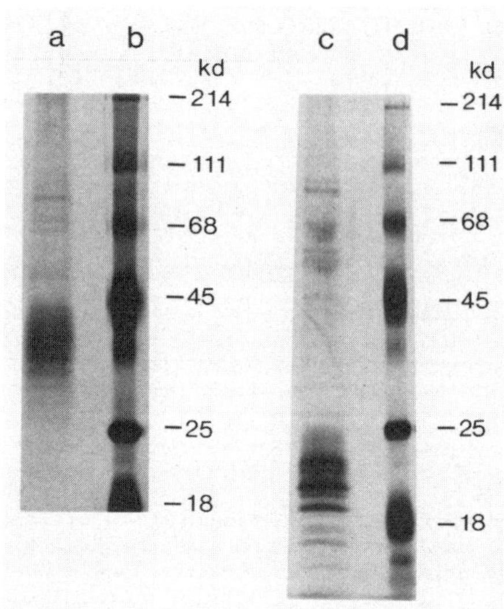

Fig. 1

Analysis of affinity purified mIL-5 by SDS-PAGE. Serum free medium conditioned for 48 hrs with the mIL-5 secreting X63Ag8.653 cell line was used as a source of mIL-5. MIL-5 was purified by affinity chromatography as described by Takatsu et al., 1988. mIL-5 was either run in the absence (lane a) or presence (lane c) of 2-mercapto-ethanol. Proteins were visualized by silver staining.

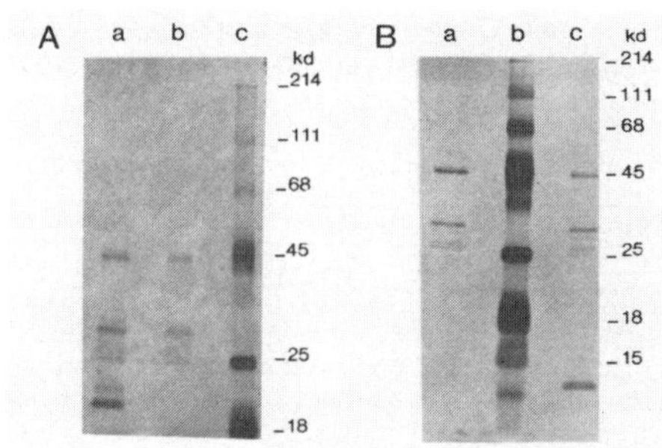

Fig.2

Analysis of Endoglycosidase F treated mIL-5 by SDS-PAGE. Samples were run under nonreducing, and reducing (Gel B) conditions and proteins (Gel A) were visualized by silver staining. Gel A: lane a, Endoglycosidase F treated mIL-5: lane b, Endoglycosidase F; lane c, markers. Gel B: lane a, Endoglycosidase F; lane c, Endoglycosidase F treated mIL-5.

were in the position to purify large quantities of mIL-5 to apparent homogeneity. SDS-polyacrylamide gel electrophoresis of the affinity-purified mIL-5 from culture supernatants of serum-free media conditioned for 24 to 72 hours with the mIL-5-secreting X63.Ag8.653 cell line indicates that mIL-5 is reasonably pure (Figure 1). Its apparent molecular weights under nonreducing (40-45 kD) and reducing (19-25 kD) conditions and the multitude of bands detected by silver staining in these molecular weight ranges indicate that purified mIL-5 is a dimer which is variably glycosylated. The purified mIL-5 had a specific activity of 1.5×10^7 units/mg protein (Table 1). The activity of the dimer was only partially lost upon boiling in SDS. Endoglycosidase F reduced the apparent molecular weight of the dimer to 19-22 kD and the monomer to 12-14 kD (Figure 2). The monomer, glycosylated or deglycosylated, obtained under reducing conditions, was inactive (Table 1).

Table 1

The effects of different treatments on the biological activity of mIL-5

Treatment of affinity purified mIL-5 with	Specific activity* (U/mg)	Loss of specific activity in %
-	1.5×10^7	-
2-mercaptoethanol (1 mM)	$> 1 \times 10^5$	>99
0.1% Sodium-dodecylsulfate and boiling	$\sim 1 \times 10^7$	5-10
Endoglycosidase F	$\sim 1 \times 10^7$	5-10
Endoglycosidase F and 1 mM 2-mercaptoethanol	$> 1 \times 10^5$	>99

* One unit is defined as the amount of mIL-5 needed to give half maximal proliferation of the IL-5 dependent B13 cell line.

A cell line has been established in long-term culture which grows in response to either IL-3 or IL-5. This cell line, called B13 (kindly given to us by Dr. R. Palacios of our Institute), when grown in IL-3, could be used to bind I^{125}-radiolabelled mIL-5 to determine the affinity(ies) and the nature of mIL-5 receptors. These binding studies are shown in Figure 3. They reveal high and low affinity receptors for mIL-5 on B13 cells, with a K_d for the high affinity form of $0.5\text{-}1 \times 10^{-11}$ M and a K_d of $1.5\text{-}3 \times 10^{-8}$ M for the low affinity form. From these measurements it can be estimated that a B13 cell expresses about 4000 high and about 50,000 low affinity receptors on its surface.

mIL-5 bound to its receptors can be covalently crosslinked with the receptor molecules through bifunctional agents such as disuccinineidyl suberate. Under nonreducing conditions one major band of 75-80 kD is detected by SDS-PAGE, whereas under nonreducing conditions this complex has an apparent molecular weight of about 100 kD (Fig. 4). Thid indicates that the polypeptide to which the mIL-5 is crosslinked after binding has apparent molecular weight of around 50 kD. Essentially identical results have been obtained with other mIL-5-binding cell lines by Takatsu and his colleagues (Takatsu et al., 1988).

Receptors for mIL-5 have now also been detected on normal B cells activated by Ig-specific antibodies and α factors (data not shown). Together with the two monoclonal antibodies raised against the mIL-5 receptors (Rolink, A. et al. manuscript in preparation) we should be able to determine the structure of the

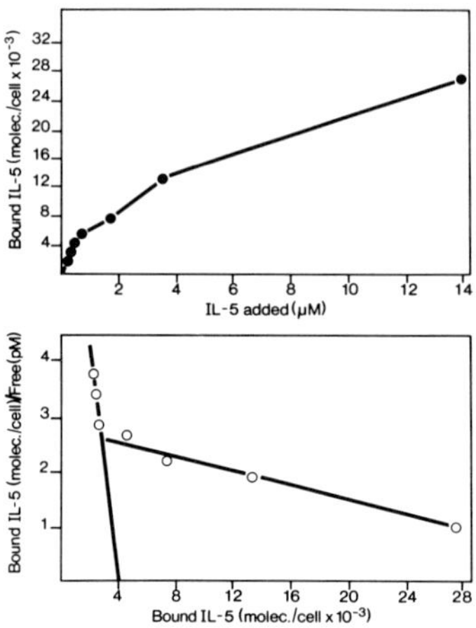

Fig. 3

Specific binding of mIL-5 to B13 cells and Scatchard plot analysis of these data. Affinity purified mIL-5 was ^{125}I labeled with the Bolton and Hunter reagent. Specific binding was determined by subtraction of the binding obtained in the presence of a 100-fold excess of non-labeled mIL-5. Binding studies were performed at 37°C for 45 min.

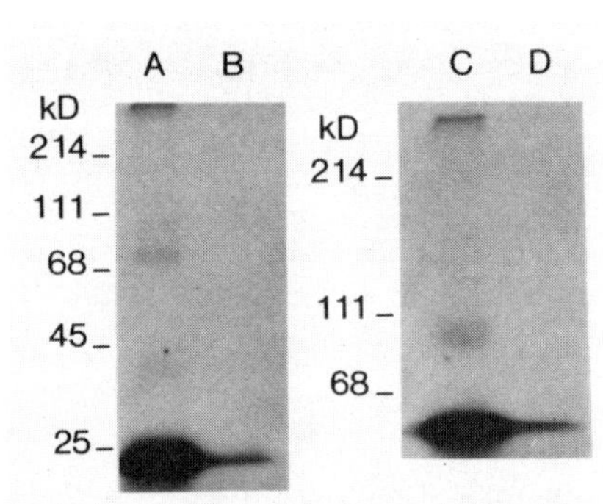

Fig. 4

Autoradiography of mIL-5 crosslinked to its receptor via DSS.
B13 cells were incubated for 45 min at 37°C with ^{125}I-mIL-5 in the absence (lane A and C) and presence (lane B and D) of a 100-fold excess of nonlabeled mIL-5. Thereafter the cells were washed mIL-5 was crosslinked to its receptor with 1 mM DSS for 30 min at room temperature. Cells were lysed with 2% NP40 and cell lysates were analyzed by SDS-PAGE under reducing (lane A and B) and nonreducing conditions (lane C and D).

receptors on normal cells, and to investigate the role of these receptors in the cell cycle control of B cells.

THE MULTIPLE ACTIONS OF MULTIPLE CYTOKINES

One helper T cell can produce several cytokines, although the spectrum of cytokines produced by T_{H1} (IL-2, IL-3, IγIFN) is different from T_{H2} (IL-3, IL-4, IL-5 IL-6?) (Mosmann and Coffman, 1987). Both types of T_H cells, therefore, produce a β-type B cell growth factor activity. The spectrum of cytokines produced by macrophages is, again, different with IL-1, α-factors, IL-6, and other growth factors such as Endo GF, FGF, and TNF-α and β (Oppenheim et al., 1986; Bazin and Lemieux, 1987; Lernhardt et al., 1987).

Two cytokines can act at the same restriction point in the cell cycle of a B cell, as IL-2 and IL-5 exemplify. It remains to be shown whether one and the same B cell is responsive to both IL's, or whether two subpopulations exist, responding to either IL-2 or IL-5.

One cytokine can be produced by more than one type of cell. The production of IL-3 by T_{H1} and T_{H2}, and the possible production of IL-6 by T_{H2} and by macrophages are examples, which are related to helper T cell-dependent activation of B cells.

Finally, one cytokine can act on more than one type of differentiated cell. IL-2 acts on several subpopulations of T cells (T_H, T_{killer}, T suppressor?) and on B cells, all of which are induced to proliferation. IL-5 acts on B cells and on eosinophils. The production of IL-3 and IL-4 by the antigen-specific, MHC-restricted interaction of T cells and A cells spreads the effects of antigen-activated cytokine production to many cells of the hematopoietic hierarchy. IL-3 has been called pan-hematopoietic, since it acts on progenitors such as CFU-S, as well as on progenitors of the T and B lineages, and it acts as an alternate cytokine to GM-CSF in the production of mature monocytes and granulocytes. This alternate use of two types of cytokines in the development of early progenitors and of myeloid cell lineages might indicate that hematopoiesis of these types of blood cells can be controlled T cell-independently, i.e. maybe endogenously, or T cell-dependently, i.e. stimulated by immune recognition of a foreign invader.

ACKNOWLEDGEMENTS

The able techinical assitance of Annick Peter and Denise Richterich-Guex is gratefully acknowledged. The Basel Institute for Immunology was founded and is supported by F. Hoffmann-La Roche, Ltd. Co., Basel, Switzerland.

REFERENCES

Abramson, S., Miller, R.C. and Phillips, R.A. (1977). J. Exp. Med. 145, 1567-1579.

Andersson, J., Schreier, M.H. and Melchers, F. (1980). Proc. Natl. Acad. Sci. USA 77, 1612-1620.

Bazin, R. and Lemieux, R. (1987). J. Immunol. 139, 780-787.

Chesnut, R.W. and Grey, H.M. (1986). Adv. Immunol. 39, 51-70.

Dick, J.E., Magli, M.C., Auszar, D., Phillips, R.A. and Bernstein, A. (1985). Cell 42, 71-79.

Erdei, A., Melchers, F., Schulz, T. and Dierich, M.P. (1985). Eur. J. Immunol. 15, 184-188.

Fleischmann, R.A., Custer, R.P. and Mintz, B. (1982). Cell 30, 351-359.

Harada, N., Takahashi, T., Matsumoto, M., Kinashi, T., Ohara, J., Kikuchi, Y., Koyama, N., Severinson, E., Yaoita, Y., Honjo, T., Yamaguchi, N., Tominaga, A. and Takatsu, K. (1987). Proc. Natl. Acad. Sci. USA, 84, 4581-4587.

Karasuyama, H. and Melchers, F. (1988). Eur. J. Immunol. 10, 97-104.

Karasuyama, H., Rolink, A. and Melchers, F. (1988). J. Exp. Med. 167,
Keller, G., Paige, C., Gilboa, E. and Wagner, E.F. (1985). Nature 318, 149-154.
Kikuchi, Y. and Yamaguchi, N. (1988). Immunol. Rev. 102, 107-134.
Lanzavecchia, A. (1985). Nature 314, 537-539.
Lernhardt, W., Karasuyma, H., Rolink, A. and Melchers, F. (1987). Immunol. Rev. 99, 241-262.
Melchers, F. (1988). In: Immunoglobulin Genes (eds. T. Honjo, F.W. Alt and T. Rabbits). Academic Press, in press.
Melchers, F. and Andersson, J. (1986). Ann. Rev. Immunol. 4, 13-25.
Melchers, F. and Lernhardt, W. (1985). Proc. Natl. Acad. Sci. USA 82, 7681-7690.
Melchers, F., Andersson, J., Lernhardt, W. and Schreier, M.H. (1980). Eur. J. Immunol. 10, 679-689.
Melchers, F., Erdei, A., Schulz, T. and Dierich, M.P. (1985). Nature 317, 264-267.
Micklem, H.S., Ford, C.E., Evans, E.P. and Gray J. (1966). Proc. Roy. Soc. London 165, 78-102.
Mosmann, T.R. and Coffman, R.L. (1987). Immunol. Today 8, 223-227.
Oppenheim, J.J., Kovacs, E.J., Matsushima, K. and Durum, S.K. (1986). Immunol. Today 7, 45-46.
Schreier, M.H., Andersson, J., Lernhardt, W. and Melchers, F. (1980). J. Exp. Med. 151, 194-206.
Steinmetz, M. (1986). Genetic Engineering 5, 116-158.
Takatsu, K., Tominaga, A., Harada, N., Mita, S., Matsumoto, M., Takahashi, T.,
Unanue, E.R. and Cerottini, J.C., (1970) J. Exp. Med. 131, 711-725.
Wu, A.M. (1967). J. Cell. Physiol. 69, 177-184.
Wu, A.M., Till, J.E., Siminovitch, L. and McCulloch, E.A. (1968). J. Exp. Med. 1968, 458-463.

The Colony Stimulating Factors: Discovery to Clinical Applications

DONALD METCALF

Cancer Research Unit, Walter and Eliza Hall Institute of Medical Research, P.O. Royal Melbourne Hospital 3050, Victoria, Australia

ABSTRACT

The four glycoprotein colony stimulating factors regulating the production of granulocytes and macrophages in mouse and man have been purified and their actions characterized. The cloning of cDNA's for each has led to the mass-production of recombinant CSF's and preliminary clinical trials indicate their effectiveness in stimulating granulocyte and monocyte formation and functional activity.

KEY WORDS

Colony stimulating factors: granulocyte formation: macrophage formation: clinical trials of colony stimulating factors.

DISCOVERY OF THE COLONY STIMULATING FACTORS

The colony stimulating factors were discovered in the course of an analysis of the active factors responsible for the proliferation in vitro of colonies of differentiating murine and human neutrophilic granulocytes and monocyte-macrophages. In these cultures, it was obvious that granulocytes and macrophages could not proliferate unless stimulated but proliferation was able to be achieved by the use of underlayers containing various cells or tissues and later by the addition of media conditioned by such tissues (Metcalf, 1984).

Based on the known existence of a single regulator, erythropoietin, able to control the proliferation of erythroid cells, it was assumed initially that a single active molecule, termed "colony stimulating factor (CSF)," might be responsible for controlling the proliferation of granulocytes and macrophages. Human urine was found to contain a factor able to stimulate colony formation by murine cells and, because of its convenience and low protein content, human urine was used as the source material in the original purification studies. The active molecule (now known as macrophage colony stimulating factor (M-CSF or CSF-1)) was eventually purified and found to stimulate the formation primarily of macrophage colonies. Murine M-CSF (molecular weight, 70,000) was subsequently purified from mouse L-cell conditioned medium.

Meantime it was becoming obvious that medium conditioned by a number of murine tissues, e.g. lung, muscle, kidney, salivary gland, also contain CSF but the active molecule appeared to be of smaller size (23,000 molecular weight) and to stimulate the formation of both granulocytic and macrophage colonies. This molecule was ultimately purified from medium conditioned by lungs from mice preinjected with endotoxin and is now known as granulocyte-macrophage colony stimulating factor (GM-CSF). Towards the completion of these studies it was recognized that yet another CSF was present in post-endotoxin serum and medium conditioned by tissues from endotoxin-injected mice, characterized by an ability to stimulate the formation almost exclusively of granulocytic colonies. This molecule (molecular weight, 25,000) was eventually purified from mouse lung conditioned medium and named granulocyte-colony stimulating factor (G-CSF). By this time, it was becoming clear that at least one other CSF must exist since medium conditioned by WEHI-3B myelomonocytic leukemic cells or lectin-stimulated lymphocytes stimulated a wide variety of hemopoietic colonies to develop - not only granulocyte and macrophage colonies but also colonies of megakaryocytes, eosinophils, erythroid and mast cells and the proliferation of certain continuous hemopoietic cell lines. Fractionation studies showed that, surprisingly, all of these activities were ascribable to a single molecule (molecular weight, 23 - 28,000) which was termed multipotential colony stimulating factor (Multi-CSF) or by other workers interleukin-3 (IL-3) (Metcalf, 1987).

With the exception of murine G-CSF, the murine molecules have no stimulating action for human granulocyte and macrophage precursors. Subsequent studies succeeded in isolating and purifying the human equivalents of GM-CSF and G-CSF. The human equivalent of murine Multi-CSF (IL-3) was eventually identified and characterized following cloning of a primate cDNA having homology with both murine and human Multi-CSF.

The molecular control of granulocyte and macrophage formation is therefore reasonably complex with four distinct CSF's involved and it may be that other CSF's exist that are also able to exert actions on these populations.

CHEMICAL NATURE AND GENETIC ARRANGEMENT OF THE CSF's

The four-year period from 1983 to 1987 witnessed a series of major advances in work on the CSF's since, during this period, cDNA and genomic clones for all four CSF's of both mouse and man were isolated and the complete amino acid sequences for each polypeptide established. From biochemical studies, the CSF's were known to be glycoproteins with a high carbohydrate content that was not necessary for biological action, at least in vitro. The polypeptides were known to be held in a configuration necessary for biological activity by mandatory disulfide bridges. Three of the CSF's were known to be monomeric (GM-CSF, G-CSF and Multi-CSF) while M-CSF was a homodimer of two polypeptide chains. The amino acid sequencing data revealed that the four CSF's exhibited no sequence homology with one another and had quite different predicted secondary structure. This was a surprising finding in view of the close functional similarities between the four molecules (see review, Metcalf, 1988).

Two sets of observations now indicate a relatedness between these four differing glycoproteins (a) unique single genes encode each CSF but these have a chromosomal location that is not random. GM-CSF and Multi-CSF are closely adjacent (within 9 Kb) on chromosome 11 in the mouse and on chromosome 5 in man. In man, the genes for M-CSF and its receptor (c-fms) are also located nearby on chromosome 5 as is the gene for eosinophil CSF (EDF or IL-5). Similarly in the mouse, the gene for G-CSF is on chromosome 11 (chromosome 17 in man) as is the gene for the myeloid leukemia inhibitory factor (LIF). There is some suggestion from an analysis of gene structure that common signal regions exist at least for GM-CSF and Multi-CSF and that, on the basis of gene structure, the CSF genes may indeed be derived from a common ancestral gene. (b) Unique membrane receptors exist for each CSF and most granulocytic and macrophage cells simultaneously express receptors for three or more CSF's. The number of receptors per cell varies but in general is small (a few hundred per cell). Despite this, the receptors, at least on murine cells, are functionally linked in a hierarchic sequence Multi-R→GM-R→M-R. Thus, occupation by Multi-CSF of its receptors leads to down-modulation of receptors for GM-CSF, G-CSF and M-CSF while occupation by GM-CSF of its receptors does not influence Multi-CSF receptors but does down-modulate G-CSF and M-CSF receptors etc. (Walker et al, 1985).

From these two sets of observations, it is apparent that the CSF's are designed to be produced and to act in a coordinated manner, permitting considerable flexibility and subtlety in the control system.

FUNCTIONAL ACTIONS OF THE CSF's

Stimulation by one or other of the four CSF's is required for every cell division of granulocyte-macrophage precursor cells. The CSF's are the only known direct proliferative stimuli for these populations and the concentrations required are low (10^{-10} to 10^{-12}M). The concentration of CSF determines the average length of the cell cycle and the total number of mature cells produced by individual progenitor cells. Because individual progenitors exhibit receptors for more than one CSF, the combined use of two CSF's results in additive or superadditive proliferative responses.

In addition to their role as mandatory proliferative stimuli, the CSF's also exhibit three other types of action on responding granulocytic and macrophage populations (a) they permit maintenance of membrane integrity and thus prolong, or are necessary for, the survival of cells at all stages of maturation (b) where progenitor cells are bipotential, CSF's can commit progenitors irreversibly to the exclusive formation of granulocytes or monocytes (c) the CSF's stimulate the functional activity of mature granulocytes and macrophages as measured by many parameters e.g. adherence, display of membrane markers, phagocytosis, cytotoxicity responses for microorganisms or tumor cells, and the synthesis of many biologically-active products such as superoxide, PGE, IL-1, TNF, plasminogen activator etc. (Metcalf, 1988).

The somewhat redundant nature of the CSF control system is therefore balanced by an economy of design in which individual CSF's exhibit a multiplicity of measurable actions on the target populations.

RESPONSES IN VIVO TO THE CSF's

With the cloning of cDNA's for each CSF, an opportunity became available to determine the effects of injecting CSF in vivo - studies not previously possible because of the minute amounts of native CSF able to be purified from even the richest tissue sources. Regardless of the expression system used - bacterial (non-glycosylated CSF) or yeast or mammalian (glycosylated CSF), careful in vitro analysis showed that the recombinant CSF's exhibited the same range of biological actions as the corresponding native CSF's and essentially similar specific activities per mg protein.

With this background of information, studies were performed on the effects of injecting CSF into adult mice. These studies showed that the half-life of intravenously injected CSF's was relatively short - the initial fall having a half-life of 1 to 3 minutes with the second phase fall a half-life of 1 to 3 hours. Injection intraperitoneally or subcutaneously achieved more sustained elevations of serum CSF levels due to the slower entry of the injected material into the circulation. Major organs degrading injected CSF appeared to be the liver and kidney.

Injection of from 2 to 200 ng of GM-CSF, Multi-CSF or G-CSF intraperitoneally three times daily to adult mice for 6 days resulted in obvious dose-related increases in the number of granulocytes and macrophages (and eosinophils in the case of GM-CSF and Multi-CSF both of which were known also to have direct proliferative effects on eosinophils in vitro). The pattern of responses differed for each CSF. G-CSF was markedly superior to the other two CSF's in elevating blood neutrophil levels whereas GM-CSF was the most effective agent in elevating peritoneal cell counts, the major cell type responding being the macrophage (Metcalf et al, 1986; 1987; Metcalf, 1987). Combination of two CSF's, as in vitro, potentiated the observed responses but preserved the characteristic responses elicited by each agent alone. In addition to rises in granulocyte numbers in the bone marrow and spleen, rises in macrophage and neutrophil numbers were also observed in non-hemopoietic tissues such as the liver and lung, suggesting that the additional cells formed following CSF stimulation were also capable of reaching peripheral tissues and thus of being available to respond to local infections.

As was the case with the in vitro studies, evidence was obtained that the injection of CSF also increased the functional activity of appropriate mature cells, indicating that the injection of CSF can result in significant enhancement of resistance using existing mature cells quite apart from increment to the mature cell population resulting from CSF-induced proliferative stimulation.

ROLE OF THE CSF's IN RESISTANCE TO INFECTIONS

Cells known to be able to synthesize one or more of the CSF's are widely distributed in the body and include lymphocytes, macrophages, fibroblasts, endothelial cells and at least some epithelial cells. Often CSF production by such cells requires inductive signalling and the present information may markedly underestimate the number of cell types able under appropriate conditions to synthesize CSF (Metcalf, 1988).

Certainly the cells known to produce CSF are those likely to make early contact with microorganisms or their breakdown products. Since induction of CSF synthesis is a rapid event, CSF levels rise within hours of induction.

A variety of evidence indicates that exposure to microorganisms is the strongest naturally-occurring inductive signal for CSF synthesis. Thus circulating levels of CSF are very low in germfree animals, low in specific pathogen-free mice, higher in conventionally reared mice and are grossly elevated during acute infections. Similar elevations of CSF have been observed in acute infections in man although not all infected persons exhibit such responses.

Even though the natural response to infections is to elevate rates of production and circulating levels of one or more CSF, it may well be that such responses do not elicit the maximum possible activation of existing granulocytes and macrophages and do not stimulate the maximum possible elevation in the production of these cells. It can be proposed therefore that the injection of CSF to animals should enhance resistance to infections. The clearest evidence documenting that this indeed occurs was obtained from a study of mice rendered leukopenic by an injection of the myelotoxic drug cyclophosphamide, followed by challenge infection with a variety of organisms. Mice injected with G-CSF exhibited a thousand-fold rise in resistance to organisms including pseudomonas and candida - organisms commonly involved in secondary infections in similar situations in man (Matsumoto et al, 1987).

These observations indicate that the injection of CSF into patients, particularly those with marrow damage, would be expected to result in a similar enhancement of resistance to life-threatening infections.

RESPONSES IN MAN TO THE INJECTION OF CSF

Following studies on the response of primates to the injection of either GM-CSF or G-CSF in which clear dose-response elevations in blood neutrophils were observed, a series of Phase I studies has been made of the effects of injecting GM-CSF or G-CSF into patients.

These studies were designed to establish whether progressive elevations of blood neutrophil levels and functional activation of such cells could be achieved by the injection of increasing doses of CSF and whether dose-limiting toxicity would be observed.

In the case of G-CSF, patients injected so far in doses of up to 60 μg/kg/day for 18 days have not exhibited dose-limiting toxicity and a marked dose-related rise in neutrophils up to 80,000 per μl was observed. Furthermore, use of G-CSF in these cancer patients shortened the period of neutropenia following chemotherapy (Morstyn et al, 1988).

Comparable studies of GM-CSF in AIDS patients with leukopenia (Groopman et al, 1987), in patients with myelodysplastic syndromes (Vadhan-Raj et al, 1987) or patients receiving autologous marrow transplants have documented the ability of GM-CSF to elicit comparable elevations in neutrophil levels to those achieved using G-CSF with suggestions that in the marrow transplant patients the frequency of fever and infections was reduced by the GM-CSF. High doses of GM-CSF in the 30 to 60 μg/kg/day range did elicit some toxic effects and this agent may possess dose-limiting toxicity, but at doses considerably in excess of those required to achieve adequate circulating levels of granulocytes.

These initial trials indicate that both G-CSF and GM-CSF should be valuable agents in patients with leukopenia either due to natural disease states or following the use of cytotoxic therapy. It remains unclear whether the CSF's will have a useful role in the management of secondary infections and leukopenia of AIDS patients or whether the CSF's might induce increased levels of HIV virus production because of monocyte activation.

POSSIBLE TOXIC EFFECTS OF THE CSF's

Past studies with agents such as γ-interferon, IL-1 or IL-2 have shown that these have severe toxic side effects despite the fact that they are normal body products. Indeed, early production of these agents in acute infections may be the basis for the toxic effects suffered during the acute phase of infections. G-CSF seems essentially to be without such side effects although GM-CSF at very high doses may produce some similar toxic effects.

Two types of possible medium to longterm toxic or undesirable consequences of the use of CSF's could be postulated on theoretical grounds: (a) a serious depletion of hemopoietic progenitor cells. These cells are the primary targets of the CSF's and since they are not self-renewing, excess stimulation of these cells to produce differentiating progeny might deplete the progenitor pool leading to a leukopenic phase. This hypothetical sequence has not been observed either in animals or man and it seems likely that compensatory production of new progenitor cells by stem cells is able to sustain progenitor cell numbers during CSF therapy. (b) Because the CSF's stimulate mature cells to produce a number of biologically-active molecules, CSF stimulation might lead eventually to tissue damage mediated by such products. For example, GM-CSF can stimulate monocytes to produce IL-1, γ-interferon and TNF and these might, in a cascade effect, damage tissues.

A possible example of such a sequence has been observed in transgenic GM-CSF mice that constitutively express elevated circulating GM-CSF levels 40 - 50-fold above normal levels. Such mice die prematurely in early middle age with lesions including macrophage destruction of the retina, focal inflammatory foci in muscle tissue leading to wasting and paralysis and fibrotic nodules in the peritoneal and pleural cavities (Lang et al, 1987). The enlarged macrophages in these lesions not only produce GM-CSF but IL-1, TNF and possibly other toxic factors. This model is of course complex since it involves CSF-induced changes during crucial developmental remodelling of organs by macrophages - a situation not encountered in an adult patient. Nevertheless the transgenic mouse may indicate an extreme version of what might occur following the longterm use of high doses of CSF.

It needs to be pointed out that injected CSF's can clearly elevate leukocyte levels in man to unnecessarily high levels e.g. 60 to 80,000/μl. It is extremely improbable that any significant clinical benefit would be achieved by having such abnormally high white cell levels in any infection. Commonsense indicates that these powerful agents need only to be administered in doses inducing the formation of moderately elevated white cell levels to serve their purpose and at these dose levels the risk of cascade-induced damage is likely to be minimal.

REFERENCES

Groopman, J.E., Mitsuyasu, R.T., De Leo, M.J., Oette, D.H. and Golde, D.W. (1987). N.Engl.J.Med. 317, 593-598.

Lang, R.A., Metcalf, D., Cuthbertson, R.A., Lyons, I., Stanley, E., Kelso, A., Kannourakis, G., Williamson, D.J., Klintworth, G.K., Gonda, T.J. and Dunn, A.R. (1987). Cell 51, 675-686.

Matsumoto, M., Matsubara, S., Matsumo, T., Tamura, M., Hattori, K., Nomura, H. Ono, M. and Yokota, T. (1987). Infect.Immun. 55, 2715-2720.

Metcalf, D. (1984). The hemopoietic colony stimulating factors. Elsevier. Amsterdam.

Metcalf, D. (1987). Proc.R.Soc. Lond. B 230, 389-423.

Metcalf, D. (1988). The molecular control of normal and leukemic blood cells. Harvard University Press. Boston.

Metcalf, D., Begley, C.G., Johnson, G.R., Nicola, N.A., Lopez, A.F. and Williamson, D.J. (1986). Blood 68, 46-57.

Metcalf, D., Begley, C.G., Williamson, D.J., Nice, E.C., DeLamarter, J., Mermod, J-J., Thatcher, D. and Schmidt, A. (1987). Exp.Hematol. 15, 1-9.

Morstyn, G., Souza, L.M., Keech, J., Sheridan, W., Campbell, L, Alton, N.K., Green, M., Metcalf, D. and Fox, R. (1988). Lancet 1, 667-672.

Vadhan-Raj, S., Keating, M., Le Maistre, A., Hittelman, W.N., McCredie, K., Trujillo, J.M., Broxmeyer, H.E., Henney, C. and Gutterman, J.U. (1987). N.Engl.J.Med. 317, 1545-1552.

Walker, F., Nicola, N.A., Metcalf, D. and Burgess, A.W. (1985). Cell 43, 269-276.

Characterization of the Mouse Interleukin 3 Receptor System

ATSUSHI MIYAJIMA[1], HOLANDA SCHREURS[1], HUEY-MEI WANG[1], KAZUO MARUYAMA[1], DAN GORMAN[1], SHIGEO KOYASU[2], ICHIRO YAHARA[2], JEAN Y. J. WANG[3], YUMIKO OHTA[4], and KEN-ICHI ARAI[1]

[1] *DNAX Research Institute of Molecular and Cellular Biology, 901 California Avenue, Palo Alto, CA 94304, USA*

[2] *Tokyo Metropolitan Institute of Medical Science, Honkomagome, Bunkyo-ku, Tokyo 113, Japan*

[3] *University of California San Diego, La Jolla, CA 92023, USA*

[4] *Nippon Roche Research Center, 200 Kajiwara, Kamakura-shi, Japan*

SUMMARY

Interleukin 3 is a T cell derived lymphokine that regulates the proliferation and differentiation of hemopoieic cells. We have shown that IL-3 exerts its biological effects through a specific membrane receptor which is linked to a tyrosine kinase, as indicated by the fact that IL-3 dependent cell can be converted, in a temperature dependent manner, to IL-3 independence by infection with a retrovirus carrying the temperature sensitive v-abl tyrosine kinase. This model is further substantiated by the finding that IL-3 induced the tyrosine phosphorylation of a number of specific proteins, including a membrane glycoprotein. A comparison of the signals generated by IL-3 and by other growth factor receptors carrying a tyrosine kinase provides information about the uniqueness or commonality of the pathways which trigger proliferation. We introduced the EGF receptor cDNA into an IL-3 dependent cell line. The transfectants expressed the EGF receptor and EGF substituted for IL-3, however, EGF-dependent proliferation was only transient, suggesting that the EGF signalling pathway partially overlaps with that of IL-3. To determine whether the IL-3 receptor is a typical growth factor receptor carrying a tyrosine kinase such as the EGF receptor, we analyzed the structure of the IL-3 receptor by cross-linking assays. Binding of IL-3 to various IL-3 dependent cells revealed several IL-3 binding proteins with molecular weights of 150, 120 and 70 kd. The inter-relationship between these molecules is unclear, they may be a complex of proteins which constitute the receptor or degradation products of the larger species. Two models for the IL-3 receptor are proposed: a) one of the IL-3 binding components has an intrinsic tyrosine kinase or b) the tyrosine kinase activity is extrinsic to but is a molecule closely associated with the IL-3 binding protein. To further characterize the IL-3 receptor, we have identified a monoclonal antibody against the IL-3 receptor from a panel of monoclonal antibodies derived from autoimmune mice. This antibody stimulates the growth of IL-3 dependent cells, stimulates tyrosine phosphorylation, and blocks IL-3 binding.

INTRODUCTION

Upon antigen stimulation helper T cells secrete a set of protein mediators called lymphokines, that play a vital role on the inflamatory response by regulating the proliferation and differentiation of T cells, B cells, and hemopoietic cells. IL-2 stimulates T cells, whereas, IL-3 and GM CSF stimulate hemopoietic cells. A class of molecules including IL-4, -5, and -6 regulate the growth and differentiation of B cells. Therefore T cells can be regarded as a signalling relay, receiving antigen-specific signals and converting them into non-antigen specific mediators of the immune response (Miyajima et al. 1988).

IL-3, initially defined as a factor that induces 20a-steroid dehydrogenase in thymus-deficient mice, has numerous other biological activites including mast cell growth factor (MCGF),Thy-1 antigen induction, and multi-colony formation (multi-CSF (Ihle et al. 1983). The multi-CSF activity of Il-3 indicates that IL-3 acts on the multipotential stem cells of the bone marrow to generate a variety of cell lineages. The mouse Il-3 cDNA was isolated from a cDNA library made from activated T cells based on MCGF activity (Yokota et al. 1984). It encodes a polypeptide of 166 amino acids including a signal sequence. There are four potential N-linked glycosylation sites and the natural IL-3 is a glycoprotein of about 28 KDa. Recombinant IL-3 expressed in heterologous host-vector systems has a similar spectrum of biological activities to that of mammalian IL-3 and has been used to characterize the mechanism of action of IL-3 (Miyajima et al. 1987) Since IL-3 exerts its multiple biological actions through a specific receptor on the target cell, characterization of the IL-3 receptor and its signal transduction machinery is important. We describe here the recent progress of our studies on the structure and function of the mouse IL-3 receptor.

SIGNAL TRANSDUCTION PATHWAY OF IL-3

Growth factors have been classified into two groups in the fibroblast model: those that act on cells resting at the G stage (competence factors and those that are required for the transition from G to S phase (progression factors). In T cells and B cells, antigen stimulation provides the competence signal that brings the resting cells into the G phase permitting cellular proliferation in response to lymphokines, such as IL-2 or B cell growth factors. In contrast to T and B cells, it is still not clear whether factor-dependent myeloid cells have a resting G stage. These cells proliferate in vitro for long periods of time in the presence of lymphokines,such as IL-3 and GM-CSF; in the absence of lymphokines, these cells rapidly die. To better understand the nature of myeloid cell proliferation, we are studying the function of IL-3 and GM-CSF using the factor-dependent cell line, IC2, which has many features in common with mast cells (Koyasu et al. 1985). This cell line proliferates in response to IL-3, IL-4, and GM-CSF. However, there are differences in the efficacy of these various factors; IL-3 and GM-CSF can maintain IC2 cells for months, whereas IL-4 supports cell growth only transiently.

Growth factor dependency can be abrogated by different mechanisms, including an autocrine mechanism in which the cell makes one of the factors required for growth. Non-autocrine mechanisms of factor abrogation require some alteration of the growth factor receptor or its downstream pathways. Therefore studying the nonautocrine mechanism of factor abrogation should provide information about the signal transduction pathway of lymphokines. Since oncogenes having a tyrosine kinase such as v-abl or v-src can abrogate IL-3-dependence (Pierce et al. 1985, Watson et al. 1987), we tested the possibility that tyrosine phoosphorylation is required for the abrogation of factor dependence. Two different approaches were used; a) an analysis of the effects of mutant Abelson leukemia virus having a temperature-sensitive tyrosine kinase and b) a direct analysis of tyrosine phosphorylated proteins.

A retrovirus containing a temperature-sensitive tyrosine kinase (Kipreos et al. 1987) was used to infect IL-3-dependent IC2 cells,producing IC2RK5 cells which expressed the v-abl tyrosine kinase. The temperature-sensitivity of the tyrosine kinase was tested by Western Blotting using anti-phosphotyrosine and anti-v-abl protein antibodies (Fig.1). The 160 kD v-abl protein was detectable independent of the temperature, however, the tyrosine phosphorylated 160 kD protein was found only at the low temperature. Concordantly, the factor dependence of the v-able infected IC2 cells was altered; the parental cells died in the abscence of IL-3, independent of temperature, whereas, the virus-infected cells grew in the absence of IL-3 at the low temperature, but not at the high temperature (Fig.1). This indicates that the tyrosine kinase is involved in the factor-independent growth of Abelson leukemia virus-infected cells and is consistent with the idea that tyrosine phosphorylation plays an important role in the IL-3 or GM-CSF signal transduction pathway.

Since IC2 cells proliferate in response to either IL-3 or GM-CSF, it is not clear with which signal transduction pathways v-abl interacts. To address this question we analyzed the signals produced by the interaction of these lymphokines with their respective receptors. To detect proteins phosphorylated at tyrosine residues, we immunoprecipitated ^{32}P labelled proteins with a polyclonal anti-phosphotyrosine antibody. Using this system we detected a membrane-bound ^{32}P-labelled 150 kD molecule which appeared only when cells were stimulated with IL-3, but not with IL-4 or GM-CSF (Koyasu et al. 1987). Tyrosine phosphorylation was induced by IL-3 within a minute, suggesting that the kinase is closely associated with the receptor. Western blotting with a different anti-phosphotyrosine antibody revealed a different set of IL-3-induced tyrosine-phosphorylated proteins of M_r of 160, 90, 70 and 55 kD (Morla et al. 1988). IL-4 induced tyrosine phosphorylation of a 170 and 110 kD proteins, whereas GM-CSF had only a weak ability to stimulate tyrosine phosphorylation. Thus it is more likely that the v-abl protein interacts with the IL-3 signal transduction pathway rather than that of GM-CSF. This leads us to another issue; Is the IL-3 receptor similar to other growth factor receptors such as EGF or PDGF?

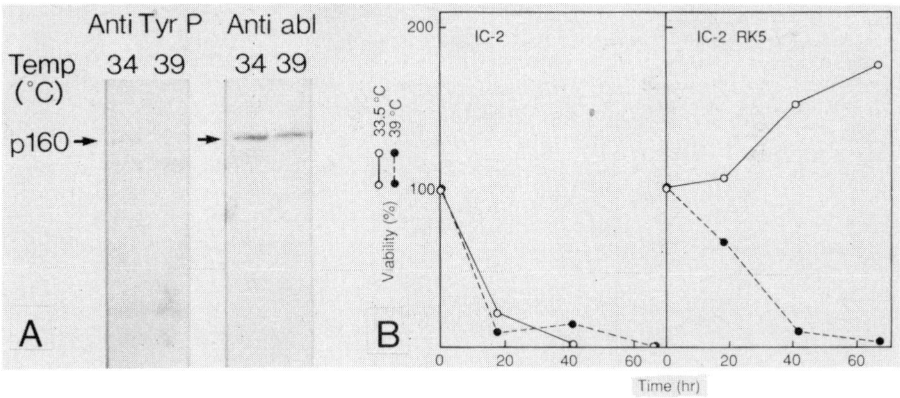

Fig. 1. Abrogation of IL-3 dependence by the temperature-sensitive Abelson leukemia virus. Panel A, Cell extracts were prepared from IC2RK5 (virus-infected IC2) grown at either 34 C and separated by SDS-PAGE. Proteins transferred to a nitrocellulose filter were incubated with anti-phosphotyrosine antibody or anti-v-abl protein antibody followed by a second stage incubation with ^{125}I-protein A. Panel B IC2 and IC2RK5 grown in the medium containing IL-3 were washed and resuspended in the medium with or without IL-3 (1nM). Cells were incubated at either 34 or 39 C and cell viability was measured by colorimetric assays using MTT.

RECEPTOR EXCHANGE EXPERIMENTS

If IL-3 shares a common signal transduction pathway with the other growth factors such as EGF or M-CSF, the IL-3 requirement for cellular proliferation may be replaced with another growth factor if its receptor is expressed on IL-3 dependent cells. Based on this idea, we attemped to introduce various growth factor receptor cDNAs into IL-3 dependent cells. Of particular interest are growth factor receptors carrying a tyrosine kinase, because the IL-3 receptor is linked to a tyrosine kinase.

The EGF receptor cDNA in the DOL vector (constructed by M Collins and R. Mulligan, Collins et al. submitted) was introduced into IC2 cells, thereby producing the 1D4 cell. The EGF receptor cDNA is transcribed from the LTR and the neo gene is transcribed from the SV40 promoter. The parental cell, IC2 has no EGF binding site, whereas 1D4 cells have high (17,000 sites/cell) and low (210,000 sites/cell) affinity binding sites for EGF. EGF stimulates the growth of ID4 cells but not the parental IC2 cell line (Fig. 2). However, the growth stimulation by EGF is transient and EGF cannot maintain the viability of the cells for more than 2 days at which time the cells start to die. These results indicate that EGF only partially substitutes for IL-3 in IC2 cells (Wang et al. in preparation). Interestingly, the result obtained with T cells was quite different from that seen using the IC2 cell line. We introduced the EGF receptor cDNA into an antigen-specific mouse T cell line. The EGF receptor expressed on the T cells showed characteristics similar to endogenous receptors on fibroblasts; EGF bound the receptor and the receptors were phosphorylated, internalized, and down-regulated by protein kinase C. However EGF did not substitute for the proliferative requirement of IL-2 at all (Gorman et al. 1988). We are now extending this transfection experiment to the insulin, PDGF, and M-CSF receptors using the IL-3-dependent cells to compare the function of these growth factors with IL-3. We anticipate that this type of analysis will provide information about the downstream events which occur after stimulation of the IL-3 receptor.

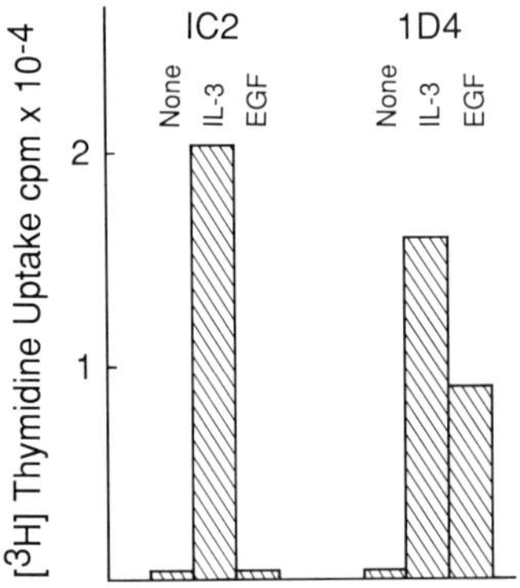

Fig. 2 DNA synthesis induced by IL-3 and EGF. IC2 and ID4 cells grown in medium containing IL-3 were washed and resuspended in medium containing 100 pM of factors as indicated. After 24 h incubation at 37 C, [^{3}H-thymidine uptake by the cells was measured.

STRUCTURE OF THE IL-3 RECEPTOR

The evidence above suggests the possibility that IL-3 receptor is a tyrosine kinase or is closely associated with a tyrosine kinase. Typical receptor tyrosine kinases are large molecules of about 150 kD, inconsistent with previous reports that the IL-3 binding protein had a molecular mass of 70-75 kD (Park et al. 1986, Nicola and Peterson 1986, May and Ihle 1986). We have reexamined this issue in extensive cross-linking assays and found that IL-3 binds several prominent proteins of M_r 150, 120 and 70 kD (Fig 3). However, it is not clear at present whether these are independent molecules or if the smaller ones are degradation products of the larger species As with many other receptors, equilibrium and kinetic assays of binding of radioactive IL-3 showed the existence of two classes of binding site with different binding affinities (Schreurs et al. in prep.). The above data leads us to the speculation that the IL-3 receptor is either a) composed on two IL-3 binding proteins with an intrinsic tyrosine kinase activity associated with the large Mr species (150 or 120 kD) or, alternatively, b) the tyrosine kinase is extrinsic to the IL-3 binding proteins (Fig. 4). However, the possibility that the 70 kD IL-3 binding molecule is a degradation product of the larger one is still open. Purification and cloning of IL-3 receptor will provide critical information about its structure.

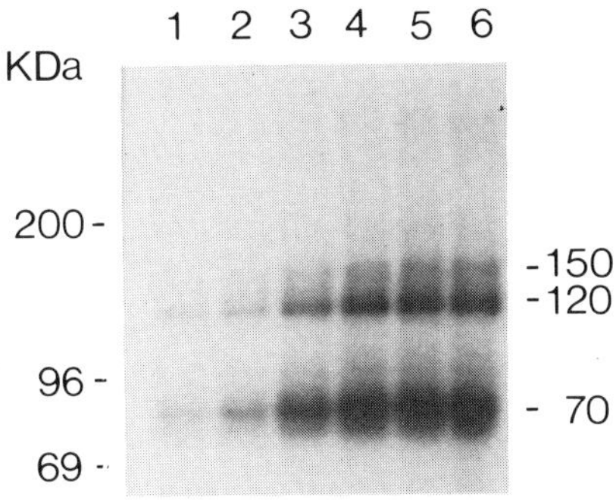

Fig. 3. Cross-linking of IL-3, MC/9 cells were incubated with various concentrations of IL-3 (lane 1; 21pM, lane 2; 63 pM, lane 3; 210 pM, lane 4; 630 pM, lane 5; 2.1 nM, 6; 6.3 nM) for 3 hrs on ice. Receptor-bound IL-3 was separated from free by centrifugation through oil, after which the cell pellet was resuspended with a 0.3 mM concentration of the cross-linker, DSS, incubated for 20 min at pH 7.1, washed and solubilized for SDS-PAGE.

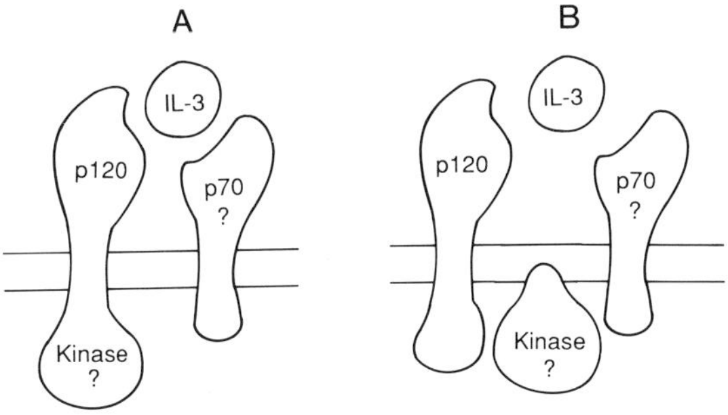

Fig. 4. Models of the association of the IL-3 receptor with a tyrosine kinase. A, the larger IL-3 binding molecule (150 or 120 kD) has an intrinsic tyrosine kinase. B, the tyrosine kinase is separated from the IL-3 binding proteins.

MONOCLONAL ANTIBODY AGAINST THE IL-3 RECEPTOR

Antibodies against the IL-3 receptor will be useful for further characterization of the protein and cloning of the gene. We have characterized candidate anti-IL-3 receptor monoclonal antibodies derived from autoimmune mice (Sugawara et al 1988). It has been known that spleen cells from MRL/1pr autoimmune mice constitutively produce an IL-3-like activity (Palacios et al. 1984), however, biochemical analysis indicated that the IL-3 itself (Ohta et al. 1988). Therefore, hybridoma cell lines secreting monoclonal antibodies with IL-3-like activity were generated using an unstimulated spleen of MRL/1pr mice (Sugawara et al. 1988). We have further characterized these antibodies by IL-3 binding and phosphorylation assays (Schreurs et al. submitted).

We first examined these monoclonal antibodies for their IL-3 agonistic activity on cell proliferation. We found that one of these antibodies, F9, stimulated the growth of all the IL-3 dependent cell lines tested. Of oncentrations of IL-3 and the F9 antibody on differentially responsive cell lines. For example, NFS60.8, a subline derived from a myeloid cell line, NFS60, required a 10-fold higher concentration of IL-3 for growth compared with that of the parental cell line. It also required a 20-fold higher concentration of the F9 antibody. The mimicry of IL-3 by the F9 by the F9 antibody was further demonstrated by F9 antibody-induced tyrosine phosphorylation detectable by Western blotting using anti-phosphotyrosine antibodies. The pattern of F9 antibody-induced tyrosine phosphorylation was almost indistinguishable from that of IL-3. This result strongly indicates that F9 recognizes the IL-3 receptor. This possibility was further supported by IL-3 binding assays using MC/9 cells which have both IL-3 and IL-4 receptors. F9 inhibits the binding of IL-3 but had no effect on IL-4 binding. Cross-linking of the IL-3 binding proteins (150, 120, 70 kD) with IL-3 was also inhibited by F9 antibody. These results strongly suggest that F9 is directed against the IL-3 receptor.

REFERENCES

Gorman, D., and Miyajima, A., (1988) J. Cellular Biochem Supplement 12A, 104.

Kipreos, E.T., Lee, G.J., and Wang, J.Y.J. (1987) Proc.Natl Acad. Sci. USA. 84, 1345-1349.

Koyasu, S., Nakauchi, H., Kitamura, K., Yonehara, S., Okumura, K., Tada, T., and Yahara, I. (1985) J. Immunol. 134, 3130-3136.

Koyasu, S., Tojo, A., Miyajima, A., Akiyama, T., Kasuga, M., Urabe, A., Schreurs, J., Arai, K., Takaku, F., and Yahara, I. (1987) EMBO J. 6, 3979-3984.

Ihle, J. Keller, J., Oroszlan, S., Henderson, L., Copland, T., Fitch, F. Prystowsky, M., Goldwasser, E., Schrader, J., Palaszynski, E., Dy, M., and Lebel, B. (1983) J. Immunol. 131, 282-287

May, W.S. and Ihle, J.N. (1986) Biochem. Biophys. Res. Commun 135, 870-879

Miyajima, A., Schreurs, J., Otsu, K., Kondo, A., Arai, K., and Maeda, S. (1987) Gene 58, 273-281

Miyajima, A., Miyatake, S., Schreurs, J., De Vries, J., Arai, N., Yokota, T., and Arai, K., (1988) FASEB J. 2, 2462-2473

Morla, A., Schreurs, J., Miyajima, A., and Wang, J. (1988) Mol. Cell Biol 8, 2214-2218

Nicola, N. and Peterson, L., (1986) J. Biol. Chem. 261, 12384-12389.

Ohta, Y., Tamura, S., Tezuka, E., Sugawara, M., Imai, S., and Tanaka, H., (1988) J. Immunol. 140, 520-525
Palacios, R. (1984) Eur. J. Immunol. 14, 599-605
Park, L., Friend, D., Gillis, S., and Urdal, D. (1988) J. Biol Chem. 261, 205-210
Pierce, J., Difiare, P., Aaronson, S., Potter, M., Humphrey, J., Scott, A., and Ihle, J. (1985) Cell 41, 685-693
Sugawara, M., Hattori, C., Tezuka, E., Tamura, S., and Ohta, Y. (1988) J. Immunol. 140, 526-530.
Watson, J., Eszes, M., Overell, R., Conlon, P., Widmer, M., and Gillis, S (1987) J. Immunol. 139, 123-129
Yokota, T., Lee, F., Rennick, D., Hall, C., Arai, N., Mosmann, T., Nabel, G., Cantor, H., and Arai, K. (1984) Proc. Natl. Acad. Sci. USA. 81, 1070-1074.

Interleukin-2 Receptor Targeted Immunosuppressive Therapy with Anti-Interleukin-2 Receptor Monoclonal Antibodies Directed against the L-Chain of the Interleukin-2 Receptor: Studies on Selectivity and Mode of Action

T. DIAMANTSTEIN[1], N. L. TILNEY[2], T. STROM[3], H. P. VAN DER MEIDE[4], H. J. HAHN[5], H-D. VOLK[6], A. P. WEETMAN[7], J. W. KUPIEC-WEGLINSKI[2]

[1] *Institute of Immunology, Klinikum Steglitz, Freie Universität Berlin, Hindenburgdamm 27, 1000 Berlin 45 FRG*
[2] *Surgical Research Laboratory and* [3]*the Harvard Thorndike Laboratory, Harvard Medical School, Boston*
[4]*TNO Primate Center Rijswijk,*
[5]*Central Institute of Diabetes "G. Katsch", Karlsburg*
[6]*Institute of Medical Immunology, Charité, Humboldt University, Berlin*
[7]*Department of Medicine, University of Cambridge Clinical School, Cambridge*

ABSTRACT

In contrast to resting lymphocytes antigen activated lymphocytes express the L-chain of the high affinity Interleukin-2 receptor. Therefore, inactivation of the L-chain bearing cells by anti-Interleukin-2 receptor monoclonal antibodies should selectively inhibit immune responses. Based on this hypothesis the effects of anti-Interleukin-2 receptor monoclonal antibodies on cell mediated immune response, on antibody formation, on allograft rejection and on organ specific autoimmune diseases previously shown to be mediated by T-lymphocytes was tested. The results revealed that cell mediated immune responses, such as delayed type hypersensitivity or local-graft versus host-reaction but not antibody formation was inhibited by such treatment. Anti-Interleukin-2 receptor monoclonal antibodies prolonged allograft survival. Prolongation of allograft survival due to antibody treatment was abolished by administration of gamma-Interferon. These results indicate that the primary target of the therapy are probably CD4+ T-lymphocytes of TH1 subtype, known to include T-cells mediating delayed type hypersensitivity and producing gamma-Interferon. Parallel application of the monoclonal antibodies directed against two distinct epitopes of the L-chain for only ten days not only prolonged but also allowed permanent acceptance of allografts. Evidences are presented indicating that allograft acceptance was mediated by CD4+ and by CD8+ T-lymphocytes with suppressive function. Similar results were obtained by short term treatment of allograft recipients with a combination of anti-Interleukin-2 receptor monoclonal antibodies and a subtherapeutic dose of Cyclosporin A. This short term treatment with antibodies and the subtherapeutic dose of Cyclosporin A also effectively abolished development of experimental autoimmune thyroiditis and cured BB-rats suffering of autoimmune diabetes.

INTRODUCTION

Activation of lymphocytes by antigens leads to a number of

sequential changes within their surface components, including the induction of cell surface molecules which are absent in the resting state. One of these activation antigens is the Interleukin-2 receptor (IL-2R), which, in contrast to other activation antigens (e.g. insulin- and transferrin-receptors) is lymphocyte specific. Recently evidence has been presented demonstrating three types of IL-2R, defined by their affinity to IL-2: low-, intermediate- and high-affinity receptors. High affinity IL-2R is a complex consisting of the low and the intermediate receptor. The gene coding for the low affinity IL-2R has been cloned, and the aminoacid sequence of the molecule deduced. It is a 55 kD glycoprotein previously named the Tac antigen, recently termed the L-chain. On the surface of cells binding IL-2 with intermediate affinity, two distinct but partially homologous 70 and 75 kD IL-2 binding proteins, termed heavy chain 1 (H1) and heavy chain 2 (H2) of yet unknown composition, could be detected (11,12). The expression of these intermediate type receptors is probably not restricted to activated lymphocytes. Apparently they are constitutive parts of the cell membrane in lymphoid cells. In contrast to the intermediate type receptor, the L-chain represents an activation antigen that due to antigenic stimulation, is transiently expressed on the activated but not on the resting lymphocytes, whereby converting intermediate affinity into high affinity receptors (Figure 1).

Figure 1: The high affinity IL-2 receptor consist of the intermediate affinity (H1 and H2) and the low affinity (L) IL-2 binding glycoproteins.

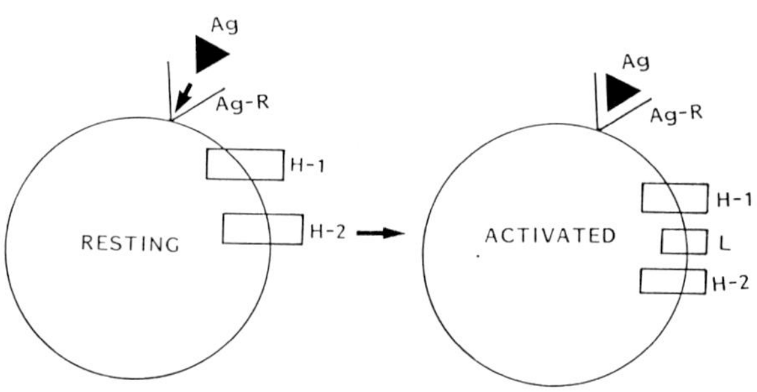

Resting T-cells express H1 and H2 chains.
Antigen activation induces L-chain expression.

Therefore, the L-chain of the receptor could serve as a target for the selective immunotherapy. The use of monoclonal antibodies (mAb) as well as toxin-derivatives of the mAb and/or toxin-derivatives of IL-2 have been envisaged as candidates for such therapeutic agents (2). We originally expected that IL-2R targeted therapy may result in an antigen-specific but transient immunsuppression.

This report summarizes the main findings obtained through the use of mAb directed against the L-chain of the IL-2R (anti-IL-2R mAb). Furthermore, experiments will be presented that allow for interpretation of the unexpected, selective, longtermed effects as well as the induction of tolerance by a short term

IL-2R targeted therapy. The effects of such a therapeutic approach on allograft rejection in various species has recently been reviewed (3,22).

1. Anti-IL-2R L-chain mAb inhibits cell-mediated immuneresponse (DTH), but not antibody formation.

That not only T-, but also B-lymphocytes activated in vitro express the L-chain, it was expected that inhibition by anti-IL-2R mAb of both cell-mediated as well as humoral immune response woul occur. However, anti-IL-2R mAb treatment inhibited in mice a delayed type hypersensitivity(DTH)-response to sheep red blood cells, but failed to affect IgM and IgG antibody production to the same antigen (8). These results (Figure 2) prompted that
1. anti-IL-2R treatment selectively affected T-, but not B-lymphocytes and
2. raised the possibility that the TH1 subset (18), known to mediate DTH rather than the TH2 (that includes TH required for B-lymphocyte help), is the target of anti-IL-2R mAb action.

Figure 2:
Anti IL-2 receptor mAb (rat anti mouse) AMT 13 inhibited DTH-response but not antibody formation.

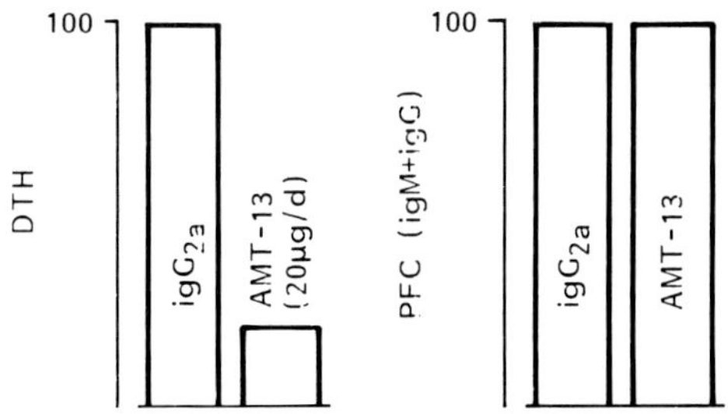

balb/c mice immunized with 10^6 SRBC. DTH tested at day 4 - 6. PFC response tested at day 7. Data taken from (8)

2. The epitope recognized by the respective Anti-IL-2R L-chain mAb is of importance, but their isotype may be not crucial for their effectivity.

The effect of four different monoclonal antibodies of the same isotype (IgG1), but recognizing four distinct non-overlaping epitopes of the IL-2R L-chain (18) of local-graft versus host-reaction (1-GVH-R) (19) and on cardiac allograft (14) rejection was tested in rats. The anti-IL-2R mAb ART-65 and ART-38 which in contrast to the anti-IL-2R mAb ART-18, do not inhibit IL-2 binding and IL-2 dependent proliferation in vitro, were effective in vivo though to a lesser degree than ART-18. On the other hand, the anti-IL-2R mAb OX-39 that inhibits IL-2 binding to the receptor in vitro was completely ineffective in vivo (Figure 3).

Figure 3:
Inhibition of clonal expansion of the IL-2 R bearing cells is not required for the in vivo action of the anti-IL-2 R antibodies.

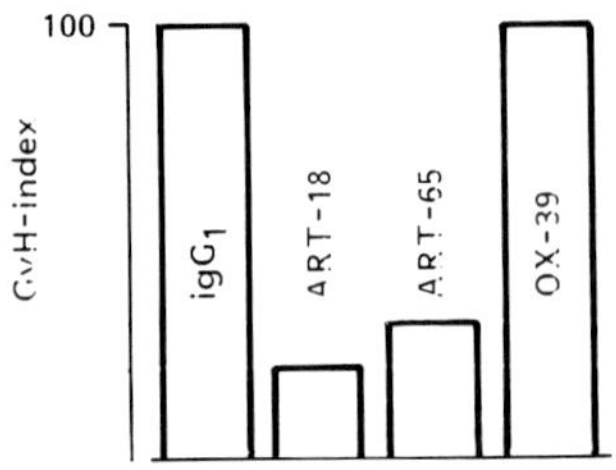

	inhibition of IL-2 binding	inhibition of IL-2 dependent proliferation
ART-18*	yes	yes
ART-65*	no	no
OX-39*	yes	no

*isotype: igG_1

Data taken from (20)

These results indicate that the antibodies act rather by inactivation (or elimination) of IL-2R+ cells, than by inhibition of their clonal expansion. A possible explanation for the inefficiency of OX-39 may be that this antibody is captured by unrelated cells as well as tissues expressing a common epitope and thereby is unable to reach the IL-2R bearing cells. It is thought that anti-L-IL-2R mAb act by eliminating the IL-2R+ cells via complement lysis or antibody dependent cell mediated cytotosicity (ADCC). If this is the case, isotype of the antibodies would be crucial in their in vivo effectivity. To test this possibility, switch variants producing IgG2b- and IgG2a- ART-18 were obtained. Comparison of the effectivity of the isotypes of the antibodies in l-GVH-R and in cardiac allograft model revealed that the ART-18 IgG isotype is not crucial for their action (15).

3. Reversal by gamma-Interferon (IFN) but not by IL-2 of prolongation of allograft rejection by the anti-IL-2R L-chain mAb ART-18.

To test the hypothesis that the target of ART-18 anti-IL-2R mAb action are the antigen activated T-cells of TH1 subset, it was investigated whether products of TH1 cells may reverse ART-18 action (Figure 4).

TH1+, but not TH2+ cells, produce gamma-IFN and IL-2 (18). Simultaneous administration of gamma-IFN and ART-18 completely abolished the prolongation of allograft rejection by ART-18 (16). IL-2 on the other hand failed to abolish ART-18 action (17). These results suggest

1. the pivotal role of gamma-IFN in allograft rejection,
2. support the hypothesis that the mAb ART-18 selectively act on a IL-2R bearing cell included in the TH1 population and
3. support the view that anti-IL-2R mAb act rather by inactivation (or elimination) of IL-2R+ cells than by inhibition of IL-2 binding to the receptor and subsequent clonal expansion of the antigen activated clone (Figure 5).

Figure 4: Reversal by g-INF of prolongatin of cardiac allograft survival by the anti-IL-2 receptor monoclonal antibody ART-18. Data taken from (16).

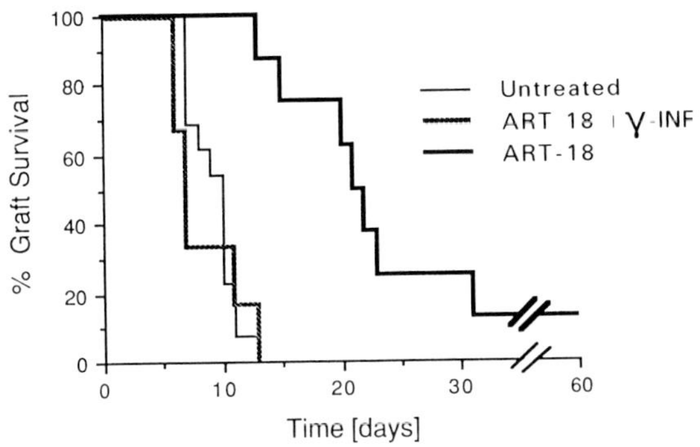

4. <u>Demonstration that ART-18 mAb treatment inactivates transferable CD4+ cells which induce acute allograft rejection and "spares" CD8+ cells with suppressive function.</u>

Rats depleted of T-cells (B-rats) do not reject an allograft. Adoptive transfer of T-cells, derived from allograft recipients, into syngeneic B-rats induce an acute allograft rejection. Using this model, it was previously demonstrated that short term treatment (10 days) of allograft recipients with mAb ART-18 depleted the rats of specific T-lymphocytes capable of inducing acute rejection when adoptively transfered into B-rats (17). On the other hand CD8+ cells derived from the spleen and lymphnodes of allograft recipients treated in an identical fashion, namely injections with ART-18 mAb on ten consecutive days starting at the day of grafting included a cell population that when transfered to a syngeneic naive (Table 1) host specificly prolonged allograft survival (17).

Table 1: Treatment of cardiac allograft recipients with two different monoclonal anti IL-2 receptor antibodies against two distinct epitops of the L-chain "spare" T-lymphocytes of different phenotype with suppressive activities. Data taken from (5)

mAb	Graft survival	Ts sparing	
		CD8+	CD4+
ART-18	21d	+	-
ART-65	16d	+	+++
OX-39	8d	N. D.	N. D.

5. Anti-IL-2R L-chain mAb directed against two distinct epitopes of the receptor ART-18 and ART-65 spare suppressors of the different phenotypes CD8+ and CD4+ respectively.

ART-65 mAb have been shown to recognize an epitope of the rat L-chain of the IL-2R distinct from that which is recognized by ART-18 mAb. When tested in the l-GVH-R (7) or cardiac allograft-model (5), ART-65 mAb were similarly effective as ART-18 though to a lesser degree. It was asked whether ART-65 applied in the same fashion as ART-18 may "spare" specific cells with suppressive function. Splenocyte and lymphnode cells derived from cardiac allograft recipients treated with ART-65, prolonged allograft survival even more effectively than the cells derived from ART-18 treated donors when adoptively transfered to naive syngeneic recipients. However, in contrast to ART-18 treatment (Table 1) predomonantly specific CD4+ cells with suppressor function were generated in ART-65 treated donors (5).

5.1. Why do anti-IL-2R mAb selectively spare phenotypically distinct T-cell subsets?

One of the possibilities currently under investigation is based on the following facts and speculations: The heavy glycosylation of the L-chain of the IL-2R molecule may explain the discrepancy between the molecular weight of the receptor calculated from the amino acid sequence (30 kD) and the actual molecular weight of the isolated receptor (55 kD). Non-random glycosylation of the L-chain of the IL-2R molecule on host lymphocytes may lead to divergent accessibility of T-cell subsets by anti-IL-2R mAb with resultant sparing of distinct T-cell subpopulations. Thus, ART-18 treatment does not affect the majority of CD8+ cells with suppressive function, but inactivates the CD4+ subset including cells with suppressive function. It is also conceivable that ART-18 and ART-65 bind to the epitopes on different L-chains of CD4+ and CD8+ cells; alternative mRNA splicing may occur.

Figure 5: Target cells of the therapy

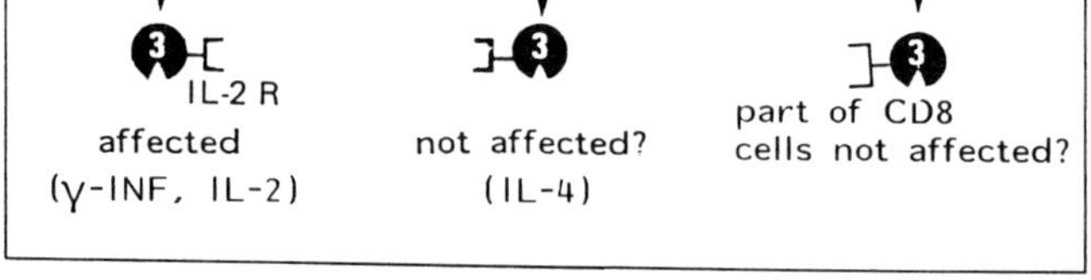

6. Simultaneous short term treatment of allograft recipients with ART-18 and ART-65 results in longterm and even permanent acceptance of the allografts.

As mentioned above, ART-18 and ART-65 mAb treatment of allograft recipients resulted in a "sparing" of two distinct cell types with suppressor functions of CD4+ and of CD8+ phenotype respectively (Table 1). ART-18 and ART-65 administered in combination caused a dramatic synergistic effect (Figure 6).

Figure 6: (LEWxBN) F1 cardiac allograft survival in LEW recipients treated with ART-18 and/or ART-65 anti- IL-2R mAb(s)

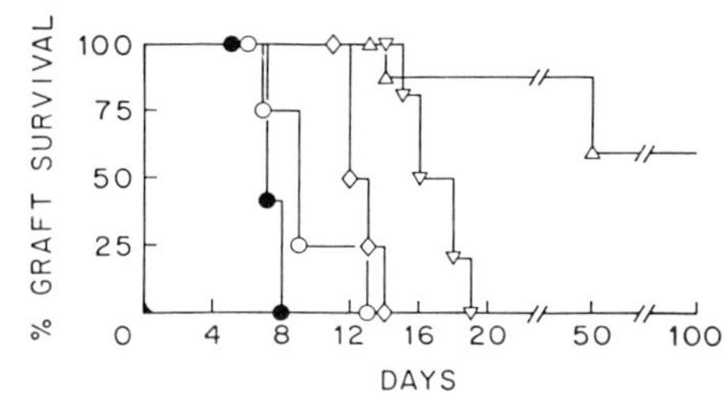

○- ART-65 (treatment for 10 consecutive post-transplant days);
◇- ART-18 (treatment for 10 consecutive post-transplant days);
▽- ART-18 (treatment for the first 5 post-transplant days) + ART-65 (treatment for the second 5 post-transplant days);
△- ART-18 + ART-65 (treatment for 10 consecutive post-transplant days;
●- untreated controls;
Daten taken from (5)

300 µg per day of either ART-18 or ART-65 for ten days prolonged graft survival up to three weeks, injection of both antibodies in much lower doses (25 µg per day for ten days) resulted not only in much longer graft survival, but even in permanent acceptance of more than 60% of the allografts (5).
If one accepts that ART-65 mAb act by sparing CD4+ and the second antibody ART-18 by sparing CD8+ cells with donor specific suppressive function, how can the dramatic synergistic action of the antibodies when administered in combination be explained? One would rather expect that they would effectively eliminate those cells spared by the other. If these donor specific cells play a role in the prevention of rejection, they should rather abolish the therapeutic effect exerted by them when administered alone. The effect could be explained in that the respective antibodies actively induce generations of either CD4+ or CD8+ cells with suppressor functions. However, experimental evidences are yet lacking for this possibility. We have alternatively to ask whether the observed "sparing" of there donor specific CD4+ and CD8+ cells with suppressor function is at all involved in the prevention of graft rejection. These are open questions requireing answers in the near future.

7. Synergistic action of anti-IL-2R L-chain mAb with irradiation

In contrast to recipients of allogeneic heart, kidney, liver and islet cell grafts in various species such as the mouse, rat monkey and man (for review see 3,22), in the mouse and the rat model anti-IL-2R mAb treatment was not successful in recipients of allogeneic skin or whole pancreas grafts. However, mild irradiation (300 r) prior to grafting, followed by a short term anti-IL-2R mAb treatment, prolonged survival of the grafted allogeneic skin in mice (6) and of the allogeneic pancreas in rats (1) significantly.

8. Cyclosporin A (CsA) potentiates the immunosuppressive effect of anti-IL-2R L-chain mAb treatment in allograft rejection.

We previously reported synergistic immunosuppressive effect of anti-IL-2R mAb and a subtherapeutic dose of CsA on 1-GVH-R (22). As recently shown ART-18 mAb treatment prolonged cardiac allograft survival. Combination of a subtherapeutic dose of CsA (1,5mg /kg per day) with an effective dose of ART-18 mAb (300µg/kg per day) for ten days was strikingly synergistic in preventing rejection: one-third of cardiac allografts survived indefinitely, the remainder rejected instead of 22 days at 50 days (3,22). Similar results were obtained through the grafting of allogeneic pancreatic islet cells (9). Pancreatic islets were grafted under the kidney capsule of streptozotocin-diabetic MHC highly incompatible rats. At the time of transplantation the animals were severely hyperglycaemic with depressed pancreatic insulin content. Hyperglycaemia reoccured in the untreated graft recipients within seven days due to rejection of the allogeneic islets. ART-18 mAb treatment alone prolonged graft survival to ca. 40 days while 30% of the recipients permanently accepted the islets. Treatment with ART-18 plus CsA in subtherapeutic doses, resulted in comparable graft prolongation. Once again 30% of the recipients maintained the grafted islets permanently. Only the combined therapy, however, produced normal glucose levels and normal glucose tolerance.
The efficiency of anti-IL-2R mAb therapy in renal allograft recipients was most recently tested in primates (21). Rejection in untreated hosts occurs within 12 days. CsA treatment (2mg per day) did not affected rejection. Anti-IL-2R mAb treatment prolonged graft survival up to 22 days. Treatment with anti-IL-2R mAb in combination with CsA prolonged graft survival and 30% of the recipients did not rejected the allograft. Almost identical results were obtained in rats grafted with allogeneic peripheral nerves (7).

9. Prevention of thyroiditis in neonatal thymectomised Buffalo rats and curing of type 1 diabetis mellitus in BB-rats by IL-2R targeted therapy.

Similar to allografts, mononuclear cells invading the target organ can be observed in experimentally induced as well as in spontaneous developing organ specific autoimmune diseases. Experimental autoimmune thyroiditis (EAT) induced by neonatally-thymectomized Buffalo rats closely resembles Hashimoto's thyroiditis. Study of the evolution of this disease is likely to increase our understanding of the pathogenesis of its human counterpart. The evolution of EAT by immunohistochemical characterisation of the thyroid infiltrate has been examined. The earliest change noted was an increased endothelial MHC class II antigen expression, associated with cellular infiltration of the thyroid at five weeks with macrophages and with equal numbers of CD8+ and CD4+ T-cells. MHC class II positive thyroid follicular cells (TFC) never preceeded the appearance of a lymphocytic infiltration. The numbers of MHC class II positive TFC was maximal (but never exceeded 10% of the total TFC) between 12 and 24 weeks. To further characterise the critical cell populations mediating the disease, depletion studies were carried out. Administration of silica, in order to impair macrophage function, resulted in decreased

thyreoglobuline antibody production, it did not prevent, but did marginally delay onset of the disease. A subtherapeutic dose of CsA (1,5mg/kg for ten days) with ART-18 mAb (1mg/kg for ten days) started at five weeks of age prevented the disease (Figure 7) in all of the treated animals (23). These results indicate that
1. MHC class II antigen positive TFC do not initiate EAT but appear following cellular infiltration of the organ prior to onset of the disease,
2. macrophages are involved in disease perpetuation and
3. disease initiation is dependent upon activated, IL-2R bearing T-cells.

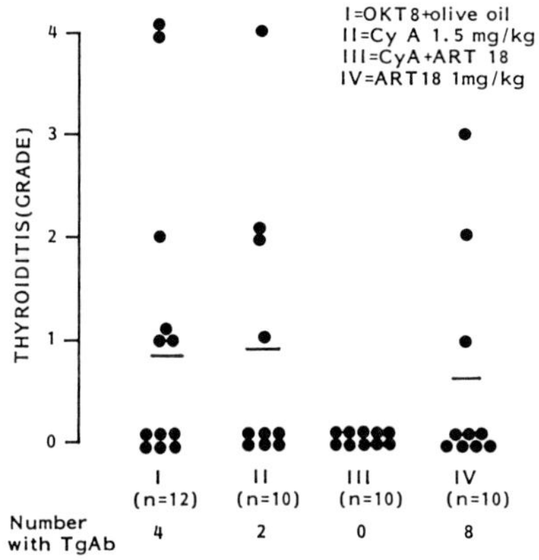

Figure 7: Prevention of experimental autoimmune thyroiditis by IL-2 receptor targeted therapy. Data taken from (23)

Similar to EAT, an intense infiltration of pancreatic islets by mononuclear cells was generally observed in diabetic BB rats, an animal model which develops spontaneously an insulin-dependent diabetes making the BB rat a chose counterpart to human subject with insulin-dependent diabetes. At the onset of the disease, the number of insulin producing ß-cells progrediently decreases. Immunohistological studies reveal that mononuclear cells invading the pancreas are concentrated within the endocrine portion of the tissue consisting of monocytes and T-lymphocytes of CD4+ and CD8+ phenotype. Some of them (less than 10%) bear IL-2R. A few IL-2R positive monocytes as well as some NK-cells were detected.
Since IL-2R targeted therapy, namely combination of a subtherapeutic dose of CsA with anti-Il-2R mAb that prevented allograft rejection and thyroiditis in Buffalo rats, it may be capable as well of not only preventing but also halting already established autoimmune diseases such as type 1 diabetes. In order to test this speculation, BB rats with mild hyperglycaemia as well as reduced ß-cells volume (less than 5% of the controls), and with only marginal insulin production, were treated with a combination of the anti-IL-2R mAb ART-18 and a subtherapeutic dose of CsA for only ten days. This treatment not only stopped the progrediance of the disease but 70% of the treated animals even recovered (10). The recovery was accompanied by an increase in ß-cell volume and in insulin production as well as a decrease of insulitis. A new stable immunological balance was established (10). Neither CsA nor the antibody when administered alone were effective. This was the first observation that IL-2R targeted immunotherapy can cure an organ specific autoimmune disease. Similar successful treatments by IL-2R targeted immunotherapy were reported in the meantime in NOD-mice and in NZB/NZW mice as well (13).

CONCLUSION

IL-2R targeted therapy selectively inhibits T-cell mediated immune response. It could be a potential alternative to the presently used conventional treatment for prevention of allograft rejection. Moreover, such a therapeutic approach may be applied in combating organ specific autoimmune diseases as well. The basis of selectivity of the action of these mAb and their mechanism of action is not yet fully understood and remains to be clarified.

REFERENCES

1. Burkhardt K., Loughnan M.S., Diamantstein T., Mandel T.E. (1988). Transpl. (in press)
2. Diamantstein T., Osawa H. (1986). Imm.Rev. 92 5
3. Diamantstein T., Osawa H., Kirkman R., Shapiro M., Strom T.B., Tilney N.L., Kupiec-Weglinski J.W. (1987). Transpl.Rev. 1 177
4. Diamantstein T., Volk H.-D., Tilney N.L., Kupiec-Weglinski J.W. (1986). Immunobiol. 172 391
5. Di Stefano R., Mouzaki A., Araneda D., Diamantstein T., Tilney, N.L., Kupiec-Weglinski J.W. (1988). J.exp.Med. (in press)
6. Granstein R.D., Goulston C., Gaulton G.N. (1986). J.Immunol. 136 898
7. Grochowicz P., Romaniuk A., Diamantstein T., Olszewski W.L. (1987). Transpl.Proc. 19 1131
8. Gross M., Volk H.-D., Eckert, Diamantstein T. (submitted)
9. Hahn H.J., Kuttler B., Dunger A., Klöting I., Lucke S., Volk H.-D., v.Baehr R., Diamantstein T. (1987). Diabetologia 30 44
10. Hahn H.J., Lucke S., Klöting I., Volk H.-D., v.Baehr R. (1987). Europ.J.Immunol. 17 1075
11. Herrmann T., Diamantstein T. (1987). Immunobiol. 175 145
12. Herrmann T., Diamantstein T. (1988). Europ.J.Immunol. (in press)
13. Kelley V.E., Gaulton G.N., Hattori M., Ikegami H., Eisenbarth G., Strom T.B. (1988) J.Immunol. 140 59
14. Kupiec-Weglinski J.W., Diamantstein T., Tilney N.L., Strom T.B. (1986) Proc.Nat.Acad.Sci. 83 2624
15. Kupiec-Weglinski J.W., Di Stefano R., Stünkel K.G., Grützmann R., Theisen P., Araneda D., Tilney N.L., Diamantstein T. (1988). Transpl.Proc. 20 272
16. Kupiec-Weglinski J.W., Di Stefano R., Stünkel K.G., van der Meide P., Tilney N.L., Diamantstein T. (1988) Transpl. (in press)
17. Kupiec-Weglinski J.W., Padberg W., Uhteg L., Ma L., Lord R., Araneda D., Strom T.B., Diamantstein T., Tilney N.L. (1987). Europ.J.Immunol. 17 313
18. Mossman T.R., Coffman R.L. (1987). Immunology Today 8 223
19. Mouzaki A., Diamantstein T. (1987). Europ.J.Immunol. 17 1661
20. Mouzaki A., Volk H.-D., Osawa H., Diamantstein T. (1987). Europ.J.Immunol. 17 335
21. Shapiro M.E., Kirkman R.L., Reed M.H., Puskas J.D., Mazoujian G. Letvin N.L., Carpenter C.B., Milford E.L., Waltman T.A., Strom T.B., Schlossman S.F. (1987). Transpl.Proc. 19 594
22. Strom T.B., Kelley V.E., Murphy J., Osawa H., Tilney N.L., Shapiro M., Kupiec-Weglinski J.W., Diamantstein T., Gaulton G., Kirkman R. (1987) in: Molecular Basis of Lymphokine Action (eds. DAvid R.Webb, Carl W.Pierce and Stanley Cohen) 371
23. Weetman A.P., Cohen S., Diamantstein T. (1988). J.Endocrinol.117 (Supplement) Abstract 268

Efficacy of Low-dose Cyclophosphamide and Interleukin-2 in Melanoma

MALCOLM S. MITCHELL, RAYMOND A. KEMPF, WILLIAM HAREL, HUNGYI SHAU, WILLIAM D. BOSWELL, SUSAN LIND, GRACE DEAN, JANE MOORE and EDWARD C. BRADLEY

Departments of Medicine, Microbiology, and Radiology, University of Southern California School of Medicine and Comprehensive Cancer Center, Los Angeles, California, and the Cetus Corporation, Emeryville, California

ABSTRACT

We have studied the effects of low-dose recombinant Interleukin-2 (IL-2) preceded by low-dose cyclophosphamide on malignant melanoma. Thirty eight outpatients, with ages ranging from 25-75 years, were treated with IL-2, 3.6 million Cetus units/m^2 i.v., daily for 5 days on 2 successive weeks beginning 3 days after 350 mg/m^2 of i.v. cyclophosphamide. This schedule was repeated at least twice more with a 1-week interval between cycles, usually at the same dosage level. Ten of the 38 patients (26.3%) had a clinically significant remission: 2 complete (5.3%), 7 partial (18.4%), and 1 ongoing, long-term (>18 mo) "minor" response (2.6%). Four others (10.5%) had shorter minor responses and four (10.5%), a mixed response. One patient with disease restricted to the skin had a complete remission, while the other patient with a complete remission had had three lung nodules and an enlarged hilar lymph node. It was gratifying that one of the major sites of disease responding to treatment was the liver. Two complete and 2 partial remissions (i.e., > 50% regressions for > 4 wk at this site) were obtained in 10 patients with liver involvement. Lung metastases also responded, in 4 of 16 patients (1 complete and 3 partial remissions). Subcutaneous nodules responded in 7 of 21 patients (2 complete, 5 partial remissions), while lymph node metastases diminished significantly in 4 of 14 patients (1 complete, 3 partial remissions). The median duration of response was 9 months (range, 1.5-20 months), with 4 patients treated for more than one year. Toxicity was moderate and controllable, and only two patients required hospitalization, both overnight. LAK cell activation was induced in 24 of 38 patients, including all 9 of the major responders. Conversely, none of 14 patients without LAK activation had a significant clinical remission. This regimen appeared to be as effective in melanoma as those involving <u>ex vivo</u> activation of LAK cells, and was more tolerable than therapy with high doses of IL-2.

KEY WORDS

Interleukin-2, Cyclophosphamide, Melanoma, Immunotherapy

INTRODUCTION

Malignant melanoma is a tumor whose incidence is increasing steadily, probably because of its association with intense, intermittent sun exposure among individuals with indoor occupations. Nearly 28,000 new cases will occur in 1988 in the United States (Silverberg and Lubera, 1988). Melanoma is therefore not a rare tumor, and with better awareness of its early signs the primary lesion is becoming more commonly recognized by internists, dentists and ophthalmologists, as well as by the patients themselves. While surgery of primary melanoma can be curative in early stages, the treatment of advanced disease is extremely disappointing. Neither chemotherapy nor radiation therapy is particularly helpful, although there have been continual reports of successful intensive chemotherapy regimens.

The report by Rosenberg and colleagues in 1985 (Rosenberg et al, 1985) of the usefulness of adoptive immunotherapy with lymphokine-activated killer (LAK) cells given together with Interleukin-2 (IL-2), in the treatment of melanoma was met with appropriate enthusiasm. IL-2 was reported by Rosenberg and colleagues to elicit LAK cells from the leukocytes of patients with melanoma when the two were incubated for 4 days in vitro. These LAK cells upon reinfusion into the patient, together with varying doses of additional IL-2 intravenously, were effective in causing 5 of 10 patients with melanoma to have significant regressions of their disease (Rosenberg et al, 1985). The strategy of ex vivo activation was necessitated by that group's findings that IL-2 given by itself was incapable of activating LAK cells sufficiently to cause clinical responses (Lotze et al, 1985). Most recently, however, the same group has reported preliminary success with high doses of IL-2 alone in vivo (Lotze et al, 1986; Rosenberg et al, 1987), although with a response rate of only 13% versus the 22% noted with LAK cell reinfusion. While the regression of a highly resistant tumor such as melanoma was highly gratifying, the toxicity of the regimens that have been described has been substantial even with modifications (West et al, 1987). In particular, elderly patients have been at a significant risk of developing interstitial edema in the lungs, as part of a diffuse capillary leak syndrome, and four deaths have been attributable to the regimen (Rosenberg et al, 1987). The cost and complexity of ex vivo activation of LAK cells are considerable, which militates against broad adoption of the technique even in modern general hospitals. Finally, in vitro incubation of leukocytes with IL-2 for several days requires extensive tissue culture facilities, and carries a risk of hepatitis.

We have investigated whether IL-2 given directly to patients with melanoma could affect the disease. Because IL-2 is known to stimulate all subsets of T cells rather than simply the T-helper and T-cytolytic cells that one might want to activate preferentially, we designed a strategy that might decrease T-suppressor cells before IL-2 was administered. This might permit the proliferation and maturation of the other subclasses unimpeded by suppressor influences. A dose of 350 mg/m^2 of cyclophosphamide was chosen for this purpose because of the work of others (Berd et al, 1984a; Berd et al, 1984b) as well as our own pilot investigations (Hengst JCD, and Mitchell MS, unpublished data) which showed that this drug at doses of 300-500 mg/m^2 selectively depleted suppressor T cells in man. We further designed a schedule of administration of IL-2 that might be given to outpatients, in a day-hospital setting that permitted close observation for 8 hours or more, and which incorporated a week's respite from therapy after each of 3 2-week cycles of treatment.

PATIENTS

Thirty-eight patients with disseminated malignant melanoma have been studied, unselected except by preestablished entry criteria. These included the presence of measurable lesions on physical examination or on X-rays or CT scans of the chest or abdomen, the absence of central nervous system involvement, a Karnofsky performance status of at least 70%, and either resistance to "standard" chemotherapy or a refusal of the patient to undergo such chemotherapy after a discussion with the referring physician. The ages of the patients ranged from 25 to 75, with eight over the age of 50. No one was excluded because of age, except for those under 18 year old. Pregnancy and lactation were also criteria for ineligibility, as were psychological or social impediments to compliance. The diagnosis was always confirmed by our pathologists after review of the original slides. A written consent form was signed by each patient, after a full explanation of the study was given by the physician. All patients to be reported here were treated with at least one full cycle of cyclophosphamide + IL-2, although the critical evaluation of a response to the treatment was performed after 3 complete cycles (1 full course).

Twenty four patients were male and fourteen were female. Sites of disease included subcutaneous and intradermal skin nodules (21 patients), pulmonary metastases (16 patients), lymph nodes (14 patients) liver metastases (10 patients), bone lesions (6 patients), pelvic mass (4 patients), adrenal metastases (4 patients), chest wall mass (1 patient), splenic metastasis (1 patient) and a renal metastasis (1 patient). The majority (26 patients) were untreated with chemotherapy. Twenty two of the 38 had received some form of immunotherapy, including fifteen who were treated with a lysate of melanoma cells and the immunological adjuvant DETOX (detoxified endotoxin and mycobacterial cell wall skeletons (Ribi et al, 1984) in a study to be reported separately (Mitchell MS et al, Cancer Res., in press, 1988). Four of the patients had had no therapy other than surgery. No therapy of any kind was permitted within the 3 weeks prior to the start of the cyclophosphamide + IL-2 regimen, during which time the patient had recovered from any side effects of previous treatment, and the disease was either stable or progressing.

REGIMEN

All treatment was administered in a day-hospital outpatient setting, where prolonged observation was possible without admitting the patient to a ward. Cyclophosphamide was given as an intravenous bolus of 350 mg/m^2 3 days before the start of the IL- 2 treatment, on a Friday morning. Beginning 3 days later, on a Monday morning, IL-2 was given as a 15 minute intravenous infusion. IL-2 was then repeated at the same level on the 2nd through 5th, and 8th through 12th days, with doses omitted on

Saturday and Sunday. The dose of IL-2 during the first 2-week "cycle" was 3.6 million units/ m^2/d. Each patient was observed for 8 h on the first day. By the fifth day the patient was permitted to go home within 1-2 hours if he or she had no serious toxicity, such as hypotension or uncontrollable fever. We found that pretreatment with acetaminophen, 650 mg, repeated every 4 hours as needed, with indomethacin 25 mg if needed, was helpful in limiting the severity of the fever although it did not entirely prevent it. Meperidine, 25 to 50 mg i.v. given once or twice p.r.n., was helpful in controlling the shaking chills that preceded the fever. Indomethacin, 25 mg was also given every 4 hours if needed for severe arthritis or fever, unless gastrointestinal toxicity became intolerable. Medicines specifically excluded were corticosteroids and type 2 antihistamines.

The 2-week cycle of cyclophosphamide + IL-2 was repeated at least twice more to complete a 3-cycle course of therapy. 3.6 million units/m^2 were most often used through all three cycles. The attending physician could, at his discretion, increase the dose to 5.4 million units/m^2 for the 2nd and 7.2 million units/m^2 for the 3rd, if the patient had tolerated earlier treatments without severe toxicity as explicitly defined by World Health Organization criteria, modified by Cetus. However, after the first 20 patients, we rarely increased the dose above the starting level. If patients had at least a minor response (see definitions of response in next section) after 3 2-week cycles, they were eligible for continuation of the treatment. Stable disease or progression after a full course of 3 cycles mandated a discontinuation of therapy. After a complete remission, two or three more cycles of treatment were given, after which treatment was stopped and the unmaintained response was followed. If patients had sustained a partial remission after 3 cycles they were treated with at least 3 more cycles or until either a complete remission or progression occurred. Maintenance therapy, of one cycle of treatment every 6 weeks, was given to those who had a stable partial remission after more intensive treatment. In one instance, a patient with a partial response of lymph nodes, but a minor response of subcutaneous lesions, was kept on this maintenance regimen, and in fact has continued on maintenance beyond 18 months.

Except for the earliest patients, most were given at least a 2-week interval after the first 3 cycles, to provide a respite from the stresses of continual treatment. The oldest patients on study and those treated for many months were often permitted a 4-week interval after each full course of 3 cycles.

CRITERIA OF RESPONSE

Standard criteria were used to judge the response to treatment. Thus, a complete remission was defined as the complete disappearance of all measured lesions for at least 4 weeks, and the failure of new lesions to appear during that time. A partial remission was defined as 50% decrease in the sum of products of the greatest perpendicular dimensions of all measured lesions, lasting for at least 4 weeks, and without the appearance of new lesions. A minor response was at least a 25% but less than a 50% diminution in the sum of the products of the perpendicular diameters of all measured lesions, or a 50% decrease in that sum that lasted less than 4 weeks. A mixed response was >50% shrinkage at one or more sites, e.g., the skin or lymph nodes, but with no change or progression at another, e.g. pelvic mass. Stable disease was no change, or a diminution of less than 25%, in the sum of the products of diameters of measured lesions. Progression was greater than 25% increase in the sum of the products of diameters of all measured lesions. "No response" to therapy, as used here, comprises both stable and progressive disease.

IMMUNOLOGICAL STUDIES

We monitored the immunological effects of our regimen in several different ways. Natural killer (NK) cells and lymphokine-activated killer (LAK) cells were measured twice before, and on the last day of, each 2-week cycle. Off-study immunological measurements were also made 72 h after completion of the final 2-week cycle. Standard assays for these cells were used (Grimm et al, 1982; Timonen et al, 1982; Pross et al, 1981) except that the cells we have termed LAK cells were tested against cultured melanoma cells resistant to NK cells, rather than against fresh tumor cells, as described in the original paper by Grimm et al (Grimm et al, 1982). With this proviso, we will refer to the cells as LAK cells. Besides melanoma, other NK-resistant tumor cells, such as Raji and Daudi B-cell lymphomas and Bachle squamous lung carcinoma cells, as well as allogeneic lymphoblasts, were also tested in randomly chosen patients. The tumor cells, but not the lymphoblasts, were found to be lysed by the cytolytic mononuclear cells, supporting their close similarity, if not identity, with bona fide LAK cells. Various ratios of effector to target cell were tested, ranging from 200:1 to 25:1 for LAK cell assays and from 40:1 to 2.5:1 for NK assays. We calculated the number of "lytic units" of each type of killer cell by best-fit regression analysis, comparing linear, logarithmic, exponential and power curves, with a computer program ("Curvefit") created by Mr. Jeffrey S. Mitchell (Epstein, Mitchell and Blackford, Computer Consultants, New Haven, CT.). The logarithmic and power curves proved most useful in this regard. The results are expressed in "lytic units" per 10 million effector cells, where one lytic unit is number of cells that can kill 30% of the target cells in 4 hours. Fisher's 2-tailed exact test was used to evaluate the statistical significance of differences between groups.

Serial measurements of concanavalin A-inducible suppressor T cells were made in 17 patients (Shou, Schwartz and Good, 1976) immediately before cyclophosphamide and then 3 and 6 days later (i.e., 3 days before IL-2 and then before the first and fourth doses).

RESULTS

Therapeutic Efficacy

Nine of the 38 patients (23.7%) sustained a partial or complete remission, and one (2.6%) has had a long-term, maintained minor remission that has lasted more than 18 months. (Table 1). There were two complete remissions, one in a patient with extensive subcutaneous metastases, and one in patient with 3 lung nodules and an enlarged hilar lymph node. There were also 7 partial remissions. One of the latter included disappearance of all lesions in the liver and skin, and of 2 of 3 lung nodules, with only a residual 1 cm pulmonary nodule. A tenth patient, a 50 year old man had a 50% decrease in the size of a large inguinal lymph node, with a lesser degree of decrease of a large number of intradermal and subcutaneous nodules. His disease, which had been inexorably progressive despite several previous types of treatment, has been entirely stable for more than 18 months on maintenance cyclophosphamide + IL-2 treatment. This long-term response has been highly significantly clinically, even though technically a "minor response".

Table 1
Results of Treatment

Complete Remissions	2	(5.3%)	23.7%	26.3%
Partial Remissions	7	(18.4%)		
Longterm Minor Response	1	(2.6%)		
Minor Responses	4	(10.5%)		
Mixed Responses	4	(10.5%)		
Progression	20	(52.6%)		
Total	38	(100%)		

Minor responses were found in a total of 5 patients (13.1%), including this patient, and mixed responses were noted in another 4 patients (10.5%).

In general, softening or flattening of skin nodules was frequently discernible after the first 2-week cycle, but optimal responses usually required 6 cycles or more.

Table 2 shows the results of treatment by sites of disease. Of most interest to us were the responses of the 5 of 11 patients with metastases to the liver, a site which in melanoma is rarely responsive to systemic treatment. There was a complete remission of 8 large liver metastases in a 42 year old woman and in approximately 12 liver metastases, including one of 5 x 4 cm, in a 45 year old man. Both of those patients also had disappearance of all of their 3-5 small skin nodules. The man had new disease in his bones, which led to discontinuation of his treatment, but has not had reappearance of liver lesions in over 9 months. The woman had 2 of 3 lung nodules disappear as well. Although overall she had only a partial remission by strict criteria, with a residual 1 cm lung nodule, we elected to discontinue her treatment after one year (15 cycles). She remained in unmaintained remission for 8 months, relapsing with brain metastases. There was no recurrence in previously responsive sites outside the central nervous system. Her total dose of IL-2 was 540 million units/m^2, the highest cumulative amount administered in our study. Two other patients had > 50% shrinkage of liver lesions, which persisted for at least 6 months. Their responses lasted nearly a year, before they too died of brain metastases.

Table 2
Results of Treatment by Site

Site of Disease	Number of Patients	Complete Remission	Partial Remission	Duration in months
Liver	10	2	2	CR: 20; 7+ PR: 13; 10;
Lung	16	1	3	CR: 8 PR: 20; 3; 2
Subcutaneous	21	2	6	CR: 20; 1.5 PR: 16; 3; 2; 2: 1; 1
Lymph node	14	1	3	CR: 8 PR: 15; 18+; 2
Bone	6	0	0	
Pelvic, Renal	5	0	0	
Adrenal	4	0	0	

Abbreviations: CR=complete remission; PR=partial remission. Durations of response are given from the date a CR was achieved, or the date therapy was begun for a PR, as per convention.

Seven of 21 patients with subcutaneous nodules responded, with 2 complete and 5 partial remissions. Two responders had long-term remissions lasting more than 18 months, on continual maintenance in one instance, and even upon discontinuation of treatment in another. A third patient was nearing a complete remission but had pernicious anorexia and depression, which forced his removal from the study despite his continuing response. There were also minor responses in 6 patients.

Metastases to the lung were also responsive in 4 of 16 patients, one of whom had a complete remission in that site. He received two further cycles of treatment, and then was observed without treatment, as per protocol. He relapsed with brain metastases after 8 months and died shortly thereafter, but his lung nodules never returned. Among the partial responders was the oldest patient on study, a 75 year old man, who tolerated 6 cycles of treatment.

Lymph node metastases responded in 4 of 14 instances, with one complete and 3 partial responses, and 4 other minor responses. The complete regression was that of a large hilar node in the patient noted above who had a complete remission of lung metastases. Three of the four responses persisted for 8 to more than 18 months, and the fourth response was limited by relapse in the brain which forced temporary discontinuation of treatment.

Unresponsive sites comprised bone, adrenal, renal and pelvic metastases, where none of 13 patients had a response. In fact, three patients developed or had exacerbations of bone pain that forced discontinuation of therapy that had beneficially affected other sites.

The median duration of complete or partial remissions is 9 months, with a mean of >10.1+ months. Four patients have had more than 12 months of remission on continued treatment.

<u>Toxicity</u>

The regimen we have described was generally well tolerated, although it was accompanied by moderate degrees of toxicity (Table 3). Severe side effects were found in 10-15% of 4 categories: fatigue, fever, nausea/vomiting and chills/rigors, and in 0 to 9% in the remaining 9 categories. Only two patients required admission to hospital as a result of the toxicity: both overnight stays either for repletion of fluids or for fatigue. Hypotension to some degree was found in two-thirds of the patients, but was usually mild to moderate. Severe hypotension (Grade III) was found in only 4 patients (10% of the entire group). Episodes of severe hypotension occurred on one occasion during the treatments of 3 patients, all of whom then continued on study at reduced levels of IL-2. An episode of hypotension also occurred early in the treatment of patient #1, who subsequently tolerated a total of 15 cycles, all at 3.6 million units/m^2. The elderly patients had the most difficulty with the regimen, requiring more encouragement to continue than did the others. Only one patient left the study because of a lack of tolerance, but diminution of dose and an increase in the interval between courses of 3 cycles were necessary for two of the oldest patients.

Table 3
Toxicity

Toxic Effect	Number of Patients Experiencing Effect	Number with Grade III Toxicity (% of entire group)	
Fatigue	40	6	(15%)
Fever	39	4	(10%)
Nausea, vomiting	38	5	(12%)
Chills, Rigors	34	3	(7%)
Hypotension	28	4	(10%)
Diarrhea	27	2	(5%)
Allergies, rash	26	1	(2%)
Fluid retention	25	2	(5%)
Dry cough, dyspnea	25	1	(2%)
Arthralgias, arthritis	24	2	(5%)
Myalgia	23	2	(5%)
Catarrhal symptoms	15	0	(0%)
Anemia	12	1	(2%)

Data on 41 patients entered onto the study are shown, including 3 not evaluable for a clinical response. World Health Organization criteria were used except for Hypotension, which was modified as described in the text, and Fluid Retention (weight gain), which was a category specifically added for IL-2 protocols by Cetus.

Shaking chills, fever to a maximum of 103 F (39.4 C), nausea and/or vomiting, and fatigue were nearly universally experienced. Fluid retention, arthralgia/arthritis, myalgia, diarrhea, dry hacking cough and rash were also common. Diuresis often ensued spontaneously over the weekend following 5 days of treatment, and in any event the fluid retention was always responsive to furosemide. The joint symptoms were severe in only one patient, and abated within a few days of cessation of a cycle of treatment. Indomethacin or ibuprofen was helpful in mitigating this symptom, but did not entirely counteract it. One patient with a previous history of rheumatoid arthritis developed an erythematous rash and a true arthritis with her first course of treatment, but on subsequent treatments only arthralgia without overt swelling or rash was noted. A dry hacking cough, responding to cough suppressants, and respiratory symptoms were also found in two-thirds of the group, which suggested an IL-2 induced bronchitis. Eosinophilia (>10% of total leucocytes) was noted in 20 patients, and 23 patients complained of myalgia. Many of the these symptoms were those one might have expected from a lymphokine active in inflammatory processes.

A mild to moderate decrease in hemoglobin was also found in 12 patients, but no significant changes in leukocytes or platelets were noted. The cyclophosphamide caused minor to moderate nausea lasting 1-3 days, in one-half the patients, and frequently caused a flareup in arthralgia. No toxic effects on hair, bone marrow or bladder were found.

Immunological Studies

An increase in LAK cell activity was significantly correlated with a clinical response ($p = 0.014$) (Table 4a). All 9 patients with a partial or complete remission had an LAK activity that was increased to a level of 10 lytic units per 10^7 cells or higher. Conversely, none of the 14 patients who failed to develop an increase in LAK activity had a clinical remission. LAK activity was also increased in 15 nonresponding patients, indicating that the induction of LAK cells was necessary but not sufficient for a remission. However, a failure to show an increase in LAK cells portended a failure to respond clinically.

In contrast, as indicated in Table 4b, NK cell activity was consistently stimulated in all patients and showed no significant correlation with clinical response ($p = 0.46$). An increase in NK activity to some degree above baseline occurred not only in the 9 responders, but also in all 29 nonresponders. Even considering those patients who had a large increase of more than 1,000 lytic units per 10^7 cells there was no significant correlation. Thus, although 7 of 9 responders had an increase of more than 1,000 lytic units per 10^7 cells, 18 of the 29 nonresponders also showed such an increase.

There were no significant preexisting levels of LAK cells measurable in the circulation. After cyclophosphamide and IL-2 those patients who had an increase usually had an incremental increase in the levels of LAK cells with successive cycles, but there was a rapid fall-off within 3 days after the end of a 2-week cycle. This characteristic requirement for the continued presence of IL-2 lent further credence to their being LAK cells rather than another type of cytolytic lymphocyte, such as a cytotoxic T cell. However, 2 patients have been shown to have an elevation of cytotoxic T cells too. One was the woman who sustained a complete remission of her liver metastases and the other was the man with a long-term minor response. The former had a level of LAK cells at the highest level in the study, nearly 5,000 lytic units, after her 15th and final cycle of treatment. Cold target competition assays performed during the last cycle of her treatment, and after the 17th month of treatment of the male patient, revealed the presence of cytolytic lymphocytes that were specifically inhibitable by melanoma cells. These cells, which are CD3 positive and can be blocked by antibodies to CD3, coexisted with LAK cells with a much broader reactivity against tumor cells.

Table 4
Immunological Correlates of Clinical Response

a) Induction of LAK Cell Activity _versus_ Response

	Response[1]	No Response	Total
LAK Increased[2]	9	15	24
LAK not Increased	0	14	14

[1] Comprises complete and partial remissions

[2] >10 lytic units maximal increase during treatment p= 0.014, Fisher's exact test

b) Induction of NK Cell Activity _versus_ Response

	Response[1]	No Response	Total
NK Increased >1,000[2]	7	18	25
NK Increased <1,000[2]	2	11	13

[1] Comprises complete and partial remissions

[2] Maximal increase in lytic units during treatment
p= 0.46, Fisher's exact test

Concanavalin-A-inducible suppressor T cells were not consistently reduced by cyclophosphamide in the 17 patients studied. In 8 of the patients there was a reduction of suppressor T cells 3 days after the cyclophosphamide, but on day 6, 3 days after IL-2 was begun, the suppressor cell activity had returned to its pretreatment level. These results contrasted with previous findings in patients who were given cyclophosphamide alone, where the decrease persisted at least until day 6 after cyclophosphamide (Hengst JCD, and Mitchell MS, unpublished data), and usually until day 28 (Ribi et al, 1984). Unfortunately, we did not have the opportunity to study patients given IL-2 alone, to determine what levels of suppressor activity would have been elicited by IL-2 had cyclophosphamide not been given.

Lack of Influence of Indomethacin or Fever on the Clinical Response

As shown in Table 5, there was no apparent influence either of high fever (temperature elevation to > 101F) or the administration of the prostaglandin antagonist indomethacin on the clinical response to the regimen. It was conceivable that each of those influences might have acted independently to mediate the effects of the regimen. In particular, antagonism of prostaglandin synthetase might have affected suppressor macrophage function and thus augmented the immunological stimulatory effects of IL-2. However, we could not find statistical evidence here that those patients who received indomethacin for high fevers or arthalgias fared differently from those who did not.

Table 5
Indomethacin or Fever >101F versus Response

Response	Indomethacin	Fever
CR	2/2	2/2
PR	5/6	6/6
Minor	4/5	5/5
None	11/17	15/17

Indomethacin: CR + PR vs Minor + None $p= 0.28$, by Fisher's exact test; $p= 0.28$ by trend analysis.

Fever: CR + PR vs Minor + None $p= >0.20$, by Fisher's exact test.

DISCUSSION

This investigation has shown that a regimen of low-dose cyclophosphamide and low-dose IL-2 was effective in the treatment of advanced melanoma, including not only subcutaneous and lymph node metastases but also more ominous sites of involvement such as the liver and the lung. The treatment was given in an outpatient setting and was generally tolerable even by elderly patients, although there were undeniably significant side effects and toxicity, particularly cumulative fatigue and arthralgias. However, most patients were able to go home within an hour after the IL-2 infusion was given. LAK cells were elicited in the circulation of these patients by the in vivo therapy.

The response of melanoma to chemotherapy is at most 20% in large series, and there is no discernible increase in the patient's survival. The regimen we have reported of low-dose cyclophosphamide and low-dose IL-2 appears to have a response rate of approximately 25% that is at least equivalent to that found in the expanded trials of IL-2 and LAK cells at the N.C.I. (Rosenberg et al, 1987) and at university centers (Parkinson D, personal communication) (19%). Our rate of remission in melanoma exceeds published rates with high-dose IL-2 given without LAK cells (Lotze et al, 1986) (13%). The duration of response to cyclophosphamide + IL-2 was also encouraging, with a median of 9 months. In particular, the long-term responses of 5 patients, 4 of them treated for at least a year, are particularly gratifying. It is worth emphasizing that that patients could be treated repeatedly with cyclophosphamide + IL-2, to attempt to improve the degree of response or to maintain stability of the disease at less than 50% of its original volume.

Various sites of disease appear to be differentially sensitive to the effects of IL-2, with subcutaneous, lymph node and pulmonary metastases most responsive in several series (Rosenberg et al, 1985; West et al, 1987). The striking response of large liver lesions in 4 patients was unique in our experience with systemically administered therapy. Two patients with liver involvement responded with complete resolution of substantial sized lesions, while durable partial remissions were achieved in 2 others. In contrast, bone disease and adrenal lesions may prove to be most resistant to this form of treatment, judging not only from the lack of responses in these sites, but also from three patients in whom persistent bone pain caused us to stop treatment that had caused regression of disease at other sites, in order to administer pain-reducing radiation therapy. Even within the same patient, we have found one site to be resistant to treatment while another was responding. In fact, our first patient on study had one lung nodule persisting relatively unchanged months after 2 other lung nodules, skin and liver lesions had all disappeared. It was also not uncommon to find several subcutaneous lesions regressing while while others were unchanged. The reasons for this sort of divergent response are not at all obvious, but the phenomenon has also been observed by others with IL-2-containing regimens (West et al, 1987).

The major cause of death in our most successfully treated patients---those who had a complete or partial remission for more than 6 months---was progression in the brain or spinal cord, with a large single metastatic lesion in the brain being the most common presentation. Regardless of its systemic effectiveness, cyclophosphamide + IL-2 cannot prevent or effectively treat lesions of the central nervous system. We are now attempting to devise a means of prophylaxis for the central nervous system in patients with a complete or stable partial remission, but the problem is not easily soluble. High-dose chemotherapy, with autologous bone marrow replacement, is a measure with potential efficacy, but has not yet been tested prophylactically in melanoma.

An improvement in survival cannot be claimed for the entire group, but it is clear that the survival of all but two of the patients with a complete or partial remission was prolonged. In addition, the patient with a long-term, maintained minor response has certainly exceeded expectations for his survival. It was possible to treat 1 patient intensively for a year, and to maintain responses with one 2-week cycle every 6 weeks for 10-18+ months in 4 other patients.

Among our 10 significant responders were 4 who had received our regimen of active specific immunotherapy (Mitchell MS, et al, Cancer Res., in press, 1988) previously, but the other 6 had never received that therapy. Nevertheless, it will be interesting to combine these two potentially complementary types of treatment particularly since cytolytic T cells are generated by active immunotherapy, and are amplified by interleukin-2, as we demonstrated in two of our patients.

Since LAK cells were elicited solely by <u>in vivo</u> administration of cyclophosphamide and IL-2, there seems little need, at least in melanoma, for <u>ex vivo</u> incubation of peripheral blood leukocytes with IL-2. Whether this will be true for other diseases such as renal cell carcinoma and breast cancer, which appear to be sensitive to IL-2 and LAK cells, remains to be determined. In any event, a relatively low dose of IL-2 has allowed us to treat even elderly patients could be treated without medical difficulties of significant proportions, although often at reduced dose levels. However, we should emphasize the necessity for strong psychological supportive care from nurses, physicians and relatives to encourage all patients complete the prescribed courses of treatment.

It remains to be proved that cyclophosphamide as we have administered it, in single low doses 3 days before each 2 week cycle, accounted for our therapeutic success with intravenously administered IL-2 in the absence of adoptive immunotherapy. Whether our hypothesis for the mechanism by which cyclophosphamide exerted its influence, via the inhibition of suppressor T cells, is correct also requires further study. Our assay for (concanavalin A-induced) suppressor T cells showed no significant change in their activity at 3 and 6 days after cyclophosphamide. Whether IL-2 alone would have stimulated even higher levels of suppressor cell activity in the absence of cyclophosphamide is uncertain.

LAK cells are easily measured, and may serve as convenient criteria for an immunological effect of IL-2, but one should not ascribe the in vivo rejection of human tumors uniquely to their activity. Cytolytic and helper T cells, macrophages, and perhaps B lymphocytes may all play important roles. IL-2, which can directly or indirectly influence all of those cells, may cause beneficial responses through effects on several types of cell at once. Nevertheless, LAK cell activation correlated well with a clinical response to therapy, and appeared to be the most important parameter to monitor as a prognostic indicator. Nearly thirty eight percent (9/24) of the patients who had a rise in LAK cell activity of at least 10 lytic units per 10^7 mononuclear cells had a remission. More importantly for prognosis, none of the 14 patients who failed to have a rise in LAK cells in response to IL-2 achieved a useful clinical remission.

Ultimately IL-2 will undoubtedly be used as an important part of a combination regimen involving not only other cytokines, but other types of biomodulators and probably chemotherapy as well. There is little doubt that several regimens involving IL-2, including the one we have described, are very useful now in the treatment of melanoma, heretofore a highly resistant form of cancer.

ADDENDUM

Just after this manuscript was completed, final data became available on the last patient on study. That patient, I.H., a 57 year old woman who had received no systemic therapy previously, had a 60% regression of disease in her right adrenal gland, the first patient to respond at that site. In addition, there was a 70% shrinkage of a pulmonary nodule and complete disappearance of breast and ear lobe masses, with only a presternal nodule remaining at 24% of its previous size, all as measured by the products of perpendicular diameters. Unfortunately, she had transient amaurosis in one eye nearly from the outset, and despite receiving only 1.8 million units/m^2 of IL-2 during cycles 2 and 3, she had continuing attacks. The toxicity forced us to abandon therapy after only 2 months. Repeat measurements at all sites performed 4 weeks after completion of treatment confirmed that a partial remission had in fact occurred.

Thus, the final figures in our study are as follows:

Complete remissions:	2	(5.1%)
Partial remission:	8	(20.5%)
Long-term "minor" response:	1	(2.6%)
Minor responses:	4	(10.3%)
Mixed responses:	4	(10.3%)
No response:	20	(51.2%)
Total:	39	(100%)

Supported by a contract from the Cetus Corporation, USPHS grant R01 CA-36233, a grant from the Concern Foundation, and gifts from Mr. Alan Gleitsman, the Morey and Claudia Mirkin Foundation, and the Lenihan Trust.

Address reprint requests to Malcolm S. Mitchell, M.D., University of Southern California Comprehensive Cancer Center, 2025 Zonal Avenue, Los Angeles, CA 90033.

REFERENCES

Silverberg, E and Lubera, J. (1988). CA- A Cancer Journal for Clinicians 1988, 38: 5-22.

Rosenberg, S.A., Lotze, M.T., Muul, L.M. et al. (1985). N. Engl. J. Med. 313, 1485-1492.

Lotze, M.T., Matory, Y.L., Ettinghausen, S.E., et al. (1985). J. Immunol. 135, 1865-1875.

Lotze, M.T., Chang, A.E., Seipp, C.A., Simpson, C., Vetto, J.T., and Rosenberg, S.A. (1986). JAMA 256, 3117-3124.

Rosenberg, S.A., Lotze, M.T., Muul, L.M. et al. (1987). New Engl. J. Med. 316, 889-897.

West, W.H., Tauer, K.W., Yannelli, J.R. et al. (1987). New Engl. J. Med. 316, 898-905.

Berd, D., Maguire, H.C., Jr. and Mastrangelo, M.J. (1984a). Cancer Res. 44, 1275-1280.

Berd, D., Maguire, H.C., Jr., Mastrangelo, M.J. (1984b). Cancer Res. 44, 5439-5443.

Ribi, E., Cantrell, J.L., Takayama, K., Qureshi, N., Peterson, J., and Ribi, H.O. (1984). Revs. Infect. Dis. 6, 567-572.

Grimm, E., Mazumder, A., Zhang, H.Z. et al. (1982). J. Exp. Med 155, 1823-1841.

Timonen, T., Reynolds, C.W., Ortaldo, J., and Herberman, R.B. (1982). J. Immunol. Meth. 51, 269-277.

Pross, H.F., Baines, M.G., Rubin, P., Shragge, P. and Patterson, M.S. (1981). J. Clin. Immunol. 1, 51-63.

Shou, L., Schwartz, S.A., Good, R.A. (1976). J. Exp. Med. 143, 1100-1110.

Anti-idiotype Modeled Peptides with Biologic Activity

W. V. WILLIAMS, D. A. MOSS, D. B. WEINER, J. A. COHEN, H. R. GUY, and M. I. GREENE

The Department of Pathology and Laboratory Medicine, and the Department of Neurology, University of Pennsylvania, Philadelphia, Pennsylvania 19104, USA; and the Laboratory of Mathematical Biology, National Cancer Institute, National Institute of Health, Bethesda, Maryland 20892, USA

ABSTRACT

We have developed synthetic peptides modeled after the hypervariable region of an anti-idiotypic/anti-receptor antibody. These peptides exhibit biologic properties identical to those of the antibody, including inhibition of DNA synthesis.

KEYWORDS

Synthetic Peptides: Anti-idiotypes: Reovirus: Receptors: Sequence Similarity

INTRODUCTION

Many biologically active substances derive their activity from their ability to interact with specific receptors. We have been studying the interaction of reovirus type 3 with its receptor(s). Reovirus type 3 inhibits DNA synthesis and proliferation of a variety of cell types (Sharpe and Fields, 1983; Fontana and Weiner, 1980). This effect is not due to infection of the host cells, as replication defective/ultraviolet inactivated reovirus type 3 particles also have this effect (Hand and Tamm, 1973). This points to receptor perturbation as the likely mechanism by which this effect is achieved.

The Reovirus Hemagglutinin

Reovirus particles interact with specific cellular receptors by means of the viral hemagglutinin (HA) (Lee, Hayes and Joklik, 1981). This protein is also responsible for determining the tissue tropism of viral infection (Fields and Greene, 1982; Weiner et al, 1977). Reovirus type 1 and type 3 bind to different receptors and display distinct patterns of tissue tropism. These properties are a function of the viral HA (Epstein et al, 1984). We have been studying the reovirus type 3 HA (or HA 3) utilizing an anti-idiotype approach (Nepom et al, 1983; Co et al, 1985), Polyclonal and monoclonal anti-idiotypic antibodies that bear the internal image of the reovirus type 3 cell attachment site have been developed (Nepom et al, 1982; Noseworthy et al, 1983). These have been utilized to characterize the reovirus type 3 receptor (Reo 3R) on a variety of cell lines (Co et al, 1985).

The Reovirus Type 3 Receptor
The Reo 3R has been demonstrated to be a 65 Kd polypeptide with a pI of 5.8-6.0 (Co et al, 1985). This protein shares many characteristics with beta-adrenegic receptors, (Co et al, 1985) and is likely to be a member of the same family of membrane bound receptors. These receptors generally transduce signals across membranes by interacting with GTP-binding (G) proteins which act as second messengers following receptor perturbation. Following this interaction, the G proteins interact with catalytic subunits (such as adenylate cyclase) leading to their activation (Gilman, 1984). Reovirus type 3 is likely to induce some of its effects on host cell metabolism by this mechanism.

Effects of Reo 3R Perturbation
Reo 3R perturbation, by reovirus type 3 or anti-Reo 3R antibodies, has been demonstrated to inhibit DNA synthesis in a variety of Reo 3R bearing cells. This includes B104 (rat neuroblastoma), L cells (murine fibroblast); and murine lymphocytes (Gaulton and Greene, submitted). This effect is dependent on receptor aggregation, as monomeric Fab fragments of anti-Reo 3R antibodies have no effect. If these Fab fragments are multimerized, inhibition of DNA synthesis is again produced (Gaulton and Greene). The essential role of receptor aggregation in this system is consistent with the multimeric form of the HA3 presented by intact virions (Joklik, 1983).

Development of Peptides
A monoclonal anti-Reo 3R antibody was developed that mimicked the reovirus HA3 (Noseworthy et al, 1983). This antibody (87.92.6) had anti-idiotypic reactivity with a neutralizing anti-reovirus HA3 antibody. 87.92.6 also competed with the HA3 for binding to specific cellular receptors (Kauffman et al, 1983). 87.92.6 inhibits DNA synthesis of Reo 3R-bearing cells. (Gaulton and Greene).

The amino acid sequences of the 87.92.6 light chain and heavy chain variable regions (V_L and V_H respectively) have been deduced (Bruck et al, 1986). Comparison of these sequences with the HA3 sequence Bassel-Duby et al, 1985), revealed amino acid sequence similarity between residues 317-332 of the HA3, and a combined determinant comprised of the V_H and V_L second complementarity determining regions (CDR IIs). The V_L CDR II in particular had striking amino acid sequence similarity with the HA3 determinant. This led as to postulate that this site comprised the receptor interaction site of the virus. To further investigate this, synthetic peptides corresponding to these sequences were utilized.

MATERIALS AND METHODS

Peptides Synthetic peptides were developed by solid-phase methods. V_L peptide dimers were coupled utilizing an added amino terminal cysteine residue as described (Williams et al, in press.). Peptides were sterilized by irradiation (10,000 rads and dissolved in RPMl medium (Gibco, Grand Island Biologicals), lmg/ml, prior to use.

Cells Murine L cells were grown adherent in (DMEM) 10% Fetal Bovine Serum (FBS) with added pen/strep. and L-glutamine (all from Gibco). Murine Rl.l cells were grown in RPMl with 10% FBS, pen/strep., L-glutamine and HEPES buffer (all from Gibco).

Reovirus Binding Inhibition
5×10^4 murine L cells were resuspended in 50 ul of 1% bovine serum albumin in phosphate buffered saline with 0.1% sodium azide (binding buffer). Peptides were added in an equal volume of distilled water for 30 minutes. Radioiodinated reovirus particles (lHA3 indicating the reovirus type 3 hemmagglutinin with all other genome segments derived from reovirus type 1 were added for an additional 30 minutes. The cells were washed 3 times and counts per minute (CPM) bound were determined. Percentage of inhibition of binding was determined by the

formula:

$$100 \times [1 - \frac{\text{specific CPM bound w/o inhibitor-specific CPM bound w inhibitor}}{\text{specific CPM bound w/o inhibitor}}]$$

Proliferation assay L cells were removed with trypsin/versene (the Cell Center, University of Pennsylvania, Philadelphia, PA), centrifuged and resuspended at 2×10^5/ml in DMEM 10% FBS. 50 ul were dispensed in the wells of 96 well flat bottom microtiter plates (Costar, Cambridge, MA). Following overnight incubation in 5% CO2, peptides were added dissolved in RPM1, 50 ul per well. The cells were incubated for 24 hours. Tritiated thymidine (1u Ci per well) was added for an additional 4-6 hours, and CPM incorporated was determined as noted above.

Percent inhibition of DNA synthesis by peptides was determined by the formula:

$$[1 - \frac{\text{(CPM without peptide) - (CPM with peptide)}}{\text{(CPM without peptide)}}] \times 100$$

RESULTS

The peptides utilized in this study were:
V_L: (C) K P G K T N K L L I Y S G S T L Q
Control: (C) N E S H V P D H D V T E E R D E
V_L peptide corresponds to the V_L CDR II of 87.92.6 (Bruck et al, 1986).

Specific interaction of peptide with the reovirus receptor
V_L peptide specifically interacts with the reovirus type 3 receptor. This can be demonstrated by its ability to inhibit binding of reovirus particles to specific receptors on murine L cells. We have demonstrated that V_L peptide inhibits the binding of reovirus type 3, but not reovirus type 1 to these cells (Williams et al, in press.). This is consistent with the observations of others indicating that these serotypes utilize distinct receptors on these cells (Epstein et al, 1984). This binding specificity is determined by the HA. Thus reassortant viron 1 HA 3 (with the type 3 HA on a type 1 background) utilizes the same receptor as reovirus type 3. V_L peptide is able to inhibit 1.HA 3 binding to L cells.

Modeling of the Receptor Interaction Site
These data indicate that this site on the 87.92.6 antibody is responsible for direct interaction with the reovirus type 3 receptor. We reasoned that this site may have conformational similarity with other known hypervariable regions. Since V_L peptide corresponds to the second complementarity determining region (CDR II) of 87.92.6, we sought other CDR II's, with known structure, that shared sequence similarity with V_L peptide. The CDR II of REI (a human light chain dimer) was quite similar:

	CDR II Sequence
87.92.6	K P G K T N K L L I Y S G S T L Q
REI	T P G K A P K L L I Y E A S N L Q

We used the known REI structure to model the 87.92.6 V_L CDR II. This model is shown in Figure 2.

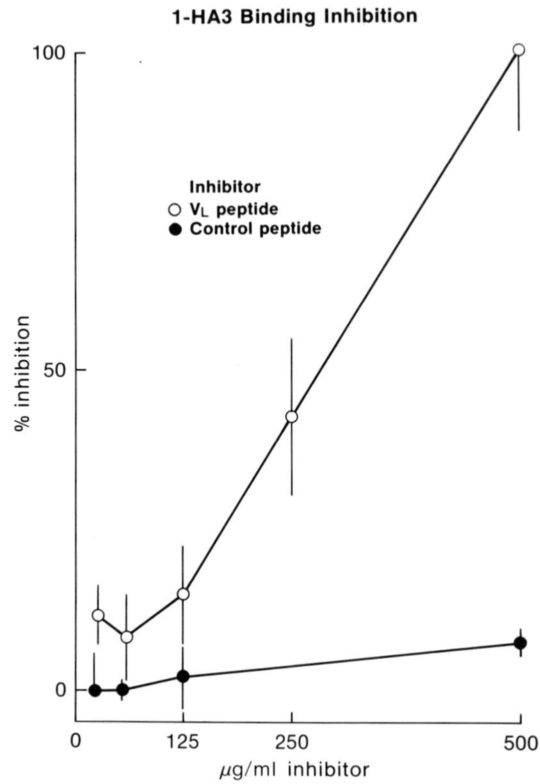

Figure 1
Specific interaction of V_L peptide with the reovirus type 3 receptor. Murine L cells were incubated with peptides, and inhibition of binding of radioactivated reovirus type 1.HA3 was determined. Percent inhibition of binding (indicating specific interaction with the reovirus type receptor) is shown versus the concentration of peptide added.

A

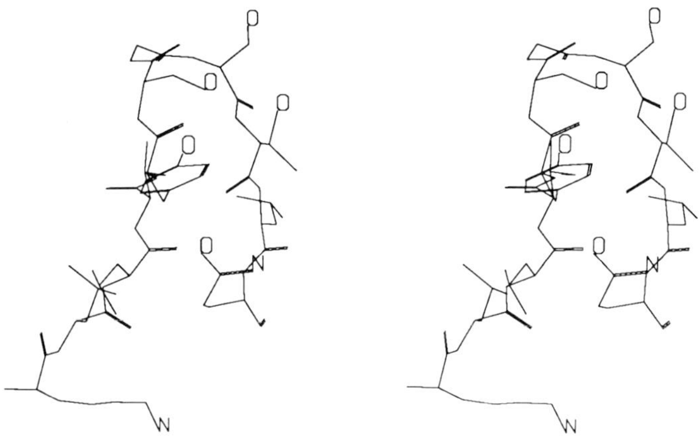

Figure 2
Stereo View of the 87.92.6 V_L CDR II modeled after the REI CDR II.

We feel that this is a useful model of this site that can be utilized to explore the role of particular residues involved in these interactions.

Peptide Inhibition of DNA synthesis
We utilized a dimeric form of this peptide to study its effects on DNA synthesis on several cell lines. As is noted in Figure 3, V_L peptide dimers markedly inhibited DNA synthesis by murine L cells.

In other studies, we have shown that this effect is dependent on dimerization of the peptide. (Williams et al, submitted). V_L peptide monomers (lacking any cysteine residues) is incapable of inhibiting this response (Williams et al, submitted.).

V_L peptide also inhibits DNA synthesis by a murine thymoma cell line (Figure 4), as well as lymphocytes in response to Con A (Williams, et al, submitted.).

These results indicate that the V_L peptide accurately reproduces the effects of both 87.92.6 (the antibody from which it was derived), and the reovirus HA3 (which is mimicked by 87.92.6). In other studies, we have demonstrated that V_L peptide specifically competes with reovirus type 3 for binding to L cells (Williams et al, in press. This indicates a specific interaction of this peptide with the Reo 3R expression on murine thymoma cells, again indicating a specific interaction. This approach of utilizing peptides modeled from antibody hypervariable loops may be useful in studying a number of receptor-ligand interactions, and in developing novel biologically active substances.

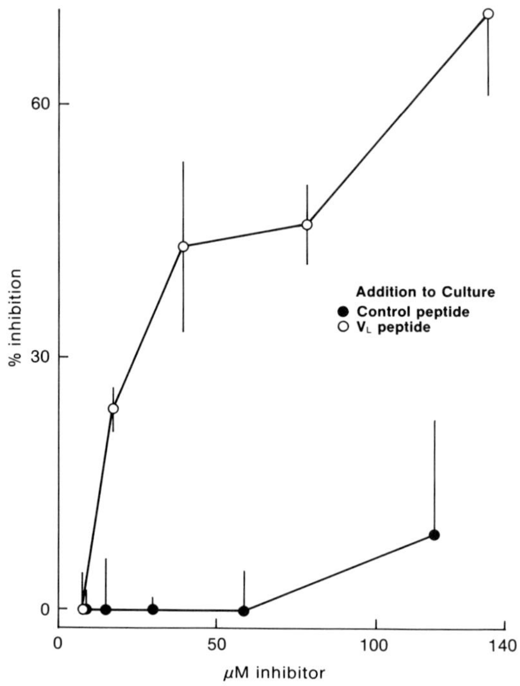

Figure 3
Inhibition of DNA synthesis by L cells. L cells were treated with peptides, as noted, for 24 hours. The DNA synthetic response was then determined. Inhibition of DNA synthesis is shown versus the concentration of peptide inhibitor. Mean +/- S. D. of triplicate wells is shown.

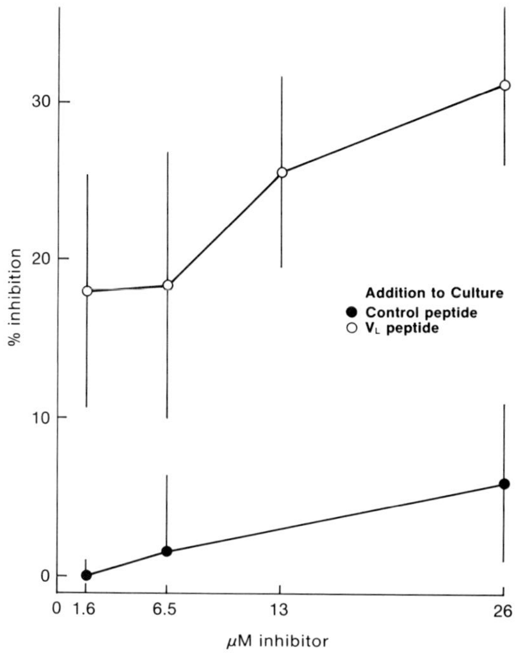

Figure 4
Peptide inhibition of murine thymoma (Rl.1) cells. Rl.1 cells were incubated with various doses of peptides. Following a 24 hour culture, the DNA synthetic response was determined. Inhibition of DNA synthesis is shown versus the concentration of peptide used. Mean +/- S. D. of triplicate wells is shown.

Conclusion

A peptide modeled after the hypervariable region of a biologically active monoclonal anti-idiotypic antibody has been demonstrated to reproduce the effects of the antibody. In addition, this peptide specifically interacted with the receptor bound by the antibody. Utilization of peptides modeled after hypervariable regions of antibodies may lead to the development of novel biologically active substances.

Acknowledgements
We would like to thank Frank Robey for supplying some of the peptides, and Glen Gaulton for his critical review.

REFERENCES

Bassel-Duby, R., Jayasuriya, A., Chatterjee, D., Sonenberg, N., Maizel, J. V., Jr., and Fields, B. N. (1985). Nature 315, 421-423.

Bruck, C., Co, M. S., Slaoui, M., Gaulton, G. N., Smith, T., Fields, B. N., Mullins, J. I., and Greene, M. I. (1986). Proc. Natl. Acad. Sci. USA 83, 6578-6582.

Co, M. S., Gaulton, G. N., Fields, B. N., and Greene, M. I. (1985). Proc. Natl. Acad. Sci. USA 82, 1494-1498.

Co, M. S., Gaulton, G. N., Tominaga, A., Homcy, C. J., Fields, B. N. and Greene, M. I. (1985). Proc. Natl. Acad. Sci. USA 82, 5315-5318.

Epstein, R. L., Powers, M. L. Rogart, R. B., and Weiner, H. L. (1984). Virology 133, 46-55.

Fields, B. N., Greene, M. I. (1982). Nature 200, (London), 19-23.

Fontana, A., Weiner, H. L., J. Immunol. 125, 2660 (1980).

Gaulton, G. N., Greene, M. I., Inhibition of cellular DNA synthesis by reovirus occurs through a receptor-linked signalling pathway which is mimicked by anti-receptor antibody. (Submitted).

Gilman, A. G., (1984). Cell 36, 577-579.

Hand, R., Tamm, I., J. Virol. 11, 223 (1973).

Joklik, W. K. (1983). In the Reoviridae. W. K. Joklik, Ed. New York: Plenum Press) 9-78.

Kauffman, R. S., Noseworthy, J. H., Nepom, J. T., Finberg, R., Fields, B. N., and Greene, M. I. (1983). J. Immunol. 131, 2539-2541.

Lee, P. W. K., Hayes, E. C., and Joklik, W. K. (1981). Virology 108, 156-163.

Nepom, J. T., Weiner, H. L., Dichter, M. A., Tardieu, M., Spriggs, D. R., Gramm, C. F., Powers, M. L., Fields, B. N., and Greene, M. I. (1982). J. Exp. Med. 155, 155-167.

Noseworthy, J. H., Fields, B. N., Dichter, M. A., Sobotka, C., Pizer, E., Perry, L. L., Nepom, J. T., and Greene, M. I. (1983). J. Immunol. 131, 2533-2538.

Sharpe, A. H., Fields, B. N., J. Virol. 38, 389 (1983).

Weiner, H. L., Drayna, D., Averill, D. R., Jr., and Fields, B. N. (1977). Proc. Natl. Acad. Sci. USA 74, 5744-5748.

Williams, W. V., Guy, H. R., Rubin, D. H., Robey, F., Myers, J. N., Kieber-Emmons, T., Weiner, D. B., and Greene, M. I. Sequence of the cell attachment site of reovirus type 3 and modeling of its three-dimensional structure. Proc. Natl. Sci. USA 74, (in press).

Williams, W. V., Moss, D. A., Cohen, J. A., Myers, J. N., Weiner, D. B., and Greene, M. I. A peptide derived from the hypervariable region of a biologically active anti-receptor antibody reproduces the biological activity of the antibody. (Submitted).

Pharmacokinetics and Organ Targeting of Monoclonal Antibodies

K. FUJIMORI and J. N. WEINSTEIN

Theoretical Immunology Section, Laboratory of Mathematical Biology, DCBD, National Cancer Institute, Bldg 10 Rm 4B-56, Bethesda, Maryland 20892, U.S.A.

ABSTRACT

In order to understand the pharmacology of monoclonal antibodies, one must consider both the global pharmacokinetics and the microscopic aspects of antibody distribution. Here we summarize calculations that identify global and local parameters affecting entry of antibody into the center of a microscopic tumor nodule. These calculations will be presented *in extenso* elsewhere.

KEYWORDS

Monoclonal antibody: diffusion: convection: pharmacokinetics: cancer.

INTRODUCTION

Both clinical and pre-clinical studies over the last several years have indicated that tumors accumulate monoclonal antibodies heterogeneously after intravenous administration. Part of that heterogeneity can be explained on the basis of uneven distribution of antigen among tumor cells and among regions of a tumor (Schlom *et al.*, 1983). Another part probably relates to nonuniform access from the bloodstream. To study the access question, we have developed a set of mathematical models that splice together global pharmacokinetics with data on microscopic processes — transcapillary passage, percolation through tumor substance, binding, cellular metabolism. The early stages of that modeling effort have been described elsewhere (Weinstein et al., 1986, 1987a, 1987b).

There are two general regimes in which the ability of antibody to percolate through tumors may become rate limiting to its effective distribution: (i) at an early stage of tumor growth, in which the nodule (or *in vitro* tumor cell spheroid) is non-vascularized and less than 1 or 2 mm in diameter; (ii) at a later stage, when the tumor has developed its own vascular supply and then has begun to outstrip it. For simplicity, we will focus on the first of those situations and will consider the tumor as a simple, uniform sphere of cells through which antibody must diffuse toward the center. The question is how uniform the concentration will be as a function of time and as a function of various parameters of the system. Elsewhere, we will describe more complex cases in which the tumor is non-uniform, in which convection dominates the transport properties (Swabb *et al.*, 1974), and in which the geometry is non-spherical — for example, in the case of tumor cords surrounding a central vessel. The problem becomes still more complex in the case of tumors large enough to develop major internal hydrostatic pressure gradients. That circumstance has been analyzed cogently by Jain (1987).

Whatever the specific geometry may be, a central issue is what we have called the "binding site barrier" — the prediction, based on quite robust calculations, being that bindable immunoglobulin will be retarded in its diffusion (or convection) through tumor by the very fact of its successful localization. The nonuniformity of distribution will tend to be exacerbated by a low diffusion coefficient, by a high density of antigenic sites, and by high affinity of the binding. For illustrative purposes we will focus here on the effect of antigen density on the distribution of IgG in a hypothetical tumor spheroid of diameter 0.6 mm (600 μm). This is about as large as such a spheroid can become before poor supply of oxygen and nutrients begins to damage cells at the center. Calculations were performed by a collocation method using computer programs and standard sets of parameter values described elsewhere (Fujimori *et al.*, 1988). Diffusion of antibody through spheroids has been analyzed mathematically by McFadden and Kwok (1988) for the special case of non-saturating, irreversible binding.

Figure 1*A* shows the radial distribution of a relatively high-affinity antibody (assumed to have $K_D = 10^{-9}$M) at a high antigen density of 10^{-6}M with respect to interstitial space. The effective diffusion coefficient is taken as 1.0×10^{-8} cm^2/sec. The antibody concentration at the outer edge of the "tumor nodule" is assumed to be in equilibrium with plasma levels after a bolus dose of 50 mg in the standard 70 kg man (Eger *et al.*, 1987). Figure 1*B* shows equivalent results for an antigen density of 10^{-7}M. Clearly, the distribution is more uniform at any given time point. Figure 1C shows the same for an antigen density of zero (*i.e.*, the case of an irrelevant immunoglobulin). The distribution to the center of the "tumor" is essentially uniform after the first several hours.

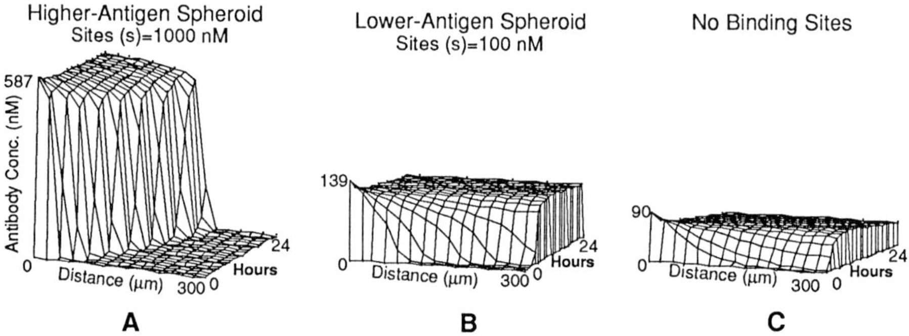

Fig 1. Calculated distribution of monoclonal IgG in a microscopic "tumor nodule" as a function of the concentration of binding sites. See text for explanation of the calculation and parameter values used. (A) High binding site density (10^{-6}M with respect to interstitial space); (*B*) Lower binding site density (10^{-7}M); (C) No binding sites (*i.e.*, the case of irrelevant IgG). The distribution clearly becomes more uniform as the binding site concentration decreases.

This small calculation serves to make a larger point: that binding sites can effectively prevent uniform distribution of antibody, and, as a consequence, that microscopic parameters related to that binding — for example, the density of binding sites — may significantly influence the efficacy of therapy with antibodies. If the aim of a therapeutic method is to reach all tumor cells individually, the binding site problem may be an important limitation; if the aim is to destroy tumor blood vessels, the process may be accelerated by avid, highly localized binding.

These calculations must be considered as predictions from a mathematically abstract situation. However, over the last few years, as stated earlier, a number of studies have demonstrated at least qualitatively the nonuniformity of percolation (Meeker, *et al.*, 1985; Abrams and Oldham, 1985; Jones, *et al.*, 1986; Sutherland, *et al.*, 1987). We will take up these issues again in more detail elsewhere.

We are grateful to Dr. David G. Covell and Dr. John E. Fletcher for their efforts in development of the computer packages used for these calculations.

REFERENCES

Abrams, P.G. and Oldham, R.K. (1985). In: Monoclonal Antibody Therapy of Human Cancer: (eds. K.A. Foon and A.C. Morgan Jr) Martinus Nijhoff. 103-120.

Eger, R.R., Covell, D.G., Carrasquillo, J.A., Abrams, P.G., Foon, K.A., Reynolds, J.C., Schroff, R.W., Morgan, A.C., Larson, S.M., and Weinstein, J.N. (1987) Cancer Res. *47*, 3328-3336.

Fujimori, K, Covell, D.G., Fletcher, J.E., and Weinstein, J.N. (In preparation)

Jain, R.K. (1987). Cancer Res. *47*, 3039-3051.

Jones, P.L., Gallagher, B.M., and Sands, H. (1986). Cancer Immunol. Immunother. *22*, 139-143.

McFadden, R. and Kwok, C.S. (1988). Cancer Res. *48*, 4032-4037.

Meeker, T.C., Lowder, J., Maloney, D.G., Miller, R.A., Thielemans, K., Warnke, R, and Levy, R. (1985). Blood *65*, 1349-1363.

Schlom, J., Colcher, D., Hand, P.H., *et al.* (1983) In: Understanding Breast Cancer: Clinical and Laboratory Concepts: (eds. M. Rich, J. Hager, and P. Furmanski) Marcel Dekker, Inc. 315-358.

Sutherland, R., Buchegger, F., Schreyer, M., Vacca, A., and Mach, J-P. (1987). Cancer Res. *47*, 1627-1633.

Swabb, E.A., Wei, J., and Gullino, P.M. (1974) Cancer Res. *34*, 2814-2822.

Weinstein, J.N., Black, C.D.V., Barbet J., Eger, R.R., Parker, R.J., Holton, O.D., III., Mulshine, J.L., Keenan, A.M., Larson, S.M., Carrasquillo, J.A., Sieber, S.M., and Covell, D.G.(1986). In: Site-Specific Drug Delivery: (eds. E. Tomlinson and S.S. Davis) John Wiley & Sons. 81-91.

Weinstein, J.N., Covell, D.G., Barbet, J., Eger, R.R., Holton, O.D. III, Talley, M.J., Parker, R.J. and Black, C.D.V. (1987a). In: Membrane Mediated Toxicity: (eds B. Bonavida and R.J. Collier) Alan R. Liss. 279-289.

Weinstein, J.N., Eger, R.R., Covell, D.G., Black, C.D.V., Mulshine, J., Carrasquillo, J.A., Larson, S.M., and Keenan, A.M. (1987b). Ann. NY Acad. Sci. *507*, 199-210.

Recent Advances in Vaccine Development

Modulation of the Immunogenic Characters of Protective Epitopes in Synthetic Vaccines

F. AUDIBERT, C. JOLIVET-REYNAUD, M. JOLIVET, and D. LISE

University of South Florida, College of Medicine, Department of Pharmacology & Therapeutics, H. Lee Moffitt Cancer Center and Research Institute, P.O. Box 280179, Tampa, Florida 33682–0179

ABSTRACT

Protective antigenic determinants can be mimicked by chemical synthesis. To become part of efficient vaccines B and T epitopes must be inserted in appropriate structures so as to elicit a strong, long lasting protective immune response. To achieve this goal synthetic peptides can be either linked to a carrier or, preferably associated within totally synthetic constructions. Adjuvants such as synthetic muramyl dipeptides can afford tools not only to enhance the level of the immune response but also to modulate its characters. These points will be illustrated using synthetic malarial vaccine models and a totally synthetic polyvalent vaccine containing B and T epitopes. Finally, a model of prevention against experimental allergic encephalomyelitis will be discussed to illustrate how the immunogenic characters of a synthetic antigen can be modulated by association with adjuvants or by suitable coupling.

KEYWORDS

Muramyl dipeptides, malarial vaccines, B and T epitopes, polyvalent synthetic vaccines, Experimental allergic encephalomyelitis prevention.

INTRODUCTION

During the last decades, the incidence of infectious diseases has decreased dramatically. Conventional vaccines have played a most important role in this event and it can be guessed that the new vaccines which are being produced will offer extra tools for a better control of viral, bacterial and parasitic infections. A series of reasons can explain the need for new vaccines: appearance of infectious agents resistant to antibiotics (viruses, bacteria) or drugs (parasites), faster spreading of epidemics and also increasing cost of sickness for the communities. Besides these reasons the emergence of AIDS has emphasized the relevance of prevention for public health. In many cases highly desirable vaccines can not be prepared using conventional approaches of purification of the protective antigen(s) since the infectious agents either can not be cultured in vitro or only under costly and/or hazardous conditions.

Two approaches for mimmicking natural protective antigenic structures currently deserve the most attention: genetic engineering and chemical synthesis.

The utilization of organic chemistry to produce vaccines implies that peptides of less than 40 and more often less than 30 amino acids constitute the key portions of the preparation which has to induce a relevant protective response. Indeed a vaccine has to evoke as early as possible a long lasting state of immunity. This response can consist in antibodies of an appropriate isotype or in cell mediated responses. Also crucial is the establishment of a strong immunological memory capable of being recalled by the natural structure if an infectious attack occurs.

These requirements have been fulfilled when successful current conventional vaccines were concerned. As shown in Figure 1 a natural vaccine contains different entities: a) antigenic determinants or epitopes, b) a structure which plays the role of carrier, indeed the word carrier covers three functions: a function of transport to vehicle the vaccine to the immune system, a function of matrix supporting the epitopes and finally the capacity of triggering T helper cells and T memory cells, c) An immunoadjuvant moiety (for example LPS or peptidoglycan). Besides these active components, conventional vaccines comprise also useless and sometimes harmful structures. Thus the aim in designing synthetic substitutes is double: 1) to obtain vaccinating preparations when conventional approaches are not workable 2) to avoid potential risks inherent to ill-defined materials.

Fig. 1

FROM CONVENTIONAL TO SYNTHETIC VACCINES.

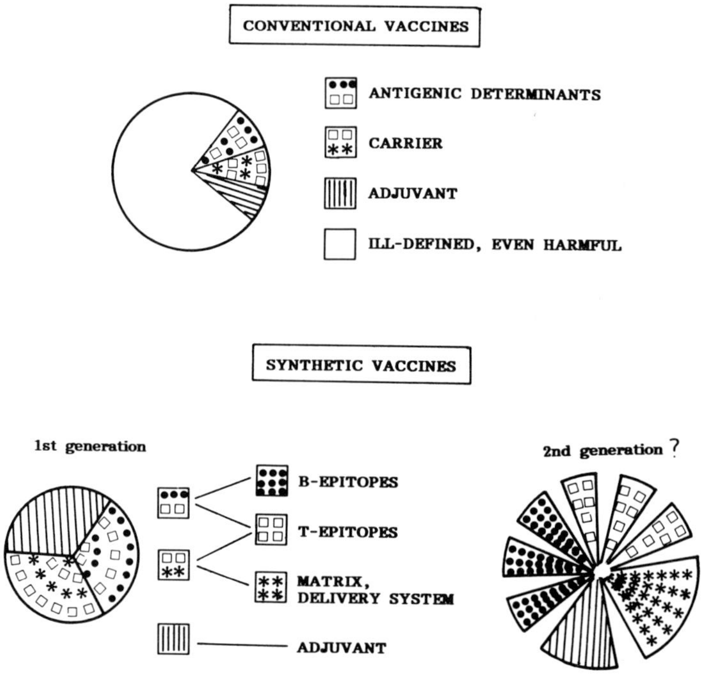

In the first studies involving synthetic antigenic determinants, attention had been mainly focused on the definition of B epitopes capable of evoking protective antibodies and several computer models have been proposed to analyze the structures most likely to represent such relevant B epitopes. The importance of T epitopes has emerged more recently. Indeed cell-mediated responses play an important role in specific immunity and as mentioned, the establishment of an appropriate immunological memory is also highly desirable. In the first generation of synthetic vaccines (Figure 1) the role of carrier had been devoted to highly immunogenic exogenous natural molecules. The use of such carriers has several limitations, such as the risk of inducing hypersensitivity reactions or of evoking epitopic suppression (Herzenberg, Tokuhisa and Herzenberg, 1980; Schutze et al, 1985) it implies also that the T helper and memory cells involved in the response do not share with B cells the specificity of the infectious agent.

Thus it seems reasonable to split the notion of carrier and to consider at first the choice of T epitopes of the appropriate specificity as has been described in several models (Cease et al, 1987; Good et al, 1987; Margalit et al, 1987; Milich et al, 1987) and then to determine how to present suitably B epitopes, T epitopes and (as seen below) adjuvant molecules to the immunocompetent cell populations. This is schematically represented in the last part of Figure 1 which indicates that the different elements to be associated in a synthetic vaccine have received better definition but also that their method of association has yet to be designed. The fulfillment of this requirement represents one of two of the main issues to be addressed in view of obtaining the second generation of synthetic vaccines.

The second issue consists in the search for adjuvants. Synthetic peptides are small and mimmicks only partially natural structures thus they are poorly immunogenic. This same problem of lack of immunogenicity exists also for most of the recombinant immunogens. The only adjuvant currently used in clinics, aluminum hydroxide is not devoid of side effects and can not induce cell mediated immunity. For these reasons other approaches have to be explored which could afford promising candidates as clinical adjuvants. Ideally adjuvants can be expected not only to amplify an immune response but to enhance preferentially the response to certain epitopes or to modify their antigenic characters. They have also the capacity of influencing the isotypes of the antibodies synthetized and of favoring either the humoral or the cell mediated responses. The adjuvants studied in this report will be muramyl dipeptides which are analogs of Nac-Mur-L-Ala-D-isoGln or MDP (Ellouz et al, 1974; Kotani et al, 1975). MDP is a synthetic glycopeptide which represents the smallest subunit of the bacterial cell walls capable of substituting for mycobacteria in Freund's complete adjuvant (FCA). The immunopharmacological activities of MDP and of its analogs have been already extensively described (Audibert, Leclerc and Chedid, 1985; Warren, Vogel and Chedid, 1986). One of the analogs murabutide is currently in clinical trials (Telzak et al, 1986).

Three models utilizing synthetic peptides as immunogens will be considered to exemplify how the lecture of the different epitopes by the immune system can be modified by appropriate covalent linkage of the peptides and by the use of adjuvants.

SYNTHETIC ANTI-MALARIA VACCINES

Circumsporozoite proteins from the different species of Plasmodium have been found to contain repetitive sequences which represent most generally immunodominant structures. A synthetic peptide, PK26: Tyr-(Gln-Ala-Gln-Gly-Asp-Gly-Ala-Arg-Gly-Gln-Pro)$_2$-Cys copying such a structure of *Plasmodium knowlesi* circumsporozoite protein (Godson et al, 1983, Schlesinger et al, 1984) has been conjugated to tetanus toxoid. When murabutide in saline was administered with the conjugate it enhanced preferentially the synthesis of biologically active antibodies (Clough et al, 1985) as shown by their capacity of inducing a positive circumsporozoite precipitation reaction. In contrast, although the conjugate elicited higher titers of binding antibodies when given in FCA, these antibodies were shown to display a lower neutralizing activity. The same peptide and an amphiphilic derivative of murabutide were covalently linked to the same carrier. Under these conditions the immune response to the peptide was greatly enhanced while the response to the carrier was decreased (Clough et al, 1985). Similar results showing that MDPs can modulate the relationships of dominance between epitopes have been reported also in a totally synthetic model using (Tyr-Glu) repeats linked to a multi-L-Ala-poly-L-Lys backbone (T,G-A--L) with or without MDP-Lys (Abehsira-Amar et al, 1987).

Fig 2

IMMUNOGENIC PROPERTIES OF $(NANP)_8$ HOMOPOLYMERIZED OR CONJUGATED TO TETANUS TOXOID AFTER ADMINISTRATION TO DIFFERENT STRAINS OF MICE.

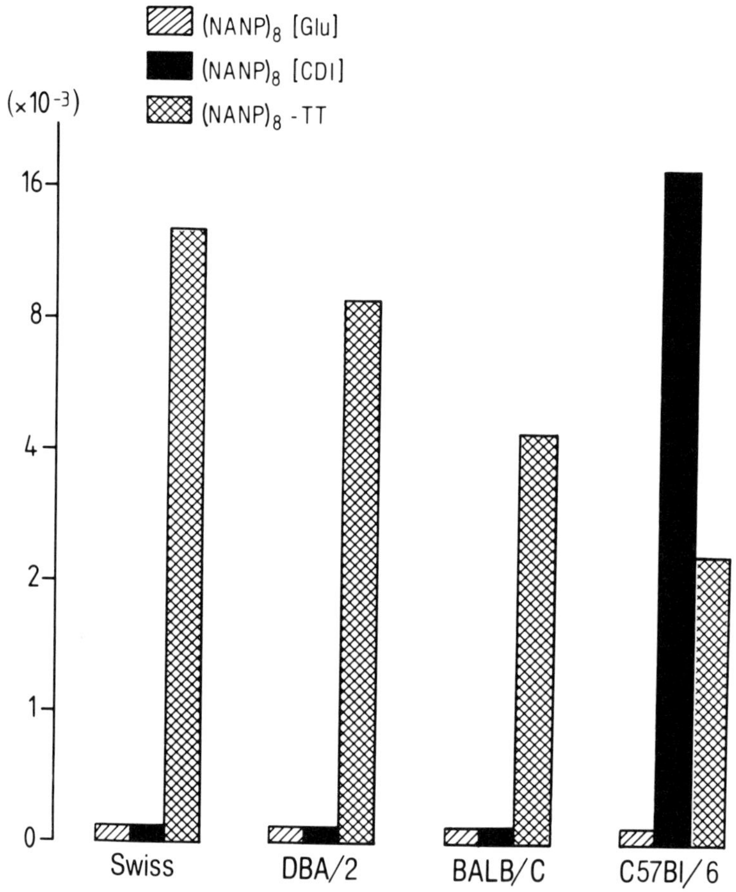

Another Plasmodium peptide has been used in the following studies. Arg-Ala-Arg-Pro (NANP) is repeated 37 times along the structure of Pl. falciparum circumsporozoite protein and represents its immunodominant motive (Dame et al, 1984). Using a $(NANP)_8$ peptide we have observed that the immunogenic characters of a synthetic antigen can be modified according to the method of construction used to prepare a synthetic vaccine. These results are reported on Figure 2.

We have compared the response to $(NANP)_8$ either conjugated to tetanus toxoid or homopolymerized using carbodiimide $(NANP)_8$ [CDI] or glutaraldehyde $(NANP)_8$ [GLU]. The three preparations (100 ug) have been administered subcutaneously in FCA to Swiss, DBA/2, BALB/c or C57Bl/6 mice. After one month animals were boosted by the different immunogens in absence of adjuvant. Results show that if the T epitopes belong to a carrier (such as tetanus toxoid) which is not submitted to a genetic control antibodies against the NANP hapten can be obtained in Swiss mice as well as in the three inbred strains of mice. In contrast, only the good responder mice to NANP, C57Bl/6, haplotype H-2b (Del Giudice et al, 1986) made antibodies in response to the construct obtained by using carbodiimide and no response was observed against the glutaraldehyde polymer. These results indicate that $(NANP)_8$ contains at least a B epitope and a T helper epitope which is available on the carbodiimide construct but has been masked when glutaraldehyde has been used as polymerizing agent. They emphasized also the critical importance of a potential genetic restriction when peptides are being inserted in a synthetic vaccinating preparation.

POLYVALENT SYNTHETIC VACCINE.

In the previous example we have seen that a totally synthetic homopolymer can evoke antibodies under appropriate conditions of polymerization and genetic control. In the following example another totally synthetic vaccine has been built by associating in the same molecular structure four peptides of different specificities (Figure 3).

Fig. 3.

SEQUENCE OF THE PEPTIDES CONTAINED IN THE POLYVALENT VACCINE.

S34 = ASN -PHE- SER- THR- ALA- ASP- SER- ALA- LYS- THR- LEU- GLU- ALA- GLU- LYS- ALA- LEU- ALA- -ALA -ARG -LYS -ALA -ASP -LEU -GLU -LYS -ALA -LEU -GLU -GLY -ALA

HBS(99-121) =
ASP- THR- GLN- GLY- MET- LEU- ILE- PRO- GLY- SER- SER- THR- THR- SER- THR- GLY- PRO- CYS

D(AA-186-201) =
ALA- ALA- CYS- ALA- GLY- ASN- ARG- VAL- ARG- ARG- SER- VAL- GLY- SER- SER- LEU- LYS- CYS

PK26 =
TYR (GLN- ALA- GLN- GLY- ASP- GLY- ALA- ARG- GLY- GLN- PRO) $_2$ CYS

S34 represents a repetitive structure of the M protein of Streptococcus Pyogenes strain 24 (Beachey et al, 1981); Hbs (99-121) belongs to the S antigen of the Hepatitis B virus (Tiollais, Charnay and Vyas, 1981; Audibert et al, 1981a); D(A-A-186-201) is the N terminal loop sequence of the diphtheria toxin, two Ala have been added to its N terminal end (Audibert et al 1981 b). PK 26 copies a repetitive structure of the circumsporozoite protein of Pl. knowlesi, one Tyr has been added to its N terminal end and one Cys to its C terminal end (Godson et al, 1983; Schlesinger et al, 1984).

We have previously shown that mice or guinea pigs immunized with this heterocopolymer either with FCA or with murabutide in saline develop high titers of biologically active antibodies against all four specificities (Jolivet et al, 1987). The immune response of guinea pigs has been further studied to determine if one or several peptides contained at least a T epitope. Results are summarized on Table 1.

Table 1.

SPECIFICITY OF THE ANTIBODY AND T CELL PROLIFERATIVE RESPONSES INDUCED BY A SYNTHETIC POLYVALENT VACCINE.

Antigenic Specificity	Antibodies binding the parental natural structure	T cell proliferation against the peptide
S-34	++++ *	--
Hbs (99-121)	++++	++++
D (AA-86-201)	++++ *	--
PK 26	++++ *	--
Polyvalent conjugate	Not tested	++++

* These antibodies have been shown to be endowed with biological activity.

Only one peptide, HBS (98-121) was capable of inducing the proliferation of T cells present in the lymph nodes of hyperimmunized animals and thus played the role of carrier for the different B epitopes involved. This T epitope was shown to be available in the polyvalent construct. In this model, peptides from different microorganisms have been associated and it demonstrates the feasibility of a totally synthetic polyvalent vaccine containing functional B and T epitopes. Indeed different peptides could be copies of amino acid sequences from the same parental structure or structures belonging to one given virus, bacteria or parasite. Thus an appropriate choice of peptides and of methods of coupling should lead to an efficient synthetic vaccine devoid of the limitations linked to the use of an exogenous carrier.

EXPERIMENTAL ALLERGIC ENCEPHALOMYELITIS (EAE).

EAE (Paterson, 1966) can be induced in guinea pigs by the administration in FCA of BP, myelin basic protein (Freund, Stern and Pisanti, 1947; Morgan, 1947; Kabat, Wolf and Berzer, 1947) or of a synthetic peptide copying a fragment of BP residues 114-122 (Westall et al, 1971; Hashim and Sharpe, 1975). This model is considered as relevant to study the multiple sclerosis disease, MS (Lassman, 1983; Paterson, Day and Whitacre, 1981; Sabin, 1974). In EAE, the clinical signs appear after 2 to 3 weeks, they are loss of weight, paralysis of the hind footpads, weakness and death. At first it is not obvious that EAE fits into a report on synthetic vaccines. Nevertheless it can be argued that the model described here is a perfect example of efficacy for an association peptide-adjuvant. Moreover the sickness can be prevented by achieving an appropriate immunization against a synthetic peptide.

1-EAE INDUCTION.

It has been reported by Nagai et al, 1978) that the nonapeptide (representing the encephalitogenic structure of BP) when administered even with low dosages of MDP in a water in oil emulsion can induce the sickness even better than in FCA. Indeed although the nine amino acids are necessary to induce the sickness when FCA is used, an heptapeptide lacking the two first amino acids is encephalitogenic after administration in Freund's Incomplete Adjuvant (FIA) containing MDP. These two peptides are depicted on Figure 4. The hexapeptide lacking Trp was never shown to be active.

Fig. 4.

SYNTHETIC ENCEPHALITOGENIC NONAPEPTIDE, HEPTAPEPTIDE AND HEXAPEPTIDE COPYING SEQUENCES OF THE HUMAN BASIC PROTEIN.

NONAPEPTIDE	PHE-SER-TRP-GLY-ALA-GLU-GLY-GLN-LYS
HEPTAPEPTIDE	TRP-GLY-ALA-GLU-GLY-GLN-LYS
HEXAPEPTIDE	GLY-ALA-GLU-GLY-GLN-LYS

Furthermore, we have shown that some MDP derivatives are even more active than MDP to serve as an adjuvant in this model. We have also observed that derivatives which are the most powerful for inducing a delayed type hypersensitivity are equally very efficient to induce the sickness. Results summarized in following Table 2 show for example that MDP-L-Ala-glyceryl-mycolate (MDP-L-Ala-Glyc-Myc) was very active.
In separate experiments we have shown that this compound increased highly the cell mediated response (Parant et al, 1980).

Table 2.

INDUCTION OF EAE BY SYNTHETIC NONAPEPTIDE AND HEPTAPEPTIDE USING MDP OR ANALOGS IN FIA.

Immunogen (10 ug)	Adjuvant			
	FCA	MDP	MDP-L-Ala-Glyc-Myc	MDP (decyl methyl)
BP	+	+	++	--
Nonapeptide	+	+	++	--
Heptapeptide	-	+	++	--
Hexapeptide	-	-	--	--

Animals treated with the nonapeptide as well as with the heptapeptide died in less than 10 days. In contrast MDP (decyl) methyl which is only adjuvant active vis a vis the humoral immunity was shown to be inefficient.

2-EAE PREVENTION.

Several attempts have been already reported to prevent the disease by inducing a state of suppression in animals.

It has been shown that if BP is administered in (FIA) no clinical signs are observed and moreover animals are protected against a further challenge by BP or by the nonapeptide in FCA (Alvord et al, 1965; Einstein et al, 1968; Lebar and Voisin, 1974). These results have been reproduced as shown on Table 3.

Table 3.

DISEASE PREVENTION BY PRETREATMENT WITH BP

Pretreatment	Challenge	EAE Induction
BP + FIA	BP + FCA	0
BP + FIA	Nonapeptide + FCA	0
-	BP + FCA	+++
-	Nonapeptide + FCA	+++

In the experiments reported here, we have used the synthetic nonapeptide to build an "anti EAE synthetic vaccine". The peptide had been conjugated through its terminal carboxyl to tetanus toxoid (TT) using carbodiimide. The conjugate (100 ug) has been administered in FCA to guinea pigs. Animals did not develop any signs of sickness. After two weeks half of the animals have been sacrificed their lymph node cells harvested and tested in a specific proliferation assay. Results are shown on Table 4.

Table 4.

LYMPHOCYTE PROLIFERATIVE RESPONSE TO THE NONAPEPTIDE OF LYMPH NODE CELLS OF GUINEA PIGS TREATED WITH THE NONAPEPTIDE - TT CONJUGATE IN FCA

Animal Treatment	Proliferative response to the Nonapeptide	
	10 ug	100 ug
Nonapeptide (100 ug)	3.2	2.3
Nonapeptide-TT (100 ug)	1.0	1.0

Guinea pigs were immunized by the footpad route. 10^6 cells were used, the proliferation index has been calculated as cpm in the assay/cpm in controls nontreated by the antigen.

It can be seen that administered free the peptide can sensitize T cells which proliferate upon stimulation. In contrast after coupling it does not induce the same response. The second half of the animals of the group treated with the conjugate and animals treated with the carrier alone in FCA were challenged with BP (100ug) in FCA one month after the pretreatment. Not one of the nine animals treated with the conjugate developed any EAE, in contrast animals treated with TT develop a severe sickness.

The humoral response to BP and to the nonapeptide free or conjugated to TT was also tested after administration in FCA (Table 5). It was observed that the 114-122 structure when inserted in the parental structure can not induce a measurable amount of anti-nonapeptide antibodies.

Nevertheless it has been shown above that BP administered in FIA can produce a suppressive response against a further challenge by the free peptide given with FCA. It was observed also that this free nonapeptide which is encephalitogenic and induce a T cell proliferative response cannot evoke a humoral response. In contrast the peptide conjugated to TT induced antibodies and prevented the establishment of EAE after further challenge by BP in FCA.

Table 5.

HUMORAL RESPONSE TO BP, NONAPEPTIDE AND NONAPEPTIDE-TT ADMINISTERED IN FREUND'S COMPLETE ADJUVANT (FCA).

Immunization	Anti-BP Antibodies*	Anti-Nonapeptide Antibodies*
BP (100 ug)	404,396	<100
N (50 ug)	<100	<100
N-TT (100 ug)	ND	57,300

BP, nonapeptide and nonapeptide-TT were injected into the foot pads.
*ELISA titers of sera pooled on day 21.

These results show that when conjugated to TT the immunogenic characters of the nonapeptide have been totally modified. It lost its encephalitogenic properties and did not induce a cell mediated response. In contrast it induced a humoral response and protected against a further challenge by an encephalitogenic stimulus. Further experiments which will be reported separately have demonstrated in strain 13 guinea pigs that suppressive T cells have been sensitized by the nonapeptide-TT conjugate.

CONCLUDING REMARKS.

In these experiments we have shown that totally synthetic constructs endowed with vaccinating properties can be prepared. We have seen also that the coupling of the peptides and the use of adjuvants can modify deeply the immunogenic characters of the different epitopes. Thus a better understanding of the relationships between the efficacy of potential vaccinating preparations and their molecular structure is necessary to design the future candidate vaccines.

REFERENCES

Abehsira-Amar, O., Uzan, M., Audibert, F., Jolivet, M., Theze, J. and Chedid, L.A. (1987) Molec. Immunol. 24 945-951.

Alvord, E.C., Deshaw, C.M., Hruby, S. and Kils, M.W. (1965) Ann N.Y. Acad. Sci. N.Y. 122., 333-345.

Audibert, F.M., Przewlocki, G., Leclerc, L.D., Jolivet, M.E., Gras Masse, H.S., Tartar, A.L. and Chedid, L.A. (1981a) Infect. Immun. 45, 261-266.

Audibert, F.M., Jolivet, M., Chedid, L., Alouf, J.E., Boquet, P., Rivaille, P. and Siffert, O. (1981b) Nature (London) 31, 88-99.

Audibert, F., Leclerc C. and Chedid L.A. (1985). In Biological Response Modifiers P.F. Torrence ed. Academic Press Inc., Orlando. 307-327.

Beachey, E.H., Seyer, J.M., Dale, J.B., Simpson, W.A., and Kang, H.A. (1981) Nature (London) 289, 457-459.

Cease, K.B., Margalit, H., Cornette, J.L., Putney, S.D., Robey, W.G., Ouyangi, C., Streicher, H.Z., Fischinger, P.J., Gallo, R.C., Delisi, C. and Berzofsky, J.A. (1987). Proc. Natl. Acad. Sci. USA 84, 4249 - 4252.
Clough, E.R., Jolivet, M.E., Audibert, F.M., Barnwell, J.W., Schlesinger, D.H., Arnon, R., and Chedid, L.A. (1985a) Infect. Immun .48, 839-892.
Clough, E.R., Jolivet, M.E., Audibert, F.M., Barnwell, J.W., Schlesinger D.H. and Chedid L.A. (1985b). Biochem. Biophys. Res. Com. 131, 70-76.
Dame, J.B., Williams, T.L., McCutchan, T.F., Weber, T.L., Wirtz, R.A., Hockmeyer, W.T., Maloy, W.L., Haynes, T.D., Schneider, I., Roberts, D., Sanders, G.S., Reddy, E.P., Diggs, G.L. and Miller, L.H. (1984). Science 225, 593-599.
Del Giudice, L., Cooper, G., Merino, J.A., Verdini, A.S., Pessi, A., Togna, R., Enders, H.D., Gorradin G. and Lambert, P.H. (1986) J. Immunol. 137, 2952-2995
Einstein, E.R., Sejtey, J., Davis, W.T. and Rauch, H.C. (1968) Immunochem. 5, 567-575.
Ellouz, F., Adam, A. Ciorbaru, R. and Lederer, E., (1974) Biochem. Biophys. Res. Commun., 1317-1325
Freund, J., Stern, E.R. and Pisanti, T.M. (1947) J. Immunol 57, 179-194.
Godson, G.N., Ellis, J., Schlesinger D.H. and V. Nussenzweig (1983) Nature London 305, 29-31.
Good, M.F., Malloy, W.L., Lundl, M.L. Margalite, H., Cornette, J.L., Smith, G.L., Moss, B., Miller, L.H. and Berzofsky, J.A. (1987) Science 235, 1059 - 1064.
Jolivet, M., Audibert, F., Gras-Masse, H. Tartar, A., Schlesinger, D.H., Wirtz, R. and Chedid, L.A. (1987) Infect. Immun. 55, 1498 -1502.
Hashim, G.A. and Sharpe, R.O. (1975) Naturel (London) 255, 484-485.
Herzenberg, L.A., Tokuhisa, T. and Herzenberg, L.A. (1980). Nature (London) 285,664-666.
Kabat, E.A., Wolf A. and Berzer A.I. (1947) J. Exp. Med. 855, 117-129.
Kotani, S., Watanabe, Y. Shimono, T., Narita, T., Kato, K., Stewart-Tull, D.E.S., Kinoshita, F., Yokogawa, K., Kasumoto, S., Shiba, T., Kasumoto, S. and Tarumi, Y. (1974) Z. Immun Forsh 149, 302-319.
Lassman, H. (1983). In "Comparative Neuropathology of Chronic Experimental Allergic Encephalomyelitis and Multiple Sclerosis", Springer Verlag, Berlin p. 9-21.
Lebar, R. and Voisin, G.A. (1974) Int. Arch Allergy 46, 82-103.
Margalit, H., Spouge, J.L., Cornette, J.L., Cease, K.B., Delisi, C. and Berzofsky, J.A. (1987) J. Immunol. 138, 2213 - 2219.
Milich, D.R., McLachan, A., Moriarty, A. and Thorton, G.B. (1987) J. Immunol. 138, 4457-4462.
Morgan, I.M. (1947) J. Exp. Med. 85, 131-140
Nagai, Y.A., Kiyama, K., Suzuki, K., Kotani, S., Watanabe, Y., Shimono, T., Shiba, T., Kusumoto, S., Ikata, F. and Takeda S. (1978) Cell Immunol. 35, 158-167.
Parant, M., Audibert, F., Chedid, L., Level, M., Lefrancier, P., Choay, J. and Lederer E. (1980) Infect. and Immun. 27, 826-831.
Paterson, P.Y. (1966) Adv. Immunol. 5, 131.
Paterson, P.Y., Day E.D. and Whitacre, E.C. (1981) Immunological Review 55, 89-120.
Sabin, A.B. (1974) Adv. Neurol 6, 133-140.
Schlesinger, D.H., Cochrane, A.H. Gwadz, R.W., Godson, G.N., Metton, R.S., Nussenzweig, R.S. and Nussenzweig, V. (1984) Biochemistry 23, 5665 - 5669.
Schultze, M.P., Leclerc, C., Jolivet, M., Audibert, F. and Chedid, L. (1985) J. Immunol. 135, 2319-2322.
Telzak E., Wolff, S.M., Dinarello, C.A., Conlon, T., Elkholy, A., Bahr, G.M., Choay, J.P., Morin, A. and Chedid, L. (1986) J. Infect. Dis. 153, 628-633.
Tiollais, P., Charnay, P., and Vyas, G.N. (1981) Science 213, 406 - 409.
Warren, H.S., Vogel, F.R. and Chedid, L.A. (1986) Ann. Rev. Immunol 4, 369-388.
Westall, F.C., Robinson, A.B., Caccam, J., Jackson, J. and Eylar, E.H. (1971) Nature 229, 22-29.

Current Status of Malaria Vaccines: The Need for Safe and Effective Adjuvants

W. A. SIDDIQUI and L. Q. TAM

Department of Tropical Medicine and Medical Microbiology, John A. Burns School of Medicine, University of Hawaii, Honolulu, HI 96822

ABSTRACT

Two P. falciparum sporozoite vaccines, adjuvanted with alum, have recently been shown to be safe in humans, but have had limited immunogenicity and protective success. Defined merozoite proteins and epitopes have been shown to be partially or completely protective in monkeys, when given in Freund's complete adjuvant (FCA). However, a synthetic polymer of three peptides had only limited success in humans, when given in alum. Sporozoite and merozoite epitopes which have been shown to be protective in animals when given in FCA have had only limited success in humans when given in alum. The experience of malariologists is that clinically effective vaccines will not be available until safe and effective adjuvants are developed, despite the successful identification and characterization of protective epitopes.

KEYWORDS

P. falciparum, vaccine, adjuvant, monkey vaccination, clinical trial

INTRODUCTION

Malaria is a threat to almost half the world's population. It is estimated that 300 million cases occur each year in the tropics, while the annual mortality in Africa alone is estimated at one million. The resurgence in malaria is due to the development of resistance of the malaria parasite P. falciparum to antimalarial drugs and of its mosquito vector to insecticides. The development of malaria vaccines is viewed as a supplement to existing control measures. Malaria is introduced by mosquito bite. Sporozoites enter the blood stream and invade liver hepatocytes within minutes. Sporozoite malaria vaccines are directed at blocking entry of sporozoites into liver cells. Sporozoites mature within hepatocytes. The liver cells release merozoites, which invade erythrocytes, thus initiating the asexual blood stage cycle. Merozoite malaria vaccines are aimed at blocking invasion of erythrocytes.

SPOROZOITE VACCINES

X-irradiated sporozoite of a mouse malaria parasite were shown to induce protection against sporozoite challenge (Nussenzweig et al, 1969). Similar evidence showed that small numbers of human volunteers were protected against malaria by immunization with attenuated, X-irradiated sporozoites (Clyde et al, 1973). The sporozoite surface is covered by a circumsporozoite (CS) protein. The immunodominant epitope of the P. falciparum CS protein is a repetive sequence of the four amino acids asparagine-alanine-asparagine-proline (NANP). Clinical tests for safety and immunogenicity of two sporozoite vaccine were conducted recently in humans. A 12 amino acid synthetic peptide $(NANP)_3$ was conjugated to tetanus toxoid, adjuvanted with alum, and administered in three doses at monthly intervals to 35 individuals. The vaccine was safe and no adverse reactions were noted (Herrington et al, 1987). Seroconversion against NANP was detected in 10 or 14 individuals receiving the highest dose of the vaccine. The three individuals having the highest antibody titers and four non-immunized controls were challenged with sporozoites. All four controls developed parasitemia. The mean period before parasites were detected in the blood was 8.5 days. Two of the three immunized volunteers developed parasites on day 11, suggesting that antibodies to the NANP epitope had been effective in reducing the number of sporozoites infecting the liver. The third individual remained completely free of parasites for the 29 day period of observation.

The other sporozoite vaccine tested recently in humans is a recombinant polypeptide containing the NANP repeat 32 times and linked to 32 amino acids of the tetracycline resistance gene ($R32tet_{32}$). The vaccine was adjuvanted in alum and administered to fifteen volunteers. Twelve of the 15 volunteers seroconverted, and six individuals with the highest antibody titers and two non-immunized controls were challenged by mosquito bite. Two volunteers had delayed onset of parasitemia and one volunteer remained completely free of parasites (Ballou et al, 1987). Both clinical trials showed that humans can be protected from sporozoite-induced malaria by immunization with the NANP repeat structure. Delayed parasitemias occured only in those individuals having the highest antibody titers, indicating that a fully effective vaccine may be possible if higher and more sustained antibody titers can be achieved. Thus, significant progress has been made in defining protective sporozoite epitopes; however, it does not appear that the full protective value of this epitope has been obtained in humans using alum as adjuvant.

ASEXUAL BLOOD-STAGE VACCINES

In 1981, Holder and Freeman at the Wellcome Laboratories demonstrated that monoclonal antibody isolated proteins on the surface of merozoite and in the apical rhoptry organelles could protect mice against P. yoelii malaria infection. Subsequent experiments have shown that P. falciparum merozoite surface and rhoptry proteins can protect susceptible Aotus (owl) and Saimiri (squirrel) monkeys against lethal infections of the human parasite. Three antigens on the merozoite surface (83K, 42K, and 19K polypeptides) are processing fragments derived from a glycosylated precursor protein having molecular weight 195,000 (gp195). The precursor protein partially protected squirrel monkeys (Hall et al, 1984; Perrin et al; 1984) and completely protected owl monkeys (Siddiqui et al, 1987). In the later experiment, we could not find parasites in thick blood films of monkeys given a lethal challenge of virulent parasites. Each of the experiments employed native gp195 given in FCA. These experiments have shown that gp195 can protect monkeys against the blood stage; however, a fully protective epitope has not yet been identified. Perrin's group has immunize a second set of squirrel monkeys with a synthetic peptide representing amino acids 24 to 66 of the gp195 sequence (conserved region) and obtained partial protection (Cheung et al, 1986). Other N-terminal synthetic peptides were reported to be poorly protective (Patarroyo et al, 1987b).

The rhoptries are two flask-shaped, electron dense organelles at the apical end of merozoites. Merozoite invasion of erythrocytes is thought to occur via two steps. First, merozoite attach to erythrocyte surface. Second, the merozoite re-orients itself until the apical rhoptries point inward. The contents of these electron dense organelles are then emptied locally onto the erythrocyte surface as the merozoite pushes in and is enveloped by the erythrocyte membrane. A native 41K rhoptry protein strongly protected squirrel monkeys (Perrin et al, 1985). The ring erythrocyte surface antigen (RESA) originates in the rhoptries and ends on the surface of newly invaded ring-stage parasites. Although the native RESA protein has not been isolated, the gene encoding RESA has been cloned (Coppel et al, 1984) and recombinant RESA polypeptides have been shown to partially protect owl monkeys (Collins et al, 1986).

Recently, a provocative experiment has been reported from the laboratory of Patarroyo in Colombia. Instead of culturing parasites in vitro, this group obtained parasite antigens directly from the blood of parasitized humans living in malaria endemic areas. Whereas, the availability of owl monkeys is limited to researchers, Patarroyo trapped native Colombian owl monkeys and performed a large number of vaccination experiments. Partial protection was obtained with 83K, 55K, and 35K proteins (Patarroyo et al, 1987a). The Colombian group then sequenced the N-terminus of these proteins and found that the 83K protein was the N-terminal processing fragment of gp195. Synthetic peptides were then prepared based on the N-terminal sequences. None of the peptides alone protected owl monkeys; however, the onset of parasitemias was delayed. Therefore, a vaccine consisting of a combination of the thre N-terminal peptides was tested. Complete protection was observed in three of six owl monkeys given the peptides in FCA (Patarroyo et al, 1987b).

The Colombian group has recently completed the first human trial of a blood-stage P. falciparum vaccine based on these synthetic peptides (Patarroyo et al, 1988). The three synthetic peptides (83.1, 55.1, and 35.1) along with the sporozoite NANP repeat were synthesized as a hybrid molecule consisting of 45 amino acids. Thirty blocks of the four determinants were polymerized into a 150,000 molecular weight polypeptide, adsorbed to alum, and used to immunize five graduate volunteer soldiers of the Colombian military. By ELISA two of the volunteers (W.G. and L.C.) appeared to have pre-immune antibodies and prior immunity to malaria. Following challenge with a wild Colombian P. falciparum strain, these two individuals and a third volunteer not having pre-existing antibodies controlled their parasitemias. The remaining two individuals developed parasitemias above 0.5% and were treated with chloroquine. All four non-immunized controls developed parasites and were drug-treated. A second group of four volunteers were not protected with a different synthetic polymer consisting of 20 blocks of four other determinants (epitope 83.18 from the N-terminal sequence of gp195, the CS NANP epitope, 18 residues comprising a T-helper cell epitope for the CS repeat, and the 5' repeat of RESA). The 100K synthetic polypeptide was poorly immunogenic, and Patarroyo reported that non of the individuals made antibodies to NANP or RESA, when alum was used as the adjuvant. Although two of the four individuals in this group delayed the appearance of parasites in the blood, all required drug therapy. Overall, Patarroyo found no correlation between humoral or cellular immunity and protection. Nevertheless, this was the first human trial of a blood-stage malaria vaccine.

ADJUVANTS

In each of the monkey experiments in which defined P. falciparum antigens have induced protective immunity, FCA was employed. In our experience with native gp195, strong adjuvants have been necessary. Beginning in 1977, our first demonstration of protective immunity in owl monkeys was with a crude antigen preparation given with two courses of FCA (Siddiqui, 1977). Later, when gp195 was purified with monoclonal antibody, we found that three courses in FCA induced protective immunity; whereas, three courses using MDP(Lys)L18 in intralipid was not protective (Siddiqui et al, 1986). Complete protection was again achieved with gp195 given three times in FCA (Siddiqui et al, 1987). Thus, we believe that gp195 requires an adjuvant as powerful as FCA. We have used the combination of immunomodulators B30-MDP, LA-15-PH, and TDM in liposomes and found high antibody levels in rabbits nearly comparable to levels induced with three courses in FCA. B30-MDP is a lipophilic MDP derivative undergoing clinical evaluation. LA-15-PH is a synthetic lipid A analog, corresponding to the major structure of non-toxic monophosphoryl lipid A of RIBI Immunochem. Trehalose dimycolate (TDM) is a cell component of the Corynebacteria, Nocardia, and Mycobacteria group shown to act synergistically with monophosphoryl lipid A (Ribi et al, 1986). Sporozoite vaccines are also being evaluated with stronger adjuvants. Alving and co-workers have shown that R32tet$_{32}$ adsorbed to alum and presented in liposomes containing lipid A produce strong primary and secondary antibody responses in rabbits and monkeys (Richards et al, 1988). NANP synthesized with hydrophic feet and presented in proteosomes consisting of a B-cell mitogen from the outer membrane of *Neisseria meningitidis* ellicits high antibody titers in mice (Lowell et al, 1988).

CONCLUSION

The NANP epitope of the circumsporozoite protein has been shown to be weakly immunogenic when given in alum, but capable of inducing protective immunity in few individuals in clinical trials. Merozoite proteins have shown great promise in monkey experiments, and a combination of three synthetic peptides has shown some effectiveness in humans. While protection has been demonstrated in animals using FCA, only limited clinical success has been achieved in humans using alum. The identification of protective *P. falciparum* epitopes has provided only half an effective vaccine. A fully protective malaria vaccine will also require the development of a safe and effective adjuvant capable of replacing FCA.

REFERENCES

Ballou, W. R., J. A. Sherwood, F. A. Neva, D. M. Gordon, R. A. Wirtz, G. F. Wasserman, C. L. Diggs, S. L. Hoffman, M. R. Hollingdale, W. T. Hockmeyer, I. Schneider J. F. Young, P. Reeve, and J. D. Chulay (1987). Lancet i, 1277-1281.

Cheung, A., J. Leban, A. R. Shaw, B. Merkli, J. Stocker, C. Chizzolini, C. Sander and L. H. Perrin (1986). Proc. Natl. Acad. Sci., USA, 83, 8328-8332.

Clyde, D. F., H. Most, V. McCarthy and J. P. Vanderberg (1973). Am. J. Med. Sci., 226, 166-177.

Collins, W. E., R. F. Anders, M. Pappaioanou, G. H. Campbell, G. V. Brown, D. J. Kemp, R. L. Coppel, J. C. Skinner, P. M. Andrysiak, J. M. Favalaoro, L. M. Corcoran, J. R. Broderson, G. F. Mitchell and C. C. Campbell (1986). Nature, 323, 259-262.

Coppel, R. L., A. F. Cowman, R. F. Anders, A. E. Bianco, R. B. Saint, K. R. Lingelbach, D. J. Kemp, and G. V. Brown (1984). Nature, 310, 789-792.

Hall, R., J. E. Hyde, M. Goman, D. L. Simmons, I. A. Hope, M. Mackay and J. Scaife (1984). Nature, 311, 379-381.

Herrington, D. A., D. F. Clyde, G. Losonsky, M. Cortesia, J. R. Murphy, J. Davis, S. Baqar, A. M. Felix, E. P. Heimer, D. Gillessen, E. Nardin, R. S. Nussenzweig, V. Nussenzweig, M. R. Hollingdale, and M. M. Levine (1987). Nature, 328, 257-259.

Holder, A. A. and R. R. Freeman (1981). Immunization against blood-stage rodent malaria using purified parasite antigens. Nature, 294, 261-264.

Lowell, G. H., W. R. Ballou, L. F. Smith, R. A. Wirtz, W. D. Zollinger and W. T. Hockmeyer (1988). Science, 240, 800-802.

Nussenzweig, R. S., J. Vanderberg and H. Most (1967). Nature, 216, 160-162.

Patarroyo, M. E., P. Romero, M. L. Torres, P. Clavijo, D. Andreu, D. Lozada, L. Sanchez, P. del Portillo, C. Pinilla, A. Moreno, A. Alegria and R. Houghten (1987a). In: F. Brown, R. Channock and R. Lerner (eds) Vaccines 87, pp. 117-124.

Patarroyo, M. E., P. Romero, M. L. Torres, P. Claviho, A. Moreno, A. Martinez, R. Rodriquez, F. Gusman and E. Cabezas (1987b). Nature, 328, 629-632.

Patarroyo, M. E., P. Amador, P. Claviho, A. Moreno, F. Guzman, P. Romero, R. Tascon, A. Franco, L. A. Murillo, G. Ponton and G. Trujillo (1988). Nature, 332, 158-161.

Perrin, L. H., B. Merkli, M. Loche, C. Chizzolini, J. Smart and R. Richle (1984). J. Exp. Med., 160, 441-446.

Perrin, L. H., B. Merkli, M. S. Gabra, J. W. Stocker, C. Chizzolini and R. Richle (1985). J. Clin. Invest., 75, 1718-1721.

Ribi, E., J. Cantrell, T. Feldner, K. Myers and J. Peterson (1986). Microbiology 1986, 9-13.

Richards, R. L., M. D. Hayre, W. T. Hockmeyer and C. R. Alving (1988). Infect. Immun., 56, 682-686.
Siddiqui, W. A. (1977). Science, 197, 388-389.
Siddiqui, W. A., L. Q. Tam, S.-C. Kan, K. Kramer, S. E. Case, K. L. Palmer, K. M. Yamaga and G. S. N. Hui (1986). Infect. Immun., 52, 314-318.
Siddiqui, W. A., L. Q. Tam, K. H. Kramer, G. S. N. Hui, S. E. Case, K. M. Yamaga S. P. Chang, E. B. T. Chan, and S.-C. Kan (1987). Proc. Natl. Acad. Sci. USA 84, 3014-3018.

ACKNOWLEDGEMENT

Gratitude is expressed to the U.S. Agency for International Development for their continuous research support and the University of Hawaii Foundation.

Immunoadjuvants for Vaccine

I. AZUMA* and Y. YAMAMURA**

*Institute of Immunological Science, Hokkaido University, Sapporo 060, and
**Osaka University, Suita 565, Japan

ABSTRACT

It is well recognized that the combination treatment of vaccine with potent immunoadjuvant is essential for the effective application of vaccine. In this symposium, the recent advances in the field of immunoadjuvants, especially of synthetic adjuvants, are reviewed. The immunological properties of synthetic adjuvants, especially muramyldipeptide (MDP) derivatives, trehalose dimycolate (TDM) analogs, lipid A and chitin derivatives are described. The nonspecific stimulation of host resistance with immunoadjuvants against infection was also discussed.

KEYWORDS

Immunoadjuvants, Bacterial fractions, Synthetic adjuvants, MDP derivatives, TDM, Lipid A derivatives, Chitin derivatives

INTRODUCTION

In last decade, the great advance has been made in the field of vaccine dvelopment, especially in the component vaccine and recombinant vaccine which were develolped by the biochemical and immunological studies and the application of genetic engeneering technology. The chemical syntheses of antigenic determinants of vaccines were attempted and the synthetic peptides were being applied for the vaccination in experimental model. For the effective application of these component vaccine, recombinant vaccine and chemically synthetic peptide vaccine to human, the development and combination of active immunoadjuvant will be essentially required.

Immunoadjuvants have also been applied for the nonspecific stimulation of host against the infections with bacteria, fungi, viruses and parasites. In this symposium, the recent results of the development of immunoadjuvants, especially chemically synthetic adjuvants in our laboratory will be summarized, and the possibility of the application of these immunoadjuvants to vaccine development will be discussed.

1) Bacterial Cell Walls, N-Acetylmuramyldipeptide and Their Acyl Derivatives

The heat-killed mycobacterial cells suspended in mineral oil were known to be the most potent immunoadjuvant as "Freund's complete adjuvant (FCA)" for the induction of cell-mediated immunity and humoral antibody formation (Freund, 1956). In 1971, we have cleary shown that the cell-wall skeleton (CWS) fraction was the adjuvant-active principle of the cells of mycobacteria and related bacteria (Azuma *et al.*, 1971). The chemical structure of CWS of *Mycobacterium bovis* BCG and its biological activities, especially adjuvant and antitumor activities, were examined in detail (Azuma and Yamamura, 1979). Furthermore, we have also reported the purification and chemical structures of the CWS fraction of *Nocardia rubra* (Azuma *et al.*, 1976; Yamawaki *et al.*, 1978), *Propionibacterium acnes* (Azuma *et al.*, 1979) and *Listeria monocytogenes* (Kamisango *et al.*, 1982), and their usefulness as immunoadjuvants were also examined. In 1974, Ellouz *et al.* (1974) reported that the minimal adjuvant-active subunit of bacterial cell walls including BCG-CWS, *N. rubra*-CWS, *P. acnes*-CWS and *L. monocytogenes*-CWS was *N*-acetylmuramyl-L-alanyl-D-isoglutamine (MurNAc-L-Ala-D-isoGln, MDP), and their biological activities of MDP were reported by several laboratories (Adam and Lederer, 1984). The variety of MDP analogs and derivatives has been synthesized, and their adjuvant activities were examined (Fig. 1). Although MDP and its analogs have potent adjuvant activities *in vivo* when they were administered as water-in-oil emulsion together with antigen, MDP exhibited only limited adjuvant activity when it was administered as aqueous solution *in vivo*, due to its rapid excretion into urine. Therefore, we synthesized several hydrophobic (acyl) derivatives of MDP analogs (Kusumoto *et al.*, 1978). Among these acyl-MDP derivatives, three synthetic compounds, B30-MDP derivative for the vaccine adjuvant, and two kinds of stearoyl MDP derivatives as the adjuvants for the nonspecific stimulation of host against bacterial and viral infections, were selected.

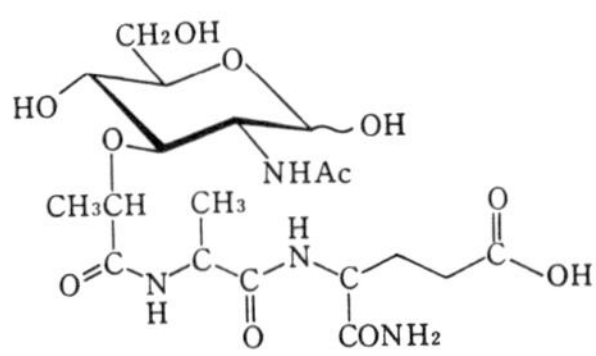

N-acetylmuramyl-L-alanyl-D-isoglutamine (MDP)

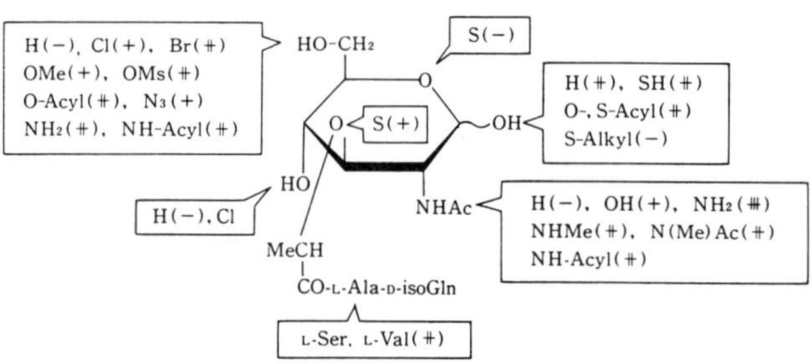

Fig. 1. MDP and its adjuvant activity—structure relationship.

In this conference, the typical example of the application of acyl-MDP derivatives for the potentiation of component vaccine was shown by Dr. Okuma and his coworkers. They reported the preparation of the liposome (MDP-virosome) consisted of B30-MDP, cholesterol and influenza virus antigen (purified haemagglutin-neuraminidase) (Fig. 2) (Workshop 20). The MDP-virosome thus prepared has 100 nm in diameter enhanced both the circulating antibody response and the induction of cell-mediated immunity against the antigen molecule locating on its surface. In the challenging experiment with influenza virus, significant survival rates were determined in mice group immunized with MDP-virosome vaccine. These results suggest that the liposome containing B30-MDP will be useful as the aduuvant-active vehicle for the component vaccine or recombinant vaccine.

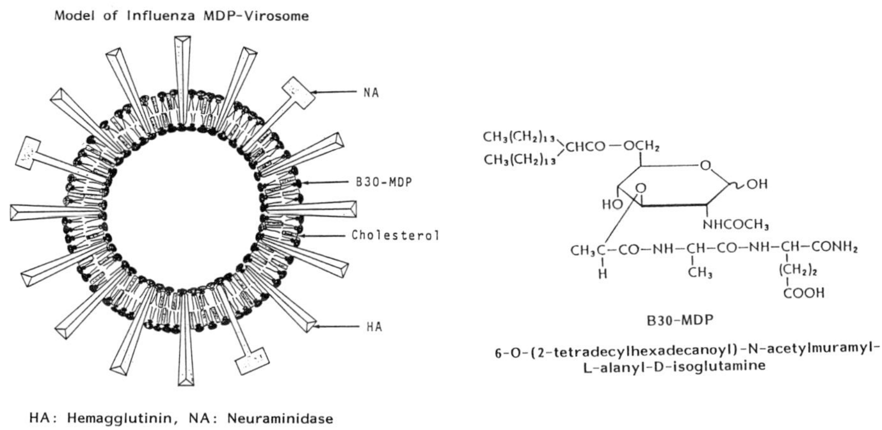

Fig. 2. B30-MDP and B30-MDP-virosome.

2) Effects of Acyl-MDP Derivatives on Host Resistance against Bacterial and Viral Infections

It is well recognized that the nonspecific host-stimulation with immunostimulants is one of the most important factors for the treatment of immunosuppressed host such as cancer patients. Chedid *et al*. (1977) have reported that MDP and its derivative stimulated host-resistance against *Klebsiella pneumoniae* infection in mice. Several MDP derivatives and related compounds such as murabutide, stearoyl-MDP derivatives, MTP-PE (Schumann, 1987), FK-565, FK-156 (Goto and Aoki, 1987) and R.P. 40 639 (Floc'h *et al*., 1987) have been reported to have host-stimulating activities against bacterial infections in experimental models. Matsumoto *et al*. (1981a, 1981b, 1983) have also examined 64 acy-MDP derivatives as adjuvants for the stimulation of host-resistance against nonspecific bacterial infection by using sepsis type infection model with *Escherichia coli* in mice, and selected 2 candidates, L18-MDP and MDP-Lys(L18) (Fig. 3). The stimulatory effects of both stearoyl-MDP derivatives were examined in detail (Matsumoto *et al*., 1987). Both stearoyl-MDP derivatives were shown to be effective for stimulation of host-resistance against infection with *E. coli*, *Staphylococcus aureus*, *Pseudomonas aeruginosa* and *Candida albicans*, but not effective for infections with *Salmonella typhimurium* and *Listeria monocytogenes*. It was also shown that both steraoyl-MDP derivatives stimulated the immunosuppressed mice, rats and guinea pigs. Both stearoyl-MDP derivatives were shown to have a synergistic effect on combination with antibiotics such as cephazolin, gentamicin and amphotericin B. On the mechanism of stimulation of the host with stearoyl-MDP derivatives, Osada *et al*. (1982) have shown that functions such as migration, phagocytosis and production of superoxide of polymorphonuclear cells were stimulated by the administration of stearoyl-MDP derivatives. We have also shown that both L18-MDP and MDP-Lys(L18) are effective for host-stimulation against opportunistic infection with Corynebacterium kutuscheri infection in mice (Ishihara et al., 1984).

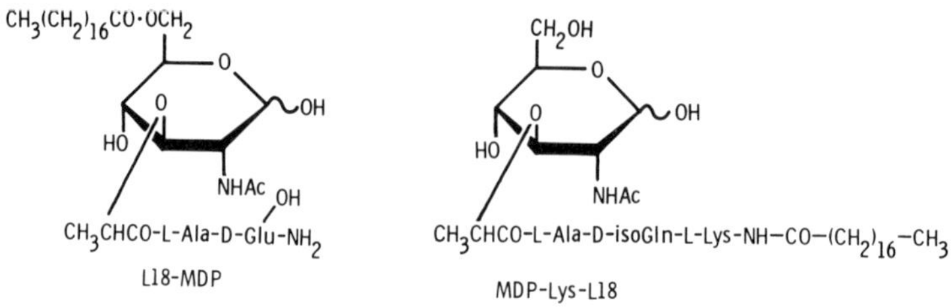

Fig. 3. Stearoyl-MDP derivatives.

We have established models for the host-stimulation with immunoadjuvants against viral infection by using Sendai virus and herpes simplex type 1 virus in mice (Ishihara et al. 1985). Intrannsal pretreatment with MDP, L18-MDP and MDP-Lys(L18) dissolved in PBS augmented the nonspecific resistance to intranasal infection with Sendai virus in mice. Intranasal administration of MDP-Lys(L18) (10 μg) 3 days and 1 day before intranasal challenge with Sendai vrius resulted in 100% survival rates; however, administration of MDP-Lys(L18) 1 day after the infection showed no effect in this experimental system in this experimental condition. It was also shown that intranasal administration of 10 μg and 1 μg of MDP-Lys(L18) was effective, but the 0.1 μg of MDP-Lys(L18) was not effectivce. The intranasal, intraperitoneal and intravenous administrations of MDP-Lys(L18) were effective, however, subcutaneous administration of MDP-Lys(L18) was not effective for the protection against Sendai virus infection in this model. The action mechanism of MDP-Lys(L18) for the protection of Sendai virus infection was investigated and discussed by Ishihara et al. (1987), and it was concluded that the growth of Sendai virus was suppressed by the treatment with MDP-Lys(L18) only at the early nonspecific phase of the infection, and that macrophages and interferon are the important elements activated by the MDP-Lys(L18) treatment. More recently, we have also shown that MDP-Lys(L18) was also effective on host resistance against herpes simplex virus (HSV) type-1 infection in cyclophosphamide-treated mice.

Dr. Furuta and his coworkers (1986) have synthesized acyl derivatives of N-acetylglucosaminyl-β(1→4)-N-acetylmuramyl tri- and tetrapeptides and their pyrogenicity in rabbits and protective activity against Pseudomonas aeruginosa in ddY mice were examined. These acyl derivatives of disaccharide tri- and tetrapeptides are more hydrophilic than L18-MDP or MDP-Lys(L18) in their physicochemical properties. Among these disaccharide peptide derivatives, both stearoyl derivatives, GM-40 and GM-53, were shown to be effective as MDP-Lys(L18) for the host stimulation against Sendai virus infection. However, both disaccharide tripeptide (GMP3) and disaccharide tetrapeptide (GMP4) were ineffective in this experimental condition (Iida et al., in preparation).

Multiprenyl structures are found in many biologically active compounds and multiprenyl compounds are known to act on the cell surface membrane. Previously we have studied the detail of adjuvant effect of multiprenyl compounds and multiprenylacetyl derivatives (Fukuda et al., 1981) of MDP and the effect on the prevention of Sendai vrius infection in mice by using similar experimental model described above (Azuma et al., 1988a). These TDM-232, TMD-233, TF-1031, and TF-1034 were administered i.n. in the form of liposome (MLV) and MDP-Lys(L18) was given by PBS solution. TMD-232 (20 μg) which was given 3 days before injection was as effective as MDP-Lys(L18) (10 μg) which was given 1 day bebore injection for the protection against Sendai virus, however, TMD-233 was ineffective. Both TF-1031 and TF-1034 were also ineffective in this experimental system. More recently, we have observed that dihydroheptaprenol (DHP) (200 μg) which was given intranasally as the form of micro emulsion with lecithin at a 1% concentration was effective as the administration of MDP-Lys(L18) (10 μg) for the protection of Sendai virus in mice. DHP was also shown to stimulate the host resistance against bacterial infections in mice (Tsukidate et al., Workshop 6 in this conference). These preliminary results suggest that the multiprenyl compound may have some host-stimulating activity and the conjugate of multiprenyl compounds and MDP may develop synergistic effect for the protection of Sendai virus infection in mice.

3) Trehalose Mycolates

Trehalose-6,6'-dimycolates (TDM), so-called cord foactor, was originally discovered by Bloch and his coworkers (Bloch, 1950; Noll et al., 1956) from mycobacterial toxic lipid for mice when injected as an oil emulsion. Further investigation revelaed that cord factor-like glycolipids were contained not only in mycobacteria but also in the lipid fractions of related bacteria such nocardia and corynebacteria. TDM was also shown to have a variety of biological activities such as (1) toxic activity in mice, (2) antitumor activity, (3) stimulation of host resistance against infections with bacteria, fungi, virus and parasites, and (4) synergistic potentiation of the anti-infectious and antitumor activities of bacterial fractions, such as cell-wall skeletons, lipid A derivatives and synthetic MDP derivatives (Lemaire et al., 1986). In this symposium, Dr. Siddiqui reported his approaches for the potentiation of malaria vaccine by using adjuvant containing TDM and synthetic MDP derivatives. Ribi et al. (1978) have reported that the adjuvant and antitumor activities of BCG-CWS, lipid A or synthetic MDP derivatives were potently stimulated by the combination with TDM. Recently, we have synthesized various TDM analogs (Fig. 4) to examine the detailed adjuvant activity of TDM, relationship between the chemical structure and activity of TDM and the mechanism of synergistic effect of TDM with combination of other synthetic adjuvants (Numata et al., 1985; 1986). Mycobacterial glycolipid, TDM, and its analogs TD(L30), TD(B30), TD(BH32), TD(BH48), TD(D28), TDNM and TDN(BH32), were synthesized, and their lethal and adjuvant activities were examined. TDM and TDNM were lethal 100% and 40% respectively when injected intravenously into mice at a dose of 150 μg as 9% oil-in-water emulsion, but the other analogs showed no lethal toxicity to mice at the same dose. The cytolyitc activity of mouse peritoneal macrophages against tumor cells was potentiated by intraperitoneal injection of TDM and its synthetic analogs. TDM and TD(BH32) also stimulated nonspecific host resistance against Sendai virus infection in BALB/c mice. We have also synthesized five monoesters, TMM, GlcM, GlcNAcM, AraM and GalM by use of mycolic acid isolated from *Mycobacterium tuberculosis* strain Aoyama B. A single intravenous administration of 400 μg of TMM in 9% oil-in-water emulsion killed 8 of 8 treated mice. The other analogs showed less lethal toxicity to mice at the same dose. Tumoricidal activity of mouse peritoneal macrophages was induced by intraperitoneal injection of TMM, GlcM, and GlcNAcM, respectively. Recently we have observed that 6-*O*-mycoloyl-*N*-acetylglucosamine and 6-*O*-mycoloyl-1-deoxyl-*N*-acetylglucosamine were also as effective as TDM for the mouse peritoneal macrophage activation, however, less toxic in mice than TDM. Natural TDM is the dimycolate of trehalose(α,α). More recently, we have examined the efficacy as immunoadjuvant of synthetic stereoisomers such as TDM(α,β) and TDM(β,β) of natural TDM(α,α) colaborating with Dr. Kitajima's group, Toa Kase Co., Ltd. The results indicated that synthetic TDM(α,β) and TDM(β,β) were as effective as natural TDM(α,α) for the activation of mouse peritoneal macrophage, however, less toxic than natural TDM(α,α) (Azuma et al., in preparation).

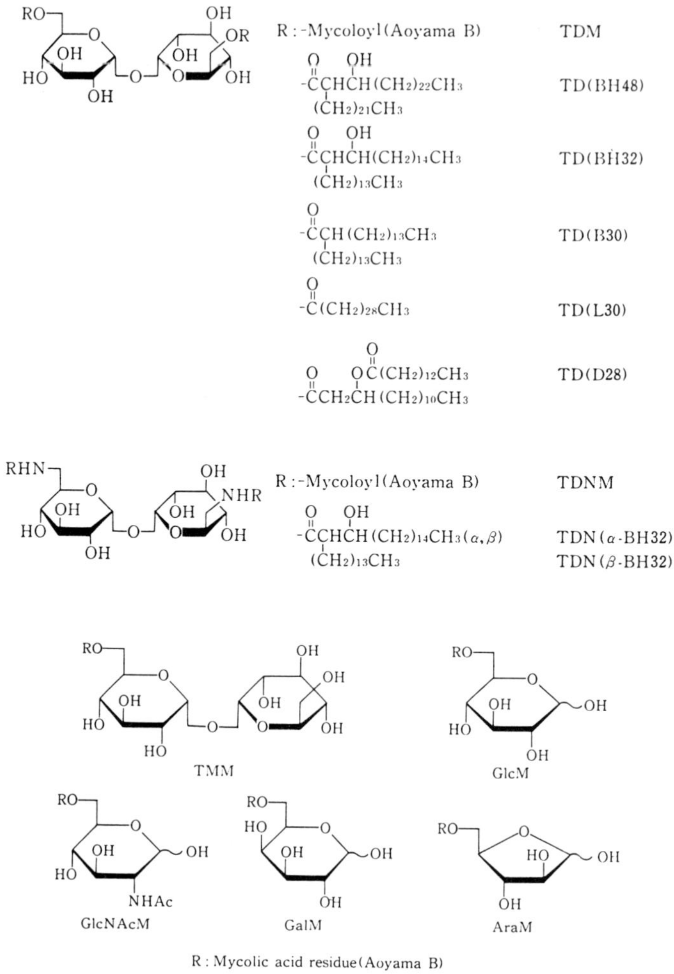

Fig. 4. TDM and related compounds.

4) Lipid A

It has been well established that lipopolysaccharide (LPS) of gram-negative bacteria carried a variety of biological and immunomodulating activities, and the active principle of LPS was shown to be lipid A moiety. Recently, the chemical structure of the lipid A was extensively studied and the lipid A of Escherichia coli LPS was elucidated by Dr. Shiba's group and other several groups, and the chemical synthesis of lipid A analogs and related compounds were reported by Dr. Shiba's group (Imoto et al., 1985) and other several groups. The chemically synthesized compound 506 (Fig. 5) and related compounds represents almost of all the biological activity of lipid A and LPS of E. coli including immunomodulating activity and lethal activity (Kotani et al., 1985; Takahashi et al., 1987).

Dr. Hasegawa and his coworkers have tried to synthesize lipid A related compounds which are adjuvant-active, but less toxic, and acylated monosaccharide derivatives, GLA-60 (Fig. 5) was selected as adjuvants (Kiso et al., 1986; 1987). Especially GLA-60 was shown to have very potent adjuvant activity for the induction of delayed-type hypersensitivity in guinea pigs, activation of mouse peritoneal macrophages, induction of serum TNF in mice after priming with P. acnes or recombinant murine interferon-γ (Saiki et al., submitted). GLA-60 was also demonstrated to have very low adverse reaction. These results suggest that the derivatives or related compounds of lipid A having low toxicity will be useful immunoadjuvants for the application to the vaccine.

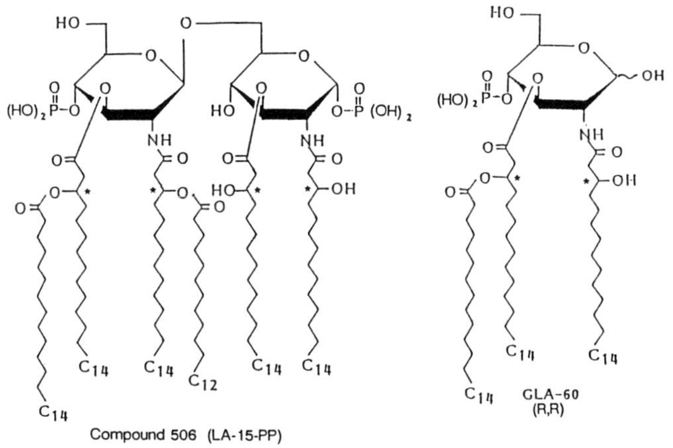

Fig. 5. Lipid A and related compound.

5) Chitin and Its Derivatives

Chitin, β-(1→4)-poly-N-acetyl-D-glucosamine having rigid crystalline structure, is widely distributed in nature. We have reported the chemical synthesis of chitin whcih was purified from queen crab shells and examined the immunological properties in detail (Tokura et al., 1983; Nishimura et al., 1984; 1985; 1986a; 1986b, 1987; Azuma et al., 1988b). Among these chitin derivatives, DAC-70 was shown to have the most potent immunoadjuvant activity on the murine macrophage activation, induction of delayed-type hypersensitivity and production of circulating antibody in guinea pig, and induction of allogeneic killer T cells, activation of natural killer (NK) cells and induction of cytokines such as IL-1 and CSF in mice. DAC-70 was also shown to have activities for the suppression of murine tumor growth, Meth A in BALB/c mice, and stimulation of host-defense mechanism against E. coli infection in mice (Iida et al., 1987).

The protective effect of chitin derivatives, DAC-70, CM-chitin, DAC-70(Me), on the Sendai virus infection was examined by using the same experimental model described above. MDP-Lys(L18) was used as positive control. Intranasal administration of DAC-70 (50 μg), DAC-70(Me) (50 μg) and MDP-Lys(L18) (10 μg) 1 day before infection was effective for the prevention against Sendai virus infection. However, intranasal administration of CM-chitin was ineffective in this experimental condition. By the dose response test, it was shown that the survival rates of mice treated with 50, 10, 1, 0.1 μg of the DAC-70 1 day before infection of the control mice were 100%, 83%, 67%, 57% and 14%, respectively. On the effect of the route of administration of DAC-70 on resistance against Sendai virus infection it was shown that intranasal or intravenous administration 1 day before the infection of DAC-70 was effective, however, intraperitoneal and subcutaneous administrations of DAC-70 (100 μg) revealed no protective activity (Iida et al., 1987).

6) Future Aspects

As reported in this symposium by Dr. Audibert, the conjugates of synthetic peptide antigen and adjuvants are very promissing approach. In this approach, synthetic adjuvants are the most useful tool.

Another approach for the potentiation of antigenicity of vaccine is the combination of adjuvant and cytokines. More recently, we have shown that the adjuvant activity determined by the ability of activation of mouse peritoneal macrophages MDP derivatives was extreamly potentiated by the combination of very low dose (1 U) of recombinant mouse interferon-γ (Saiki et al., 1988). These results suggest that suitable combination treatment of cytokine and immunoadjuvants will potentiate effectively the vaccine potency.

It should be pointed out that the development of drug delivery system is also important factor for the effective application of vaccine. We have suggested chitin derivatives such as DAC-70 and CM-chitin are adjuvant-active and biodegradable with lysozyme in the host. DAC-70 and CM-chitin are easily made to beads and microspheres having the functions of macrophage activation and cytokine production (Nishimura et al., 1987). These results suggest the possibility of chitin derivatives for the application to the slow-release drug (vaccine) carrier.

In conclusion, the development of safer immunoadjuvants is as important as that of new vaccine. Further approaches should be required.

ACKNOWLEDGMENTS

This work was supported in part by Grants-in-Aid for Cancer Research from the Japanese Ministry of Education, Science and Culture; from the Japanese Ministry of Health and Welfare for Comprehensive 10-Year Strategy for Cancer Control; and for Scientific Research and for Developmental Scientific Research (62870023) from the Japanese Ministry of Education, Science and Culture; and for Scientific Research from the Japanese Ministry of Education, Science and Culture; by the Osaka Foundation for Promotion of Clinical Immunology; by Yamanouchi Foundation for Research on Metabolic Disorders; and also by Grant-in-Aid for Special Project Research from Hokkaido University, Japan.

REFERENCES

Adam, A. and Lederer, E. (1984). Medicinal Res. Rev. 4, 111-152.
Azuma, I., Kishimoto, S., Yamamura, Y. and Petit, J.-F. (1971). Jpn. J. Microbiol. 15, 193-197.
Azuma, I., Nishimura, K. and Tokura, S. (1988a). In: Handbook of Immunotherapeutic Agetns: Clinical Immunopharmacology and Pharmacology: (ed. G. Renoux) Marcel Dekker, Inc. In press.
Azuma, I., Saiki, I., Iida, J., Fukuda, T. and Kobayashi, S. (1988b). Vaccine 7, in press.
Azuma, I., Taniyama, M., Yamawaki, K., Sugimura, K. and Yamamura, Y. (1976). Gann 67, 733-736.
Azuma, I. and Yamamura, Y. (1979). GANN Monogr. Cancer Res. 24, 121-142.
Azuma, I., Yamawaki, M., Yoshimoto, T., Saiki, I., Uemiya, M., Tanio, Y., Tokuzen, R., Yasumoto, K. and Yamamura, Y. (1979). Gann 70, 737-748.
Bloch, H. (1950). J. Exp. Med. 91, 197-217.
Chedid, L., Parant, M., Lefrancier, P., Choay, J. and Lederer, E. (1977). Proc. Natl. Acad. Sci. USA 74, 2089-2093.

Ellouz, F., Adam, A., Ciorbaru, R. and Lederer, E. (1974). Biochem. Biophys. Res. Commun. 59, 1317-1325.

Floc'h, F., Poirier, J., Fizames, G. and Woehrle, R. (1987). In: Immunostimurants: Now and Tomorrow: (eds I. Azuma and G. Jollès) Japan Sci. Soc. Press/Springer-Verlag. 183-204.

Freund, J. (1956). Adv. Tuberc. Res. 7, 130-148.

Fukuda, T., Kobayashi, S., Yukimasa, H., Terao, S., Fujino, M., Shiba, T., Saiki, I., Azuma, I. and Yamamura, Y. (1981). Bull. Chem. Soc. Jpn. 54, 3530-3535.

Furuta, R., Kawata, S., Naruto, S., Minami, A. and Kotani, S. (1986). Agric. Biol. Chem. 50, 2561-2572.

Goto, T. and Aoki, H. (1987). In: Immunostimulants: Now and Tomorrow: (eds I. Azuma and G. Jollès) Japan Sci. Soc. Press/Springer-Verlag. 99-108.

Iida, J., Une, T., Ishihara, C., Nishimura, K., Tokura, S., Mizukoshi, N. and Azuma, I. (1987). Vaccine 5, 270-274.

Imoto, M., Yoshimura, H., Kusumoto, S. and Shiba, T. (1985). Tetrahedr. Lett. 26, 1545-1548.

Ishihara, C., Hamada, H., Yamamoto, K., Iida, J. and Azuma, I. (1985). Vaccine 3, 370-374.

Ishihara, C., Mizukoshi, N., Iida, J., Yamamoto, K. and Azuma, I. (1987). Vaccine 5, 295-301.

Ishihara, C., Yamamoto, K., Hamada, H. and Azuma, I. (1984). Vaccine 2, 261-264.

Kamisango, K., Saiki, I., Tanio, Y., Okumura, H., Araki, Y., Sekikawa, I., Azuma, I. and Yamamura, Y. (1982). J. Biochem. 92, 23-33.

Kiso, M., Tanaka, S., Fujita, M., Fushishima, Y., Ogawa, Y., Ishida, H. and Hasegawa, A. (1987). Carbohydr. Res. 162, 127-140.

Kiso, M., Tanaka, S., Tanahashi, M., Fujishima, Y., Ogawa, Y. and Hasegawa, A. (1986). Carbohydr. Res. 148, 221-234.

Kotani, S., Takada, H., Tsujimoto, M., Ogawa, T., Takahashi, I., Ikeda, T., Otsuka, K., Shimauchi, H., Kasai, N., Mashimo, J., Nagao, S., Tanaka, A., Tanaka, S., Harada, K., Nagaki, K., Kitamura, H., Shiba, T., Kusumoto, S., Imoto, M. and Yoshimura, H. (1985). Infect. Immun. 49, 225-237.

Kusumoto, S., Okada, S., Yamamoto, K. and Shiba, T. (1978). Bull. Chem. Soc. Jpn. 51, 2122-2126.

Lemaire, G., Tenu, J.-P., Petit, J.-P. and Lederer, E. (1986). Med. Res. Rev. 6, 243-274.

Matsumoto, K., Ogawa, H., Kusama, T., Nagase, O., Sawaki, N., Inage, M., Kusumoto, S., Shiba, T. and Azuma, I. (1981a). Infect. Immun. 32, 748-758.

Matsumoto, K., Ogawa, H., Nagase, O., Kusama, T. and Azuma, I. (1981b). Microbiol. Immunol. 25, 1047-1058.

Matsumoto, K., Osada, Y., Une, T., Otani, T., Ogawa, H. and Azuma, I. (1987). In: Immunostimulants: Now and Tomorrow (eds I. Azuma and G. Jollès) Japan Sci. Soc. Press/Springer-Verlag. 79-97.

Matsumoto, K., Otani, T., Une, T., Osada, Y., Ogawa, H. and Azuma, I. (1983). Infect. Immun. 39, 1029-1040.

Nishimura, K., Ishihara, C., Uke, S., Tokura, S. and Azuma, I. (1986a). Vaccine 4, 151-156.

Nishimura, K., Nishimura, S., Nishi, N., Numata, F., Tone, Y., Tokura, S. and Azuma, I. (1985). Vacccine 3, 379-384.

Nishimura, K., Nishimura, S., Nishi, N., Saiki, I., Tokura, S. and Azuma, I. (1984). Vaccine 2, 93-99.

Nishimura, K., Nishimura, S., Seo, H., Nishi, N., Tokura, S. and Azuma, I. (1986b). J. Biomed. Mater. Res. 20, 1359-1372.

Nishimura, K., Nishimura, S., Seo, H., Nishi, N., Tokura, S. and Azuma, I. (1987). Vaccine 5, 136-140.

Noll, H., Bolch, H., Asselineau, J. and Lederer, E. (1956). Biochim. Biophys. Acta 20, 299-399.

Numata, F., Ishida, H., Nishimura, K., Sekikawa, I. and Azuma, I. (1986). J. Carbohydr. Chem. 5, 127-138.

Numata, F., Nishimura, K., Ishida, H., Ukei, S., Tone, Y., Ishihara, C., Saiki, I., Sekikawa, I. and Azuma, I. (1985). Chem. Pharm. Bull. 33, 4544-4555.

Osada, Y., Otani, T., Sato, M., Une, T., Matsumoto, K. and Ogawa, H. (1982). Infect. Immun. 38, 848-854.

Ribi, E., McLaughlin, C.A., Cantrell, J.L., Brehmer, W., Azuma, I., Yamamura, Y., Strain, S.M., Hwang, K.M. and Toubiana, R. (1978). In: Immunotherapy of Human Cancer (The University of Texas System Cancer Center, M.D. Anderson Hospital and Tumor Institute) Raven Press. 131-154.

Saiki, I., Saito, S., Fujita, C., Ishida, H., Iida, J., Murata, J., Hasegawa, A. and Azuma, I. (1988). Vaccine 6, 238-244.

Schumann, G. (1987). In: Immunostimulants: Now and Tomorrow (eds I. Azuma and G. Jollès) Japan Sci. Soc. Press/Springer-Verlag. 183-204.

Takahashi, I., Kotani, S., Takada, H., Tsujimoto, M., Ogawa, T., Shiba, T., Kusumoto, S., Yamamoto, M., Hasegawa, A., Kiso, M., Nishijima, M., Amano, F., Akamatsu, Y., Harada, K., Tanaka, S., Okamura, H. and Tamura, T. (1987). Infect. Immun. 65, 57-68.

Tokura, S., Nishi, N., Tsutsumi, A. and Somorin, O. (1983). Polymer J. 15, 485-489.

Yamawsaki, M., Azuma, I., Saiki, I., Uemiya, M., Aoki, O., Ennyu, E. and Yamamura, Y. (1978). Gann 69, 619-626.

Immunopharmacology of Model Cytokine, IL-6 (BSF2/IFNß2)

Interleukin 6 and its Receptor: Pathological Role in Autoimmunity and Lymphoid Malignancy

T. HIRANO, T. TAGA, K. YAMASAKI, T. MATSUDA, B. TANG, S. SUEMATSU, Y. HORII, Y. HIRATA, H. YAWATA, A. MURAGUCHI, M. KAWANO*, N. MIYASAKA**, M. SHIMIZU† and T. KISHIMOTO

Institute for Molecular and Cellular Biology, Osaka University, 1–3 Yamada-oka, Suita, Osaka 565, Japan

**Department of Internal Medicine, Research Institute for Nuclear Medicine and Biology, Hiroshima University, Kasumi 1–2–3, Minami-ku, Hiroshima 734, Japan*

***Institute of Rheumatology, Tokyo Woman's Medical College, 2–4–1, Nishi-shinjuku, Shinjuku-ku, Tokyo 163, Japan*

†Osaka-Minami National Hospital, Kawachi-nagano, Osaka 586, Japan

ABSTRACT

Interleukin 6 (BSF-2/26kD protein/IFN-β 2/HPGF/HSF) is a multifunctional cytokine produced by both lymphoid and non-lymphoid cells. Both high and low affinity IL-6 specific receptors were identified and the cDNA encoding IL-6-R was cloned. The data showed that IL-6 receptor is a member of the immunoglobulin superfamily. IL-6 was demonstrated to be an essential factor for immunoglobulin production by B cells. The results suggested that the deregulation is involved in the pathogenesis of autoimmne diseases and the oncogenesis of multiple myeloma.

KEYWORDS

Interleukin 6: BSF-2: IFN-β 2: 26kD protein: HPGF: HSF: receptor: immunoglobulin production: autoimmune disease: multiple myeloma.

INTRODUCTION

Interleukin 6 (IL-6) is a multifunctional cytokine which had previously been called by a variety of names such as, B cell stimulatory factor 2 (BSF-2), (Hirano et al, 1985 and 1986), interferon β 2(IFN-β 2) (Ziberstein et al, 1986 and May et al, 1986), 26kD protein (Haegeman et al, 1986), hybridoma/plasmacytoma growth factor (HPGF) (Van Dame et al, 1987) and hepatocyte stimulating factor (HSF) (Andus et al, 1987 and Gauldie et al, 1987) on the basis of its biological activities. Following the molecular cloning of the cDNAs encoding human BSF-2, IFN-β 2 and 26kD protein (Hirano et al, 1986; Zilberstein et al, 1986; May et al., 1986; Haegeman et al, 1986), it was found that all these molecules are identical and therefore, it has been called IL-6. Human BSF-2 (IL-6) was originally identified as a factor in culture supernatants of PHA-(Muraguchi et al, 1981) or antigen- (Teranishi et al, 1982) stimulated peripheral mononuclear cells which induced immunoglobulin (Ig)-production in Epstein-Barr virus (EBV) transformed B cell lines. The molecule involved in differentiation was found to be separable from IL-2 and B cell growth factor (Teranishi et al, 1982; Yoshizaki et al, 1982) . The establishment of human T cell hybridoma generating BSF-2 activity confirmed that BSF-2 is a distinct molecule from other cytokines (Okada et al, 1983). Subsequently it was demonstrated that BSF-2 functions in the late phase of Staphylococcus aureus Cowan I stimulated normal B cells to induce Ig-production provided other factors, such as IL-2 were available (Hirano et al, 1984; Teranishi et al, 1984). Furthermore, BSF-2 was found to act on B cell lines at the mRNA level and induce biosynthesis of secretory type Ig (Kikutani et al, 1985). It is now established that IL-6 (BSF-2/IFN-β2/26kD protein/HPGF/HSF) is a multifunctional cytokine produced by a variety of lymphoid and non-lymphoid cells. As summarized in Fig.1, the activities of IL-6 are follows: 1) induction of B cell differentiation, 2) induction of cell growth of myeloma/plasmacytoma/hybridoma cells (Van Damme et al, 1987; Kawano et al, 1988) and EBV-transformed B lymphoblastoid cell lines (Tosato et al, 1988), 3) induction of IL-2 production (Garman et al, 1987), cell growth (Lotz et al, 1988) and cytotoxic T cell differentiation (Takai et al, 1988) in T cells, 4) induction of macrophage differentiation (Miyaura et al, in press), 5) stimulation of multipotential colony formation in haematopoietic stem cells (Ikebuchi et al, 1987), 6) regulation of acute phase response (Andus et al, 1987; Gauldie et al, 1987), and 7) induction of neural differentiation (Satoh et al, in press). Furthermore, it has been demonstrated that deregulated production of IL-6 may be involved in a variety of chronic inflammatory diseases and certain lymphoid malignancies (Kawano et al, 1988; Hirano et al, 1987).

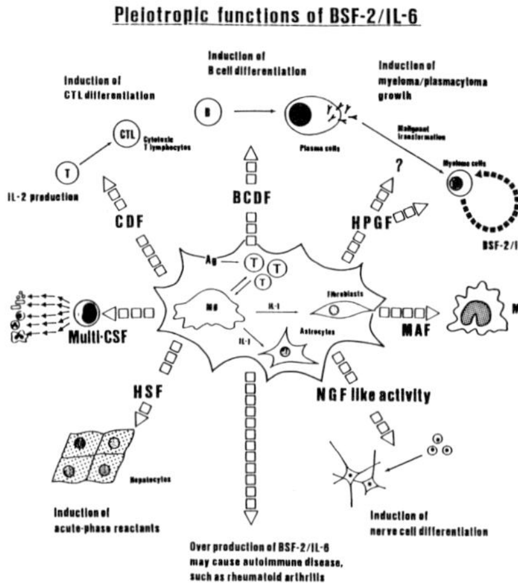

Fig. 1. Pleiotropic function of IL-6

STRUCTURE OF IL-6 AND ITS GENE.

We purifeid human IL-6 to homogeneity (Hirano et al, 1985) from the culture supernatant of a human T cell leukemia virus type I (HTLV-1) transformed T cell line and determined its partial N-terminal amino acid sequence (Hirano et al, 1987). The nucleotide sequence and deduced amino acid sequence of the cloned cDNA show that IL-6 consists of 212 amino acids including a hydrophobic signal sequence of 28 amino acids (Hirano et al, 1986). The sequence of IL-6 was compared to other known proteins. Only human G-CSF showed a significant homology with IL-6; the position of four cysteine residues of IL-6 match with those of G-CSF, suggesting a similarity in the tertiary structure of these two molecules. Furthermore, it was found that the organization of the IL-6 gene is very similar to that of G-CSF; both genes consist of 5 exons and 4 introns and the size of each exon is strikingly similar (Yasukawa et al, 1987). These findings suggest that the genes for IL-6 and G-CSF might be evolutionarily derived from a common ancestor gene.

PRODUCTION OF IL-6.

It has been found that IL-6 is produced by many different types of lymphoid or non-lymphoid cells, either constitutively or in response to various stimuli. Although we purified IL-6 from a HTLV-1-transformed T cell line (Hirano et al, 1985), there are, so far, no direct evidence that normal T cells indeed produce IL-6. In order to demonstrate that IL-6 is produced by T cells, immunocytochemical staining of cultured purified T cells was performed utilizing anti-IL-6 monoclonal antibody (MoAb) (αBSF2-166, Matsuda et al, 1988). Stimulation with PHA alone induced blast formation of $CD3^+$ T cells, but the stimulated T cells were not stained with αBSF2-166. However if $CD3^+$ T cells were stimulated with PHA in the presence of monocytes, the cells forming rosette with sheep red blood cells were specifically stained with anti-IL-6 MoAb. The data indicated that T cells produce IL-6 only in a monocyte dependent manner. The functions of monocytes could be replaced by TPA but not by IL-1. Monocytes produced IL-6 in the absence of an apparent stimulus, and the peak IL-6 mRNA expression was achieved at 5 hrs following culture, whereas that of T cells was at around 48 hrs after culture initiation, indicating that IL-6 produced by monocytes and T cells with different kinetics may exert distinct functions at different phases of the immune response.

It has been demonstrated that a variety of stimuli induces IL-6 production in a various kinds of cells. S1-mapping and primer extension analyses showed the presence of multiple initiation sites and the preferential utilization of specific initiation site in a variety of cells (Yasukawa et al, 1987), suggesting that different regulatory mechanisms may be responsible for the expression of IL-6 gene in different tissues. In fact, sequences similar to transcriptional enhancer elements such as c-fos serum response element, cAMP consensus, AP-1 binding consensus and glucocorticoid receptor consensus regions have been identified in the 5'flanking region.

IL-6 RECEPTOR IS AN IMMUNOGLOBULIN SUPERFAMILY.

The specific receptor for IL-6 (IL-6-R) was found to be expressed on lymphoid cells as well as non-lymphoid cells in accordance with the multifunctional properties of IL-6 (Taga et al, 1987). Binding of ^{125}I-IL-6 to B lymphoblastoid cell line was competitively inhibited by unlabeled IL-6 but not by IL-1, IL-2, IFN-β2, IFN-γ and G-CSF. The cells express IL-6-R are EBV-transformed B cell lines, myeloid cell lines, hepatoma cell lines, myeloma cell lines, resting normal T lymphocytes and activated normal B lymphocytes as summarized in Table 1. Scatchard plot analysis demonstrated that both high and low affinity IL-6-R with Kd value 1.7×10^{-11} and 1×10^{-9}M, respectively are expressed on a myeloma cell line, U266. The number of the high affinity receptors was about 10% of the total receptors. In order to reveal the molecular structure of the IL-6-R and analyse the mechanisms of signal transduction, attempts were made to clone the cDNA for the IL-6-R. Biotinated IL-6 and fluorescein-conjugated avidin were employed as a probe for the detection of the IL-6-R. We also employed a high efficiency COS7 cell expression system with CDM8 vector (provided by Dr. B. Seed). A cDNA clone (pBSF2R.236) was isolated and in order to characterize IL-6-R encoded by pBSF2R.236 insert cDNA, a stable transfectant, JBSF2R expressing IL-6-R was established from a human T cell line, Jurkat. Scatchard plot analysis demonstrated that JBSF2R expressed both high and low affinity IL-6-R. Northern blot analysis with the pBSF2R.236 insert cDNA showed that mRNA of approximately 6 kb long was expressed in a myeloma cell line (U266), a B lymphoblastoid cell line (CESS) and a histiocytic cell line (U937) but not in a Barkitt's cell line (BL29) and a T cell line (Jurkat). The result coincided with the data obtained by the binding study. The deduced amino acid sequence demonstrated that IL-6-R consists of 468 amino acids including a signal peptide of ~ 19 amino acids followed by a domain of ~ 90 amino acids belonging to the Ig superfamily. The cytoplasmic domain consists of ~ 82 amino acids lacking a tyrosine-kinase domain. The schematic model of IL-6-R is illustrated in Fig.2.

Table 1. Expression of IL-6-R on a variety of cells

cells	number of receptor/cell
EBV-transformed B cell lines	200 - 3,000
Barkitt's lymphoma cell lines	not detectable
myeloma cells and cell lines	100 - 20,000
hepatoma cell lines	2,000 - 3,000
myeloid leukemia cell lines	2,000 - 3,000
rat pheochromocytoma cell line	~ 1,200
resting B cells	not detectable
activated B cells	~500
resting T cells	~300

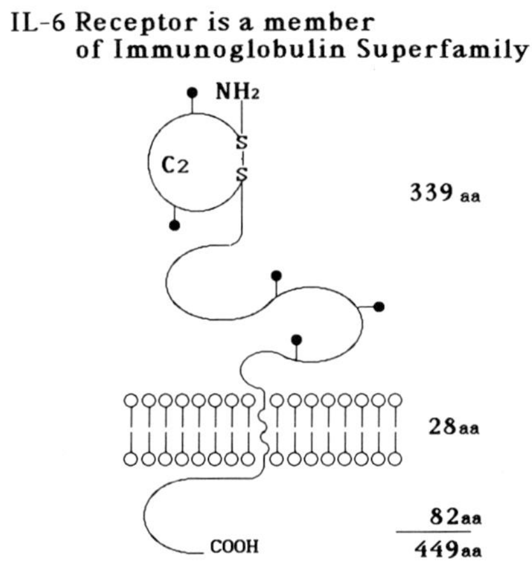

Fig. 2. Schematic model of IL-6 receptor

ESSENTIAL ROLE OF IL-6 IN THE ANTIBODY FORMATION.

In order to study whether IL-6 is obligatory for B cells to produce antibodies, the effect of anti-IL-6 antibodies on pokeweed mitogen (PWM)-induced Ig production was examined. Peripheral blood mononuclear cells (MMC) were cultured with PWM in the presence of anti-IL-6 for 8 days. As shown in Fig.3A, the PWM-induced IgG production was inhibited up to 80% by the addition of anti-IL-6 antibody. The same observation was made with the F(ab')2 fragment of anti-IL-6 antibody, indicating that the inhibition was not mediated through the Fc receptor. Furthermore, the inhibitory effect of anti-IL-6 was reversed by the addition of excess amount of recombinant IL-6. The antibody was effective even when added on day 4 of an 8 day culture. However, anti-IL-6 antibody had no effect on PWM-induced ^{3}H-TdR uptake which was measured on day 3 and 7 (Fig.3B). These results indicated that IL-6 is one of the essential late-acting factors for the Ig-induction in B cells but not responsible for the growth of mitogen-stimulated B cells.

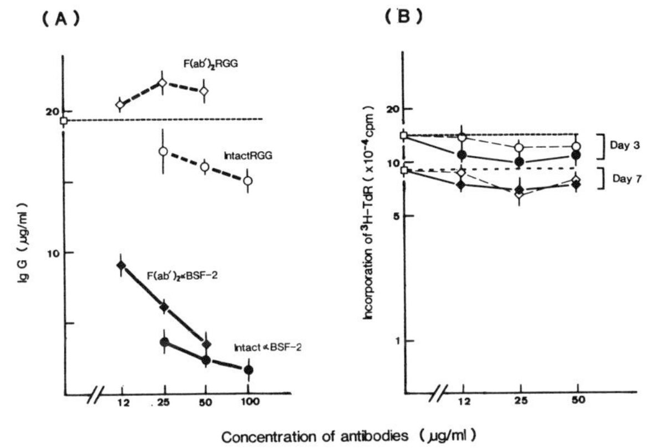

Fig.3. Effect of anti-IL-6 antibodies on PWM-induced Ig-production (A) and proliferation (B) of B cells. (A) (●—●), whole IgG of the antibodies; (◆—◆), F(ab')2 fragment of the antibodies; RGG, normal rabbit IgG. (B) (●,◆), whole IgG of the antibodies; (○,◇), normal rabbit IgG. (taken from Muraguchi et al, 1988.)

IL-6 AND AUTOIMMUNE DISEASES

Systemic autoimmune diseases are characterized by hyperactivation of B cells and the production of various autoantibodies. Several studies in murine systems suggest that the dysregulation of lymphokine production or the production of abnormal lymophokines could be responsible for the hyperactivation of auto-antibody producing B cells. Since IL-6 is responsible for Ig-induction in B cells, IL-6 may be a principle lymphokine for generalized autoimmune diseases.

One of the typical examples is cardiac myxoma, which is a benign intraatrial heart tumor and one third of the patients show autoimmune phenomenon with auto-antibody production (Sutton et al, 1980). Furthermore, these symptoms disappear upon the surgical removal of the tumor, suggesting that the myxoma itself or its products are involved in the autoimmune condition of these patients. In fact, the culture supernatants of cardiac myxoma cells were found to display high IL-6 activity (Hirano et al, 1987). Northern blot analysis with the cDNA for IL-6 confirmed the elevated expression of mRNA in cardiac myxoma cells (Hirano et al, 1986). The results strongly suggest that the overproduction of IL-6 may be responsible for autoantibody production and autoimmune phenomenon.

Then, the question to be asked is whether the overproduction of IL-6 is involved in the pathogenesis of generalized autoimmune diseases, such as rheumatoid arthritis (RA). The concentration of IL-6 in the synovial fluids from the affected joints of RA and osteoarthritis (OA) patients was measured by a RIA with anti-IL-6 antibodies. As shown in Fig.4, 22 out of 25 specimens (92%) from RA patients showed detectable levels of IL-6. The mean value of IL-6 in these 22 samples was 15.6 ± 13 ng/ml (2.6 -59 ng/ml). However, only 4 out of 17 specimens (24%) obtained from OA patients displayed detectable but low level of IL-6 (3.4 - 5.8 ng/ml). The synovial tissues (18 samples) biopsied from active

RA patients, when incubated for 24 hr, produced large amounts of IL-6 (mean value was 212 ± 165 units/ml), and the activity was completely neutralized by anti-IL-6 antibodies. These results suggest that the unregulated productions of IL-6 may play an important role in the pathogenesis of RA and explain the infiltration of synovium by a large number of plasma cells and the production of various autoantibodies including rheumatoid factor. As it was described, IL-6 functions as hepatocyte stimulating factor to induce acute phase proteins and it also could induce fever as an endogenous pyrogen (Nijstein et al, 1987). Therefore, not only local but also several of the generalized symptoms in RA patients, such as hyper γ-globulinemia, an increase in acute phase proteins and fever, could be explained by the overproduction of IL-6.

IL-6 IS AN AUTOCRINE GROWTH FACTOR FOR MULTIPLE MYELOMAS.

IL-6 was found to be an autocrine growth factor for human multiple myelomas (Kawano et al, 1988): i) IL-6 could augment the in vitro proliferation of myeloma cells in 12 out of 26 cases (Fig.5A); ii) myeloma cells constitutively produce IL-6 and express IL-6 receptor in all cases examined and iii) most importantly, anti-IL-6 antibodies inhibit the in vitro proliferation of myeloma cells (Fig.5B). Potter et al (Potter and Boyce, 1962; Nordan and Potter, 1986) demonstrated that murine plasmacytoma developed exclusively from the mineral-oil-induced epitheloid tissue composed of macrophages and neutrophils and suggested that macrophage-derived growth factors, which is now known to be identical to IL-6 (Van Snick et al, 1988), may accelerate the development of plasmacytoma. The evidence suggests that deregulated expression of the genes encoding IL-6 and/or IL-6 receptor is involved in the oncogenesis of myeloma. The results implicates that specific inhibitors of IL-6 or anti-IL-6 antibodies may be possible candidates for the specific therapy of multiple myelomas.

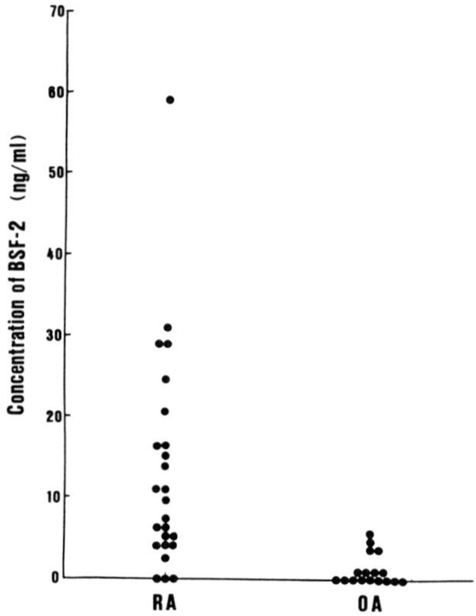

Fig. 4. Concentration of IL-6 in the synovial fluids from active RA and OA patients

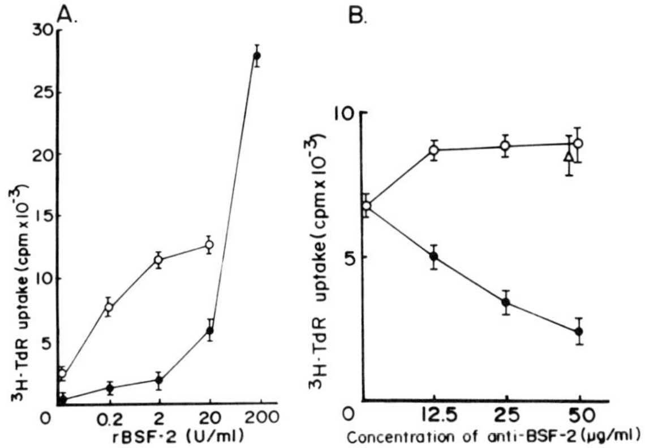

Fig. 5. (A) Augmentation of the proliferation of myeloma cells isolated from patients with multiple myeloma. Two representative cases are shown. (B) Inhibition of the in vitro growth of myeloma cells by anti-IL-6 antibody (●) and the rescue of the inhibitory effect by the addition of rIL-6 (▲). (○) represents normal rabbit IgG. (taken from Kawano et al, 1988).

CONCLUSION.

It has been demonstrated that IL-6 is a multifunctional cytokine acting on B cells, T cells, monocytes, haematopoietic stem cells, hepatocytes and nerve cells. Thus IL-6 may play a central regulatory role in host-defense mechanisms against infections, inflammations and tissue injuries. IL-6 is produced in various tissues and it has been suggested that the deregulated expression of IL-6 and/or its receptor may be involved in the pathogenesis of autoimmune diseases and multiple myeloma. Therefore, future studies on the regulation of expression of IL-6 and its receptor and the mechanisms of signal transduction through the receptor will provide critical information on the regulation of growth and differentiation of various cell types and it will also shed light on the role of IL-6 in the pathogenesis of various diseases. Furthermore, it will provide new diagnostic means and treatment approaches to these diseases.

ACKNOWLEDGEMENTS

The authors would like to thank Drs. B. Seed and T. Taniguchi for providing a cDNA library and Dr. E. Barsoumian for critical review of the manuscript. We also thank Ms. M. Harayama and K. Kubota for their secretarial assistance.

REFERENCES

Andus, T., Geiger, T., Hirano, T., Northoff, H., Ganter, U., Bauer, J., Kishimoto, T. and Heinrich, P.C. (1987). FEBS Lett. 221, 18-22.
Garman, R.D., Jacobs, K.A., Clark, S.C. and Raulet, D.H. (1987). Proc. Natl. Acad. Sci. USA. 84, 7629-7633.
Gauldie, J., Richards, C., Harnish, D., Lansdorp, P. and Baumann, H. (1987). Proc. Natl. Acad. Sci. USA. 84, 7251-7255.
Haegeman, G., Content, J., Volckaert, G., Derynck, R., Tavernier, J. and Fiers, W. (1986). Eur. J. Biochem. 159, 625-632.

Hirano, T., Taga, T., Nakano, N., Yasukawa, K., Kashiwamura, S., Shimizu, K., Nakajima, K., Pyun, K.H. and Kishimoto, K. (1985). Proc. Natl. Acad. Sci. USA. 82, 5490-5494.
Hirano, T., Yasukawa, K., Harada, H., Taga, T., Watanabe, Y., Matsuda, T., Kashiwamura, S., Nakajima, K., Koyama, K., Iwamatu, A., Tsunasawa, S., Sakiyama, F., Matsui, H., Takahara, Y., Taniguchi, T. and Kishimoto, T. (1986). Nature 324, 73-76.
Hirano, T., Teranishi, T., Lin, B.H. and Onoue, K. (1984). J. Immunol. 133, 798-802.
Hirano, T., Taga, T., Yasukawa, K., Nakajima, K., Nakano, N., Takatsuki, F., Shimizu, M., Murashima, A., Tsunasawa, S., Sakiyama, F. and Kishimoto, T. (1987). Proc. Natl. Acad. Sci. USA. 84, 228-231.
Ikebuchi, K., Wong, G.G., Clark, S.C., Ihle, J.N., Hirai, Y. and Ogawa, M. (1987). Proc. Natl. Acad. Sci. USA. 84, 9035-9039.
Kawano, M., Hirano, T., Matsuda, T., Taga, T., Horii, Y., Iwato, K., Asaoku, H., Tang, B., Tanabe, O., Tanaka, H., Kuramoto, A. and Kishimoto, T. (1988). Nature 332, 83-85.
Kikutani, H., Taga, T., Akira, S., Kishi, H., Miki, Y., Saiki, O., Yamamura, Y. and Kishimoto, T. (1985). J. Immunol. 134, 990-995.
Lotz, M., Jirik, F., Kabouridis, R., Tsoukas, C., Hirano, T., Kishimoto, T., and Carson, D.A. (1988). J. Exp. Med. in press.
Matsuda, T., Hirano, T. and Kishimoto, T. Eur. J. Immunol. in press.
May, L.T., Helfgott, D.C. and Sehgal, P.B. (1986). Proc. Natl. Acad. Sci. USA. 83, 8957-8961.
Miyaura, C., Onozaki, K., Akiyama, Y., Taniyama, T., Hirano, T., Kishimoto, T. and Suda, T. FEBS Lett. in press.
Muraguchi, A., Kishimoto, T., Miki, Y., Kuritani, T., Kaieda, T., Yoshizaki, K. and Yamamura, Y. (1981). J. Immunol. 127, 412-416.
Muraguchi, A., Hirano, T., Tang, B., Matsuda, T., Horii, K., Nakajima, K. and Kishimoto, T. (1988). J. Exp. Med. 167, 332-344.
Nijistein, M.W.N., De Groot, E.R., Ten Duis, H.J., Klasen, H.J., Hack, C.E. and Aarden, L.A. (1987). The Lancet ii, 921-921.
Nordan, P.R. and Potter, M. (1986). Science 233, 566-569.
Okada, M., Sakaguchi, N., Yoshimura, N., Hara, H., Shimizu, K., Yoshida, N., Yoshizaki, K., Kishimoto, S., Yamamura, Y. and Kishimoto, T. (1983). J. Exp. Med. 157, 583-590.
Potter, M. and Boyce, C. (1962). Nature 193, 1086-1087.
Satoh, T.S., Nakamura, T., Taga, T., Matsuda, T., Hirano, T., Kishimoto, T. and Kaziro, Y. Mol. Cell. Biol. in press
Sutton, M.G.S.J., Mercier, L., Giuliani, E.R. and Lie, J.T. (1980). Mayo Clin. Proc. 55, 371-376.
Taga, T., Kawanishi, K., Hardy, R.R., Hirano, T. and Kishimoto, T. (1987). J. Exp. Med. 166, 967-981.
Takai, Y., Wong, G.G., Clark, S.C., Burakoff, S.J. and Herrmann, S.H. (1988). J. Immunol. 140, 508-512.
Teranishi, T., Hirano, T., Arima, N. and Onoue, K. (1982). J. Immunol. 128, 1903-1908.
Teranishi, T., Hirano, T., Lin, B.H. and Onoue, K. (1984). J. Immunol. 133, 3062-3067.
Tosato, G., Seamon, K.B., Goldman, N.D., Sehgal, P.B., May, L.T., Washington, and Pike, S.E. (1988). Science 239, 502-504.
Van Damme, J., Opdenakker, G., Simpson, R.J., Rubira, M.R., Cayphas, S., Vink, A., Billiau, A. and Snick, J.V. (1987). J. Exp. Med. 165, 914-919.
Van Snick, J., Cayphas, S., Szikora, J.-P., Renauld, J.-C-., Van Roost, E., Boon, T. and Simpson, R.J. (1988). Eur. J. Immunol. 18, 193-197.
Yasukawa, K., Hirano, T., Watanabe, Y., Muratani, K., Matsuda, T. and Kishimoto, T. (1987). EMBO J. 6, 2939-2945.
Yoshizaki, K., Nakagawa, T., Kaieda, T., Muraguchi, A., Yamamura, Y. and Kishimoto, T. (1982). J. Immunol. 128, 1296-1301.
Zilberstein, A., Ruggieri, R., Korn, J.H. and Revel, M. (1986). EMBO J. 5, 2529-2537.

The Hybridoma/Plasmacytoma Growth Factor (HPGF) Activity of IL-6. Stimulation of its Secretion by Different Inducers in Various Cell Types

J. VAN DAMME°, J. VAN SNICK†, B. DECOCK, J.-P. LENAERTS, W. PUT, G. OPDENAKKER° and A. BILLIAU

Rega Institute for Medical Research, University of Leuven, B-3000 Leuven and †Ludwig Institute for Cancer Research, Brussels Branch, B-1200 Brussels, Belgium

KEYWORDS

HPGF: hybridoma/plasmacytoma growth factor; BSF-2: B-cell stimulatory factor-2; IFN-β: interferon-β; IL-1: interleukin-1; NDV: Newcastle disease virus; PolyrI:rC: polyriboinosinic-polyribocytidylic acid; LAF: lymphocyte activating factor.

INTRODUCTION

Human fibroblasts can be stimulated to produce a factor (HPGF) capable of supporting the growth of certain murine B-cell hybridomas and plasmacytomas (Van Damme *et al.*, 1987d). Natural HPGF has been purified to homogeneity and identified by NH_2-terminal sequence analysis (Van Damme *et al.*, 1987b) with T-cell-derived B-cell stimulatory factor-2 (BSF-2) (Hirano *et al.*, 1986), as well as with the fibroblast-derived interferon-β2 (IFN-β2) (Zilberstein *et al.*, 1986) or 26 kDa protein (Haegeman *et al.*, 1986). No biological activity could be ascribed to the 26 kDa protein, whereas IFN-β2 was claimed to have antiviral effect. HPGF, also identical with hepatocyte stimulating factor (Gauldie *et al.*, 1987) is now designated interleukin-6 (IL-6). Monocytes have been shown to produce a HPGF, identical to the fibroblast-derived HPGF/IL-6 (Brakenhoff *et al.*, 1987, Van Damme *et al.*, 1988). Recently, its biological activity has been extended to T-cells (Garman *et al.*, 1987; Lotz *et al.*, 1988, Baroja *et al.*, Houssiau *et al.*, 1988).

MATERIALS AND METHODS

Induction of HPGF/IL-6

Human diploid fibroblasts (strain E_6SM) and the cell lines used were cultivated in Eagle's minimum essential medium, supplemented with 10 % fetal or newborn calf serum. Confluent cultures were induced to produce HPGF/IL-6 by stimulation with different doses of pure natural IL-1β (Van Damme *et al.*, 1985), poly(rI).poly(rC) (P.L. Biochemicals Inc., Milwaukee, WI) or Newcastle disease virus (NDV). Supernatant fluids were harvested after a 48 hours induction pe-

°J. Van Damme is a research associate of the Belgian National Fund for Scientific Research, and G. Opdenakker is a senior research assistant.

riod. Samples containing virus were dialysed at pH 2.0 (for 48 hours) prior to assay.

Biological assays

B-cell hybridoma growth activity was determined on factor-dependent murine 7TD1 cells (Van Snick et al., 1986), 1 U/ml corresponding to half maximal increase in cell numbers. Plasmacytoma growth activity was measured by [^{3}H]thymidine incorporation by factor-dependent murine cell lines (Van Snick et al., 1987).

The antiviral activity of HPGF/IL-6, IFN-β, and IL-1 was detected on fibroblasts, using a standard cytopathic reduction assay (Van Damme et al., 1987c). Lymphocyte activating factor (LAF) activity was determined by [^{3}H]thymidine incorporation in murine thymocytes (Van Damme et al., 1988).

Purification procedure

HPGF/IL-6, produced by IL-1-stimulated MG-63 osteosarcoma cells, was purified to homogeneity as described (Van Damme et al., 1987b).

RESULTS AND DISCUSSION

Production of HPGF/IL-6 by fibroblasts stimulated by different inducers

IL-1 has been reported to be a potent inducer of HPGF/IL-6 in human fibroblasts (Van Damme et al., 1987a). TNF-α was found to be a weaker inducer, whereas other cytokines, including IL-2, IFN-γ, IFN-$β_1$ were only marginally inducing HPGF/IL-6.The conditions for induction of HPGF/IL-6 in fibroblasts showed similarities with those for IFN-$β_1$. For example, the double-stranded RNA polyrI:rC, which is known as a good inducer of IFN-$β_1$ in such cells, was found to be an even more potent inducer of HPGF/IL-6 (Van Damme et al., 1987a). Similarly, viruses such as Newcastle disease virus (NDV) used as IFN-inducers in mouse fibroblasts were found to stimulate HPGF/IL-6 production (Cayphas et al., 1987).

In Table 1, human IL-1β, polyrI:rC and NDV were compared for HPGF/IL-6 induction in both human and mouse fibroblasts. PolyrI:rC was found to be the best

Table 1. Dose-dependent induction of HPGF/IL-6 in fibroblasts by various inducers

Induction		Production of HPGF/IL-6[a] ($\log_{10}$ U/ml) on	
Substance	Dose	Human fibroblasts	Mouse L929
IL-1β	200 (U/ml)	3.0	< 1.0
	20	2.9	< 1.0
	2	2.7	< 1.0
	0.2	2.1	< 1.0
PolyrI:rC	100 (μg/ml)	3.8	2.8
	10	3.8	1.3
	1	3.3	< 1.0
	0.1	1.4	< 1.0
NDV	10 (HAU/ml)	3.4	3.6
	1	2.8	2.2
	0.1	1.4	< 1.0
	0.01	< 1.0	< 1.0

[a]measured by its B-cell hybridoma growth activity

inducer in human fibroblasts, whereas NDV was a better inducer in mouse L929 cells. Although human IL-1β was not active on mouse L929 cells, it can induce HPGF/IL-6 in mouse embryonic fibroblasts (data not shown). Optimal production was obtained with 10 μg/ml of polyrI:rC, 10 hemagglutination U/ml of NDV or 2-20 U/ml of natural IL-1β.

Induction of HPGF/IL-6 in different cell lines

It was verified whether the induction of HPGF/IL-6 in normal human fibroblasts could be extended to transformed cells. Table 2 shows that several human cell lines could produce HPGF/IL-6 after induction with IL-1β, polyrI:rC or NDV. The WISH amnion cells were comparable to diploid fibroblasts (E_6SM) in their response to those inducers, but did spontaneously produce some HPGF/IL-6. The MG-63 osteosarcoma cell line, developed for the production of IFN-β_1 (Billiau *et al.*, 1977), yielded high titers of HPGF/IL-6 after stimulation with IL-1β, but was less productive after treatment with polyrI:rC. The HEp-2 epidermal carcinoma cell line was only weakly responsive to IL-1β, whereas polyrI:rC was ineffective. NDV only marginally induced HPGF/IL-6 in these latter two cell lines.

No significant induction of HPGF/IL-6 by either of the three inducers was obtained with HeLa (carcinoma of cervix), HL-60 (promyelocytic leukemia) and Namalva (Burkitt lymphoma) cells. However, the Namalva cell line is known as a good producer of IFN after stimulation with NDV (Zoon *et al.*, 1978), and HL-60 cells have been described to express the receptor for IL-6 (Taga *et al.*, 1987).

Table 2. Production of HPGF/IL-6 by various human cell lines

Cell line	Production of HPGF/IL-6[a] ($\log_{10}$ U/ml) after			
	IL-1β	PolyrI:rC	NDV	Control
E_6SM	3.8	4.3	2.9	< 1.0
WISH	3.2	3.6	2.8	1.6
MG-63	3.8	2.9	1.6	< 1.0
HEp-2	2.7	< 1.0	1.6	< 1.0
HeLa	< 1.0	1.4	< 1.0	< 1.0
HL-60	< 1.0	< 1.0	< 1.0	< 1.0
Namalva	< 1.0	< 1.0	< 1.0	< 1.0

[a] measured by its B-cell hybridoma growth activity

Identification of fibroblast-derived HPGF/IL-6 with BSF-2 and IFN-β2/26kDa protein

Supernatant fluids of MG-63 cells stimulated with IL-1β were used as a source of HPGF/IL-6. The use of the highly sensitive and specific hybridoma growth assay has facilitated the purification of HPGF/IL-6 to homogeneity. Nevertheless, five different concentrations and purification steps were necessary in order to obtain pure protein (Van Damme *et al.*, 1987b). HPGF/IL-6 was first adsorbed to controlled pore glass, then chromatographed on an antibody column and subsequently fractionated by gel filtration. These three steps resulted in a 10,000-fold purification and 100-fold concentration (Table 3). The HPGF/IL-6 activity from gel filtration, eluting in a single peak with an Mr of 27,000, was further purified to homogeneity by cation-exchange chromatography and reversed-phase HPLC. The pure factor appeared as a single protein band upon SDS-PAGE with an Mr of 23,000. The molecule showed a specific activity of 10^9 U/mg in the hybridoma growth assay.

NH_2-terminal sequence analysis revealed that HPGF/IL-6 corresponds to the T-cell-derived, BSF-2 as well as to the fibroblast-derived 26kDa/IFN-β_2 protein lacking a defined function. Some heterogeneity was observed in that different NH_2-terminal positions were found for HPGF/IL-6 and BSF-2 proteins (Van Damme et al., 1987b; Hirano et al., 1987).

Table 3. Purification of fibroblast-derived HPGF/IL-6 to homogeneity[a]

Purification step	Concentration factor	Recovery of HPGF/IL-6	Purification factor
1) Adsorption to CPG	10	90	60
2) Antibody chromatography	10	90	10
3) Gel filtration	1	60	20
4) Cation exchange column (FPLC)	5	90	5
5) Reversed phase HPLC	1	100	3
Total	500	50	150,000

[a]Starting material (1500 ml at 1 mg/ml protein) contained about 10^7 units of HPGF/IL-6 (hybridoma growth activity).

Biological activities of HPGF/IL-6

Since HPGF/IL-6, strongly inducible with IL-1, was found to be identical with IFN-β2, its biological properties were compared with those of IL-1 and IFN-β1. Although IFN-β1 and IL-1 did show antiviral effect on human fibroblasts, no such activity could be detected with natural HPGF/IL-6. This finding (Van Damme et al., 1987d) is in contrast with the antiviral effect ascribed to recombinant IFN-β2 (Zilberstein et al., 1986). However, it is in agreement with the observation by others that recombinant 26 kDa protein (Poupart et al., 1987) and BSF-2 (Reis et al., 1988) did not possess such antiviral activity. In addition, HPGF/IL-6 was found not to be responsable for the antiviral activity of IL-1 since only antibody against IFN-β1 and not to HPGF/IL-6 were able to neutralize this effect (Van Damme et al., 1987c).

Table 4. Activity of human HPGF/IL-6 in various biological assays as compared to IL-1β and IFN-β1

Assay system	Biological activity (%) of		
	IFN-β1	IL-1β	IL-6
Antiviral effect	100	90	< 0.1
Thymocyte activation	< 0.1	100	5
Plasmacytoma growth	< 0.1	< 0.2	1
B-cell hybridoma growth	< 0.1	< 0.2	100

In contrast to its lack of IFN-β like activity, natural HPGF/IL-6 did possess, similarly to IL-1, lymphocyte activating factor (LAF) activity, as tested on thymocytes. Whereas IL-1β showed an identical specific activity in both the antiviral and the LAF assay, HPGF/IL-6 was less active on thymocytes than on B-cell hybridomas (Table 4).

Similarly to the HPGF/IL-6 dependent B-cell hybridomas some murine plasmacytoma cell lines can only be kept surviving in vitro in the presence of murine (Van Snick et al., 1987) or human HPGF/IL-6 (Van Damme et al., 1987d). However, more HPGF/IL-6 was needed to sustain the growth of plasmacytomas as compaired to hybridomas (Table 4). IL-1β and IFN-β1 were not active on those plasmacytomas and hybridomas, indicating the specificity of these cells as test system for HPGF/IL-6.

CONCLUSION

Hybridoma/plasmacytoma growth factor (HPGF/IL-6) can be induced in fibroblasts by various agents, such as the cytokines IL-1 and TNF-α (Content et al., 1985; Kohase et al., 1986; Van Damme et al., 1987a), the double stranded RNA polyrI:rC (Van Damme et al., 1987a) and certain viruses, e.g. NDV (Cayphas et al., 1987). Depending on the inducer substance and the cell type used different amounts of HPGF/IL-6 were found to be produced.

Fibroblast-derived HPGF/IL-6 was purified to homogeneity (Van Damme et al., 1987d) and identified with BSF-2 (Hirano et al., 1986) and 26 kDa/IFN-β2 (Haegeman et al., 1986, Zilberstein et al., 1986). However, unlike IFN-β1 natural HPGF/IL-6 does not possess antiviral activity (Van Damme et al., 1987). Like IL-1, the molecule can activate thymocytes. Hence, HPGF/IL-6 is active on both B- and T-cells. The effect of HPGF/IL-6 on T-cells has been confirmed recently in several laboratories (Garman et al., 1987; Lotz et al., 1988; Houssiau et al., 1988; Baroja, 1988).

ACKNOWLEDGMENT

We wish to thank Chris Callebaut and Odette Van Brusselen for excellent editorial help.

REFERENCES

Baroja, M.L., Ceuppens J.L., Van Damme, J. and Billiau A. (1988). J.Immunol. (in press).

Billiau, A., Edy, V.G., Heremans, H., Van Damme, J., Desmyter, J., Georgiades, J.A. and De Somer, P. (1977). Antimicrob. Agents Chemother 12, 11-15.

Brakenhoff, J.P.J., De Groot, E.R., Evers R.F., Pannekoek H. and Aarden L.A. (1987). J. Immunol. 139, 4116-4121.

Cayphas S., Van Damme J., Vink A., Simpson R.J., Billiau A. and Van Snick J. (1987) J. Immunol. 139, 2965-2969.

Content J., De Wit L., Poupart, P., Opdenakker G., Van Damme J. and Billiau, A. (1985). Eur. J. Biochem 152, 253-257.

Garman R.D., Jacobs K.A., Clark S.C. and Raulet D.H. (1987). Proc. Natl. Acad. Sci. USA 84, 7629-7633.

Gauldie J., Richards C., Harnish D., Lansdorp P. and Baumann H. (1987). Proc. Natl. Acad. Sci. USA 84, 7251-7255.

Haegeman G., Content J., Volckaert G., Derynck R., Tavernier J. and Fiers W. (1986). Eur. J. Biochem. 159, 625-632.

Hirano T., Yasukawa, K., Harada H., Taga T., Watanabe Y., Matsuda T., Kashiwamura S.-I., Nakajima K., Koyama K., Iwamatsu A., Tsunasawa S., Sakiyama F., Matsui H., Takahara Y., Taniguchi T. and Kishimoto T. (1986). Nature 324, 73-76.

Hirano T., Taga T., Yasukawa, K., Nakajima K., Nakano N., Takatsuki F., Shimizu M., Murashima A., Tsunasawa S., Sakiyama F. and Kishimoto T. (1987). Proc. Natl. Acad. Sci. USA 84, 228-231.

Houssiau F.A., Coulie P.G., Olive D. and Van Snick J. (1988). Eur. J. Immunol. in press.

Kohase M., Henriksen-DeStefano D., May L.T., Vilcek J. and Sehgal P.B. (1986). Cell 45, 659-669.

Lotz, M., Jirik F., Kabouridis P., Tsoukas C., Hirano T., Kishimoto T. and Carson D.A. (1988). J. Exp. Med. 167, 1253-1258.

Poupart P., Vandenabeele P., Cayphas S., Van Snick J., Haegeman G., Kruys V., Fiers W. and Content J. (1987). The EMBO Journal 6, 1219-1224.

Reis L.F., Le J., Hirano T., Kishimoto T. and Vilcek J. (1988). J. Immunol. 140, 1566-1570.

Taga T., Kawanishi Y., Hardy R.R., Hirano T. and Kishimoto T. (1987). J. Exp. Med. 166, 967-981.

Van Damme J., De Ley M., Opdenakker G., Billiau A., De Somer P. and Van Beeumen J. (1985). Nature 314, 266-268.

Van Damme J., Cayphas S., Opdenakker G., Billiau A. and Van Snick J. (1987a). Eur. J. Immunol. 17, 1-7.

Van Damme J., Cayphas S., Van Snick J., Conings R., Put W., Lenaerts J.-P., Simpson R.J. and Billiau A. (1987b). Eur. J. Biochem. 168, 543-550.

Van Damme J., De Ley M., Van Snick J., Dinarello C.A. and Billiau A. (1987c). J. Immunol. 139, 1867-1872.

Van Damme J., Opdenakker G., Simpson R.J., Rubira M.R., Cayphas S., Vink A., Billiau A. and Van Snick J. (1987d) J. Exp. Med. 165, 914-919.

Van Damme J., Van Beeumen J., Decock B., Van Snick J., De Ley M. and Billiau A. (1988). J. Immunol. 140, 1534-1541.

Van Snick J., Cayphas S., Vink A., Uyttenhove C., Coulie P.G., Rubira M.R. and Simpson R.J. (1986). Proc. Natl. Acad. Sci. USA 83, 9679-9683.

Van Snick J., Vink A., Cayphas S. and Uyttenhove C. (1987). J. Exp. Med. 165, 641-649.

Zilberstein A., Ruggieri R., Korn J.H. and Revel M. (1986). The EMBO Journal 5, 2529-2537.

Zoon K.C., Buckler C.E., Bridgen P.J. and Gurari-Rotman D. (1978). J. Clin. Microbiol. 7, 44-51.

Interferon-type and Other Activities of IFN-ß-2/BSF-2/HSF

M. REVEL, L. CHEN, Y. MORY, A. ZILBERSTEIN
and R. MICHALEVICZ*

*Dept of Virology, Weizmann Institute of Science, Rehovot, and *Dept of Hematology, Ichilov Hospital, Tel-Aviv, Israel*

ABSTRACT

The multiple activities of IFN-β-2 (BSF-2, IL-6, 26 Kd, HGF, HSF) suggest that this multifunctional cytokine plays a role in the various aspects of inflammation resulting from pathogenic infections.

INTRODUCTION

The cytokine IFN-β-2 was first described and cloned from ds RNA-induced human fibroblasts by its β-IFN type antiviral and antigrowth activity (Weissenbach et al,1980; Sehgal and Sagar, 1980; Zilberstein et al,1986). IFN-β-2 is induced in fibroblasts by viral ds RNA, TNF, IL-1 (Zilberstein et al,1986; Kohase et al,1986), bacterial LPS (Helfgott et al,1987) and growth stimulants (Zhang et al,1988). It was then shown to be identical to the B cell differentiation factor BSF-2 also named IL-6 (Hirano et al,1986) and to stimulate growth of plasmacytomas and hybridomas (HGF activity) (Van Damme et al,1987) and of EBV-transformed human B cells (Tosato et al,1988). IFN-β-2 is, however, a potent growth-inhibitor for tumor cells (Revel et al,1987; Chen et al,1988). The cytokine is also an HSF stimulating synthesis of the acute phase proteins in hepatocytes (Gauldie et al,1987) and it was found to induce complement factor B and C3 synthesis in fibroblasts (Katz et al,1988). Activation of T-cell functions (Takai et al,1988) and stimulation of differentiating hematopoietic colony formation (Ikebuchi et al,1987; Revel et al,1988) were also observed. This report describes some of these activities in recombinant E.coli-produced preparations of this multifunctional cytokine.

RESULTS

Direct expression of rIFN-β-2 in E.coli

The human IFN-β-2a cDNA (Zilberstein et al,1986) was fused at the PRO^{29} codon to a MET initator codon and a tryplac promoter and expressed in IPTG-induced E.coli JM101 i^q (pkkβ2/7). Nucleic acid free extracts were obtained by polyethylene imine precipitation and passage on DEAE cellulose. The effluent fractions were adsorbed onto S-Sepharose in 10 mM Na acetate pH 5 (Buffer A) and eluted by a 0-0.3 M NaCl gradient. Active fractions were pooled, dialyzed against buffer A and chromatographed on a Mono-S FPLC column eluted with a 0-0.3M NaCl gradient. Two activities were followed during purification: 1) HGF activity measured as

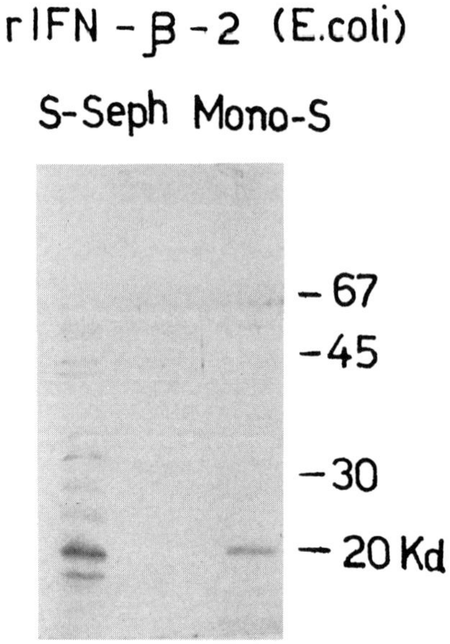

Fig 1.

Purification of rIFN-β-2 produced in E. coli (see text). Polyacrylamide gel electrophoresis in SDS after the Sulfonyl Sepharose step (2.4 μg, left) and the Mono-S FPLC step (0.4 μg, right). The middle slot contained only buffer. Coomassie blue stain.

Fig 2 (below).

Antiviral assay as described in the text. The colored wells indicate protection against virus.

ANTIVIRAL ACTIVITY OF rIFN-β2
(E.coli) ON FS11 / VSV

1 2 3 4 5 6 7 8 9 10 11

IFN standard
Mock E.coli pKK
rIFN-β-2 (E.coli)

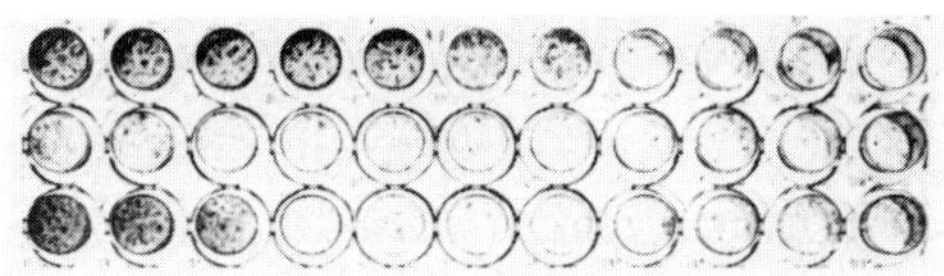

rIFN-β-2: wells 1= dil 1/100; 2=dil 1/200; 3=dil 1/400

---> TNF serial dilutions --->
0 1 2 3 4 5 6 7 8 9 10 11

Mock E.coli (dil 1/100)
rIFN-β-2 (E.coli)(dil 1/100)
No IFN

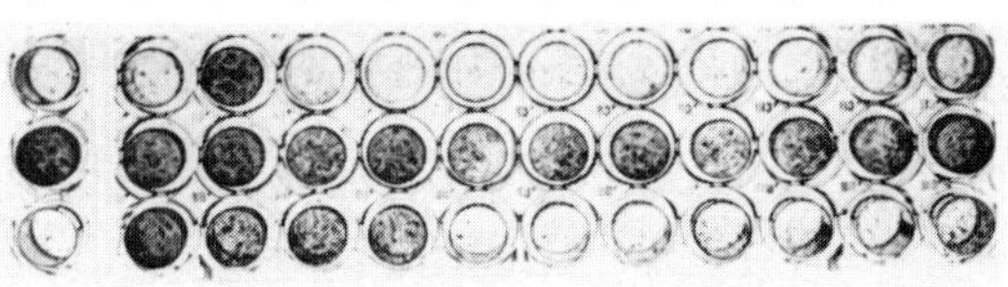

wells:	0	1	2	3	4	5	6	7	8	9	10	11
TNF U/ml:	0	25	12	6	3	1.5	0.7	0.35	0.17	0.09	0.045	0.025

increase in ^{3}H-thymidine (Td) incorporation in murine plasmacytoma cells T1165 (Dr R. Nordan, NIH) and 2) AP activity measured by inhibition of ^{3}H-Td incorporation in human breast cancer cells T47D. One unit is defined as the concentration needed for 50% of the maximal effect. HGF and AP activities were expressed at approximately the same concentration. These units are used throughout this report. The two activities co-eluted throughout the purification and coincided with the rIFN-β-2 protein on immunoblots with polyclonal antibodies against the N-terminal peptide PRO^{29}-THR^{48} of the IFN-β-2a precursor. The final preparation showed a single 20 Kd band on SDS-polyacrylamide gel electrophoresis (Fig. 1).

Activities of E.coli-produced rIFN-β-2.

a) Antiviral activity (AV). Human foreskin fibroblasts were seeded in 96-well microplate and cultured 10-12 days, the medium being changed at 7 days. The cells were exposed to serial dilutions of a rIFN-β-2 preparation titrating 12,000 HGF or BSF-2 U/ml for 24 hours infected by VSV and stained by crystal violet 3 days post-infection. Protection was observed up to a 1:400 dilution (30 HGF/AP U) of rIFN-β-2. A comparable preparation from E.coli transformed by the same plasmid without the IFN-β-2 cDNA (mock) gave no protection (Fig. 2). In 3 repeat experiments the titers varied from 1:400 to 1:1600. It is interesting to note that the cell culture conditions required for antiviral response to rIFN-β-2 (E.coli) were the same as required for the antiviral activity of TNF, which protected down to 3 cytotoxic U/ml (Fig 2.). We also examined the effects of rIFN-βII-TNF mixtures. rIFN-β-2 (120 U/ml) protected irrespective of whether or not TNF was present, whereas mock did not protect the cells against VSV with or without TNF (Fig. 2). Thus, the antiviral action of rIFN-β-2 (E.coli) on 12-day fibrocytes does no require the presence of TNF. The AV activity is, however, low compared to most other IFNs (Revel et al, 1987).

b) Antiproliferative effect (AP) We have reported that IFN-β-2 is a potent inhibitor of tumor cell growth (Revel et al,1987). Colony formation by breast ductal carcinoma cells T47D and by breast adenocarcinoma cells MCF-7 cells was inhibited 80-90% by rIFN-β-2 (E.coli) at concentrations of 10-20 (HGF) U/ml in a 15 day assay. In short-term (24 hours) assays a marked decrease in ^{3}H-Td

Table 1: NEUTRALIZATION OF THE ANTIGROWTH EFFECT OF rIFN-β-2

Additions	Antibodies	Breast Ca T47D cells [^{3}H]-Thymidine cpm x10^{-3}	Lymphoma U937 cells Cell Number x10^{-5}
None	None	95 ±2	16
IFN-β-2	None	28 ±2	10.5
IFN-β-2	Antipeptide P^{29}-T^{48}	95 ±3	18
IFN-β-2	Normal serum	24 ±1.5	10.6
IFN-β-2	McAB to IFN-β1	69 ±6	20
IFN-β-2	McAB to IFN-γ	11 ±2	12.8

IFN-β-2 (E.coli) used at 12 and 120 U/ml. Results are mean ± the standard deviation. McAB 29AB1 against IFN-β1 were used at 160 U/ml. Antibodies to the IFN-β-2 peptide (7500 U/ml for neutralization of the antiproliferative effect) were used at a 1:10 dilution. T47D cells treated for 24 hours and U937 for 3 days incorporation is observed (Table 1). Growth of the monocytic lymphoma cell line U937 was inhibited 50% after 3 days of treatment with about 20 HGF/AP U/ml (Table 1 and Chen et al,1988) and 60 U/ml completely prevented increase in number of cells. Cell death measured by trypan blue uptake was not increased. Removal of rIFN-β-2 led to resumption of growth at 1/2 the control rate. In Molt-4 T leukemia cells DNA synthesis was inhibited at the same concentrations as for U937 (Chen et al,1988). The Burkitt B lymphoma Daudi cells showed 50% ^{3}H-Td incorporation with 250 BSF-2 U/ml whereas the CESS B-lymphoblastoid cells were not inhibited. More differentiated EBV-transformed B-lymphocytes and plasmacytomas were stimulated (see below). HeLa cells and diploid fibroblasts showed 50% inhibition at 125 U/ml while murine L cells or rat leukemic RBL-1 cells were not inhibited (Chen et al,1988).

c) Hematopoietic Cell Differentiation

A 3 day treatment of U937 cells with rIFN-β-2 (E.coli about 50 U/ml) induced morphological changes (Fig. 3) and increased the monocytic surface antigens MO-1 and MO-2. The effect was similar to that caused by 10 U/ml IFN-γ. An increase in HLA-DR positive cells was also seen although smaller than that caused by IFN-γ. rIFN-β-2 appears, therefore, to trigger the monocytic differentiation of the U937 lymphoma cells as it decreases their growth. Recent studies have shown that Acute Lymphatic Leukemia cells are also stimulated to differentiate by rIFN-β-2.

We have previously reported (Revel et al,1988), that addition of rIFN-β-2 (CHO) to liquid cultures of hematopoietic stem cells from blood of hairy cell leukemia patients increases the number of colonies subsequently formed upon plating with CSFs indicating an activation of the pre-CFU cells. A similar effect is seen in normal bone marrow and blood stem cells, IFN-β-2 synergizing with IL-3 to increase colonies, e.g. erythroid bursts (BFU-E) (Table 2). Ikebuchi et al (1987) showed that IFN-β-2/IL-6 synergizes with IL-3 to increase blast cell colonies, being thought to consist of pre-CFU cells. IFN-β-2 is not by itself capable to support hematopoietic colony formation (CFUs) as IL-3 or GM-CSF. Recently, it was discovered that the murine hematopoietic factor MGI-2 is identical to IFN-β-2/IL-6 (Sachs et al, personal commun.). MGI-2 was known to increase the receptors to IL-3 and other CSFs (Lotem and Sachs,1986). The effect of IFN-β-2 in hematopoiesis could be best explained, therefore, as due to differentiation of the stem cells.

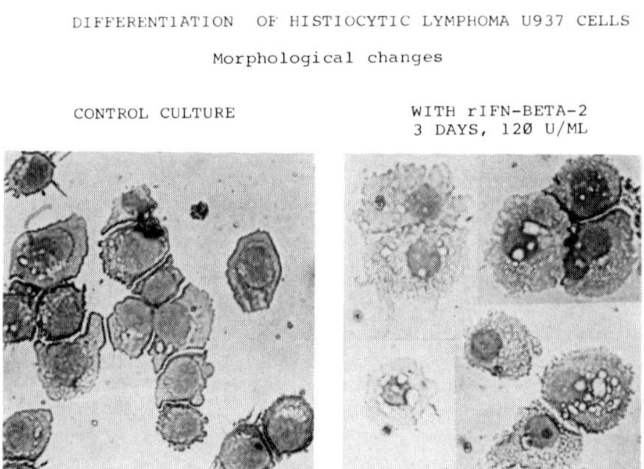

Fig 3.

Differentiation effect on U937 cells, Giemsa staining. FACS analysis showed 5-8 fold increase in cells with MO-1, MO-2 and HLA-DR antigens.

Table 2: STIMULATION BY IFN-β-2 OF HEMATOPOIETICS PROGENITORS IN LIQUID CULTURES OF NORMAL BM

Primary Stimulus	Number of secondary colonies (with LCM) CFU-Mix	CFU-GM	BFU-E	Total
None	4	5	0	9
LCM	39	15	67	111
IFN-β-2	4	21	2	27
IL-3	17	15	37	69
IL-3 + IFN-β-2	28	19	61	108
IL-1	4	4	2	10
IL-1 + IFN-β-2	0	11	0	11

Bone marrows were Monocyte and T cell depleted and 4HC-treated before liquid culture for 7 days followed by plating for colonies in methylcellulose for 15 days. CHO produced IFN-β-2 (Zilberstein et al,1986) used at 0.3 AV U/ml. IL-1 and IL-3 at 2 and 10 U/ml.

d) B-cell differentiation and plasmacytoma cell growth (BSF-2, HGF).

As first described by Hirano et al (1986), rIFN-β-2/BSF-2 stimulates immunoglobulin secretion from the human lymphoblastoid cell line CESS. With 10 U/ml of our E.coli IFN-β-2, the concentration of IgG in the medium increased from 250 to 850 ng/ml in a 3 day assay. The maximal amplitude of this effect was, however, half of that observed with a crude BCDF preparation (PHA treated adherent blood mononuclear cells) suggesting that other factors are also active to increase Ig secretion. IFN-γ has been reported to have such effects (for review, Revel,1987). Van Damme et al (1987), showed that growth of murine plasmacytomas and hybridomas is stimulated by human rIFN-β-2/BSF-2. In plasmacytoma T1165 cells, this HGF activity needed about 10 BSF-2 U/ml for maximal response, i.e. a 20 fold increase in ^{3}H-Td incorporation after 24 hours. However, crude BCDF produced up to 50 fold increases. IFN-α,β1 and γ were shown to also stimulate B cell growth (for review, Revel,1987). Human EBV-transformed B lymphocytes are growth stimulated by IFN-β-2 (Tosato et al,1988). Table 3 shows that a two-fold increase in ^{3}H-Td incorporation is observed with 125 U/ml rIFN-β-2 (E.coli). It is seen that rIFN-β1 also stimulates the growth of these cells.

e) Induction of complement and acute phase proteins.

Hepatocyte stimulation factor (HSF) was identified as IFN-β-2 (Gauldie et

Table 3: GROWTH-STIMULATION OF EBV TRANSFORMED B LYMPHOCYTES BY rIFN-β-2

Additions	TI CELLS ^{3}H-Thymidine incorporation, cpm x 10^{-3}
None	13.0
rIFN-β-2 (coli) 125 BSF-2 U/ml	21.7
Mock E.coli	13.7
rIFN-β-2 (CHO) 250 AV U/ml	21.4
rIFN-β_1 500 AV U/ml	22.0

3,000 TI cells (EBV transformed human lymphocytes) treated 24 hours and thymidine labeled overnight.

al,1987). With G. Darlington (Houston) we found that Hep3B2 hepatoma cells treated by 10 BSF-2 U/ml rIFN-β-2 show a 50 fold increase in fibrinogen, complement C3 and CRP production with a reduction in albumin secretion (Table 3). In our hands, both CHO and E.coli rIFN-β-2 also increased α_1 acid glycoprotein (not shown).

In collaboration with Dr Y. Katz and R.C. Strunk (St Louis), rIFN-β-2 (E.coli) was shown to induce the synthesis of complement C3 and Factor B in normal human fibroblasts (Katz et al, 1988). There was a 50-60 fold increase, linear with the dose of rIFN-β-2 from 0.1-100 BSF-2 U/ml. On the other hand, IFN-γ induced C2, C1R, C1S, C1I and factor H but not C3 and B. However, there was a strong synergism between IFN-γ and IFN-β-2 for factor B and C3 induction in human adult fibroblasts. Induction was seen at the mRNA level. It is of interest that the promoter of the Factor B gene (on chromosome 6 next to C2) has at -127/-138 a consensus IFN-responsive sequence AGGAAACAGAAAC found in many IFN-α, β and γ responsive genes (Wu et al, 1987; Benech et al,1987).

f) Antibodies neutralizing rIFN-β-2 activity.

The effects of various antibodies on the antiproliferative action of rIFN-β-2 (E.coli) was investigated. First, polyclonal rabbit antibodies against the N-terminal PRO^{29}-THR^{48} peptide of IFN-β-2 (antibodies 79-1-3) releaved the inhibition of ^{3}H-Td incorporation in T47D breast cancer cells and of U937 cell growth (Table 1). Control normal rabbit antiserum was without effect. Second, as found with CHO-produced rIFN-β-2 (Zilberstein et al,1986), antibodies to IFN-β1 were also capable of neutralizing the activity of E.coli-produced rIFN-β-2. We have reported (Chen et al,1988) that polyclonal rabbit antibodies against pure IFN-β1 releave the AP effect on T47D cells while anti-IFN-α did not. We have now used the neutralizing monoclonal antibody 29AB1 made against IFN-β1 (Zilberstein et al,1986) and found that it releaves the growth inhibition of rIFN-β-2 on T47D cells and on U937 cells (Table 1). A neutralizing monoclonal antibody to IFN-γ (186-5), used in comparison, did not alter the AP effect of rIFN-β-2.

This cross-neutralization by antibodies to IFN-β1 has been the basis for the designation IFN-β-2 for the new cytokine cloned along with IFN-β1 from dsRNA-induced human fibroblasts (Weissenbach et al,1980; Sehgal and Sagar,1980). However, the β-2 IFN gene (7p15-21) is not in the IFN-αs,β1 gene cluster on chromosome 9 (the same being true for IFN-γ) and the protein sequence has low homology as compared to the other members of the IFN-αs,β1 family (Zilberstein et al,1986). Nevertheless, a comparison of human and murine IFN-β-2/IL-6 with the human and murine IFN-β1 (Fig. 4) shows enough sequence conservation to support the possibility of common epitopes near the active site which could explain the cross-neutralization. The homology also suggests that the IFN-β-2

Table 4: INDUCTION OF ACUTE PHASE PROTEINS IN Hep 3B2 HEPATOMA CELLS

rIFN-β-2/BSF-2 U/ml	Fibrinogen μg/ml	C3 complement μg/ml	CRP ng/ml	Albumin μg/ml
0	0.13	0.04	--	10.3
10	7.9	0.39	3.1	5.8
20	7.8	0.49	4.7	8.9
40	9.9	0.58	3.7	7.7
80	8.3	0.54	5.2	9.6
0 (mock)	0.19	0.08	--	8.1

Hep3B with E.coli rIFN-β-2. Amounts after 24 hours. --, undetectable.

Fig 4. SEQUENCES OF HUMAN AND MOUSE IFN-Beta-1 and IFN-Beta-2

```
                                                 1
Hu B1                       MTNKCLLQIALLLCFSTTALSMSYNLLGFLQRSSNFQCQK
Mo B1                       MNNRWILHAAFLLCFSTTALSINYKQLQLQERTNIRKCQE
                                    1       oo        o   oo
Hu B2   MNSFSTSAFGPVAFSLGLLLVLPAAFPAPVPPGEDSKDVAAPHRQPLTSSERIDKQIRYI
Mo B2   MKFLSARDFHPVAF-LGLMLVTTTAFPTSQVRRGDFTEDTTPNRPVYTTSQVGGL-ITHV
--------------------------------------------------------------------

Hu B1   LLWQLNGRLEYCLKDRMNFDIPEEIKQLQQFQKEDAALTIYEMLQNIFAIFRQD
Mo B1   LLEQLNGKINL-TYRAD-FKIPMEMTEKMQKSYTAFAIQEMLQNVFLV--FRNN
        * o    * o * o o      o   o   o  oo       o  oo
Hu B2   LDGISALRKETCNKSNMCESSKEALAENNLNLPKMAEKDGCFQSGFNEETCLVK
Mo B2   LWEIVEMRKELCNGNSDCMNNDDALAENNLKLPEIQRNDGCYQTGYNQEICLLK
--------------------------------------------------------------------

Hu B1   SSSTGWNETIV--ENLLANVYHQINHLKTVLEEKLEKEDFTRGKLMSSLHLKRYYG
Mo B1   FSSTGWNETIV--VRLLDELHQQTVFLKTVLEEKQEERLTWEMSSTA-LHLKSYYW
        ooo*  *   o o o  oo         . *o    o   o   o    *o
Hu B2   II-TGLLEFEVYLEYLQNRFESSEEQARAVQMSTKVLIQFLQKK-AKNLDAITTPD
Mo B2   ISS-GLLEYHSYLEYMNNNLKDNKKDKARVLQRDTETLIHIFNQEVKDLHKIVLPT
--------------------------------------------------------------------

Hu B1   RILHY-LKAKEYSHCAWTIVRVE--ILRNFY-FINRLTGYLRN
Mo B1   RVQRY-LKLMKYNSYAWMVVRAE--IFRNFL-IIRRLTRNFQN
         o    * o  o   *       *o*  o  o     o oo
Hu B2   PTTNASLLTKLQAQNQWLQDMTTHLILRSFKEFLQSSLRALRQM
Mo B2   PISNALLTDKLESQKEWLRTKTIQFILKSLEEFLKVTLRSTRQT
--------------------------------------------------------------------
```

genes may be related to the ancestor gene which gave rise to the IFN-αs, β gene classes. IFN-β-2/BSF-2 has a similar low level of homology with G-CSF (Hirano et al,1986) and these proteins may be part of a larger gene superfamily. The other possibility to explain the cross-neutralization of IFN-β-2 be anti-IFN-β1 antibodies would be that IFN-β1 is an intermediate in IFN-β-2 action. In our work, we could find no support for this model (Zilberstein et al,1985).

DISCUSSION

An attempt to integrate the activities of IFN-β-2.

Can the mutiple activities associated with the IFN-β-2/IL-6 molecule be viewed in a way that could outline the function of this cytokine ? Synthesis of IFN-β-2 is induced in multiple cell types (e.g. fibroblasts, keratinocytes, monocytes, lymphocytes, epithelial and endothelial cells) by molecules derived from infectious agents both viral and bacterial (e.g. ds RNA and lipopolysaccharides), by inflammatory cytokines (e.g. IL-1, TNF), and by growth factors (e.g. PDGF, GM-CSF, activators of protein kinase C) (see Introduction). The activities of the cytokine are, therefore, likely to be related to infections/inflammation and to growth control. By its ability to induce components of the alternative complement pathway in fibroblasts, it could participate locally in the defense against bacterial or parasitic infection; its antiviral action could also precede or even prime that of the classical IFNs. By its action on liver cells, it would trigger the systemic acute phase response, which by the antiproteases and fibrinogen produced is essential for repair of the tissue damage. Activation and expansion of the mature B lymphocytes and plasma cells population with increase in secretion of immunoglobulin, as well as T cell activation, would contribute to the specific defense against the infectious agent. Stimulation of hematopoiesis and

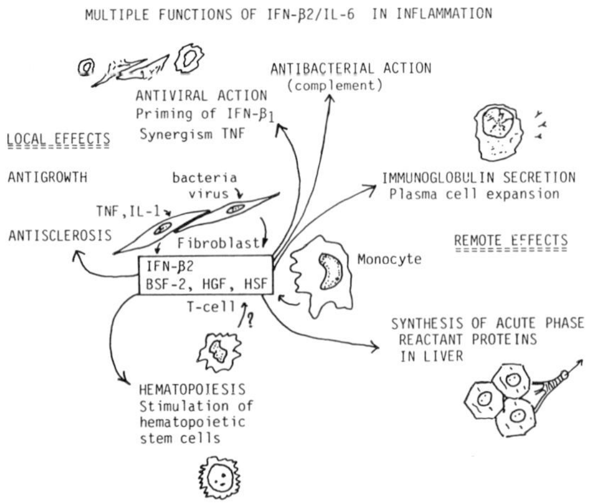

Fig 5.

differentiation of blood monomyelocytic and erythroid lineages could complete the effects of IL-1, supplying the increased number of blood cells required at the infection/inflammmation site. The potent antigrowth effect observed on various cells may be viewed as part of a mechanism to limit sclerosis of tissues damage by inflammation and to regulate the growth and differentiation of cells triggered by liberation at the site of injury of growth factors, such as PDGF, IL-1 and TNF. IFN-β-2 could play an important regulatory function in the inflammatory cytokine network as summarized in Fig. 5.

In this view, the dominant function of IFN-β-2 would be to induce the differentiated functions of many cell types, in general inhibiting their proliferation, plasma cells being the notable exception where differentiation is accompanied by growth stimulation. IFN-β-2 was discovered by its antiviral activity but many of its other activities have also been seen with the classical IFN-αs, β and γ, for example general inhibition of cell growth and stimulation of differentiation (Revel,1984), stimulation of complement synthesis (Wu et al,1987), and B cell growth and immunoglobulin production (Siegel et al,1986; Revel,1987). It seems, therefore, justified to keep it in the interferon group where it was first found and named because some of its activities are neutralized by antibodies to β IFNs. IFN-γ often acts differently than IFN-αs and β1, and so does IFN-β-2. It has now been shown that IFN-β-2 interacts with at least 3 proteins on the surface of cells and it is likely that these may be receptors (Coulie et al,1987). Other IFNs do not compete for binding to these receptors, but conversely we observed that rIFN-β-2 competes with the binding of IFN-α when added in amounts corresponding to its AV activity, indicating that some of its effect may be mediated by the type I IFN receptor (Shulman and Revel, unpublished). The IFN-γ receptors are also distinct from that of IFN-αs,β1 (Novick et al,1987). IFN-β-2 could, like TGF-β, exert its multiple effects through several different cell receptors involving different part of the protein recognized by distinct antibodies. A further complication is that IFN-β-2 undergoes processing and various post-translational modifications in mammalian cells including N- and O-glycosylation, phosphorylation etc..) (May et al,1988) and a number of different forms differing in molecular weights are detected by immunoblots even in SDS. Some of these forms are 70 Kd and could be oligomers. Interaction with different receptors and hence individual activities, could depend on these modifications which would increase or decrease individual activities. Compared at the same HGF activity, CHO-IFN-β-2 had more

AV activity than the E.coli product (Revel et al,1987,1988). Further comparison of the activities of E.coli produced rIFN-β-2 and of the various forms made by mammalian cells should help clarify whether the different activities of the cytokine are regulated by its conformation.

ACNOWLEDGEMENTS

We thank Dr M. Rubinstein and L. Sachs for help and discussions. The excellent assistance of Mrs P. Federman, R. Kaufman, Z. Marks, R. Zwang is acknowledged. Work supported in part by InterYeda, Ltd, Israel.

REFERENCES

Benech, P., Vigneron, M., Peretz, D., Revel, M. and Chebath, J. (1987) Mol. Cell. Biol. 7, 4498-4504.
Chen, L., Mory, Y., Zilberstein, A. and Revel, M. (1988) Proc. Natl. Acad. Sci. USA, in press.
Coulie, P.G., Vanhecke, A., VanDamme, J., Cayphas, S., Poupart, P., Dewit, L., and Content J. (1987) Eur. J. Immunol. 17, 1435-1442.
Hirano,T., Yasukawa,K., Harada,H., Taga,T., Watanabe,Y., Matsuda,T., Kashimura,S., Nakajima,K., Koyama,K., Iwamatsu,K., Tsunasawa,S., Sakiyama,F., Matsui,H., Takahara,Y., Taniguchi,T. and Kishimoto,T. (1986) Nature (London) 234, 73-76.
Gauldie, J., Richards, C., Harnish, D., Lansdorp, P. and Baumann,H. (1987) Proc. Natl. Acad. Sci. USA 84, 7251-7255.
Helfgott, D.C., May, L.T., Shtoeger, Z., Tamm, I. and Sehgal, P.B. (1987) J. Exp. Med. 166, 1300-1308.
Ikebuchi, K., Wong, G.G., Clark, S.C., Ihle, J.N., Hirai, Y. and Ogawa, M. (1987 Proc. Natl. Acad. SCi. USA 84, 9035-9039.
Katz, Y., Revel, M. and Strunk, R.C. (1988) EMBO J., submitted.
Kohase, M., Henrikson-Destefano, D., May, L.T., Vilcek, J. and Sehgal, P.B. (1986) Cell 45, 659-666.
Lotem, J. and Sachs, L. (1986) EMBO J. 5, 2163-2170.
May, L.T., Santhanam, U., Tatter, S.B., Bhardwaj, N., Ghrayeb, J. and Sehgal, P.B. (1988) Biochem. Biophys. Res. Commun. in press
Novick, D., Orchansky, P., Revel, M. and Rubinstein, M. (1987) J. Biol. Chem. 262, 8483-8487.
Revel, M. (1984) In: Antiviral Drugs an Interferon: The Molecular Basis of their Activity (ed. Y. Becker) Martinus Nijhoff, pp 357-433.
Revel, M. (1987) Nature (London) 325, 581.
Revel, M., Zilberstein, A., Ruggieri, R., Rubinstein, M. and Chen, L. (1987) J. Interferon Res. 7, 529-536.
Revel, M., Zilberstein, A., Ruggieri, R., Chen, L., Mory, Y., Rubinstein, M. and Michalevicz R. (1988) In: Tumor Necrosis Factor, (eds. Bonavida, B., Kirchner, H.) Karger, S., Basel, in press.
Sehgal, P.B. and Sagar, A.D. (1980) Nature (London) 288, 95-97.
Siegel, D.S., Le, J. and Vilcek, J. (1986) Cell. Immunol. 101, 380-390.
Takai, Y., Wong, G.G., Clark, S.C., Burakoff, S.J. and Herrmann, S. (1988) J. Immunol. 140, 508-512.
Tosato, G., Seamon, K.B., Goldman, N.D., Sehgal, P.B., May, L.T., Washington, G.C., Jones, K.D. and Pike, S.E. (1988) Science 239, 502-504.
Weissenbach, J., Chernajovsky, Y., Zeevi, M., Shulman, L., Soreq, H., Nir, U. Wallach, D., Perricaudet, M., Tiollais, P. and Revel, M. (1980) Proc. Natl. Acad. Sci. USA 77, 7152-7156.
Wu, L-C., Morley, B.J. and Campbell, R.D. (1987) Cell 48, 331-342.
Zhang, Y., Lin, J.X. and Vilcek, J. (1988) J. Biol. Chem. 263, 6177-6182.
Zilberstein A., Ruggieri, R., Korn, H.J. and Revel, M. (1986) EMBO J. 5, 2529-2537.
Zilberstein, A., Ruggieri, R. and Revel, M. (1985) In: The Interferon System, (eds. Dianzani, F., Rossi, G.B.) Serono Symposia No 24, Raven Press, New York, pp 73-83.

Interleukin-6: Biological Function and Regulation of the Gene Expression *in Vitro* and *in Vivo*

W. FIERS, P. BROUCKAERT, J. CONTENT*, R. CONTRERAS, B. EVERAERDT, Y. GUISEZ, C. LIBERT, D. SPRIGGS**, N. TAKAHASHI, B. TISON, P. VANDENABEELE and J. VAN SNICK***

Laboratory of Molecular Biology, State University of Gent, K. L. Ledeganckstraat 35, 9000 Gent, Belgium
**Institut Pasteur du Brabant, Brussels, Belgium*
***Dana-Farber Cancer Institute & Harvard Medical School, Boston, USA*
****Ludwig Institute, Brussels, Belgium*

INTRODUCTION

More than ten years ago, optimal conditions were established to superinduce IFN-β in fibroblast cells (Reynolds et al., 1975). This involved the induction with poly I,C in the presence of cycloheximide. The latter drug prevents the rapid degradation of the IFN mRNA. Using a library made from mRNA of induced fibroblast cells, we isolated not only the human IFN-β gene (Derynck et al., 1980), but also a cDNA which corresponded with messenger RNA translatable in an in vitro system into a 26-kDa protein (Content et al., 1982). As at that time we could not ascribe unambiguously a biological function to this protein, we continued to refer to it as 26-kDa protein. Clearly, this cDNA gene was identical to the one which had been cloned before by M. Revel and colleagues, and which they referred to as IFN-β2 (Weissenbach et al., 1979 and 1980). Like IFN-β, this 26-kDa protein/IFN-β2 was an inducible protein which contains a cleavable signal sequence and becomes glycosylated upon translation in an in vitro system in the presence of a microsome fraction. But unlike IFN-β, which requires double-stranded RNA or poly I,C for induction, cycloheximide alone was sufficient to lead to 26-kDa mRNA accumulation (Content et al., 1982). In the same publication, we also reported our failure to demonstrate either antiviral or even ppp(A2'p5')$_n$A synthetase-inducing activity (Content et al., 1982; Fiers et al., 1982). Of course, cycloheximide can hardly be considered a natural inducer, but it was subsequently found that a lymphokine identified as IL1 was able to strongly induce 26-kDa protein (Content et al., 1985).

We published the complete nucleotide sequence of the 26-kDa cDNA (Haegeman et al., 1986). It codes for a 27 amino acid signal sequence followed by a 186 amino acid long mature polypeptide, which contains two potential N-glycosylation sites. As expected, when the sequence of the IFN-β2 clone was published, it turned out to be completely identical to that of the 26-kDa protein (Zilberstein et al., 1986). But most remarkable of all was the finding that the sequence of B-cell stimulatory factor-2, of which the cDNA gene was reported by Hirano et al. (1986), was again identical, amino acid for amino acid, to our 26-kDa protein. The first realisation that 26-kDa protein and B-cell stimulation factor-2 are identical, came from the collaboration between the groups of A. Billiau and J. Van Snick. They worked, on the one hand, on a human hybridoma growth factor induced by IL1 (Van Damme et al., 1987) and, on the other hand, on a murine hybridoma-plasmacytoma growth factor named HP1 (Van Snick et al., 1987; Billiau, 1987). The N-terminal sequence of the murine HP1 was quite different from that of the human 26-kDa protein (Van Snick et al., 1986). However, cloning and subsequent characterization of the murine HP1 gene demonstrated that it is indeed the murine equivalent of the human IL6 gene (Van Snick et al., 1988).

Having now available a sensitive biological assay for the 26-kDa protein, based either on B-cell growth activity or B-cell differentiation activity, we could reinvestigate its possible relationship to IFN-β (Poupart et al., 1987). Both recombinant proteins were made in Xenopus laevis oocytes injected with the messengers synthesized in vitro from appropriate plasmids. The IFN-β had the expected specific activity of about 3 to 5 x 10^8 units/mg, while the 26-kDa protein was highly active in the B-cell growth/differentiation assay. But no antiviral activity was detectable and the specific activity must be at least one million times lower, compared with authentic IFN-β, if at all. As the 26-kDa protein could no longer be regarded as related to IFN-β, neither in structure nor in biological or immunological properties, it seemed logical to rename this protein Interleukin-6 or IL6 (in fact B-cell stimulation factor-1 had already been renamed IL4, and IL5 had also been cloned and well characterized).

The discovery by Gauldie et al. (1987) that IL6 is identical to the previously characterized hepatocyte-stimulating factor opened another Pandora box. Furthermore, IL6 not only acts on B-cells, but also activates T-cells (Garman et al., 1987; Uyttenhove et al., 1988). Moreover, in combination with IL3, it supports the proliferation of hemopoietic progenitor cells (Ikebuchi et al., 1987). Undoubtedly, this list of biological activities of IL6 is not yet complete and it is not unlikely that several other cell types will respond to the pleiotropic factor IL6.

PRODUCTION OF IL6

As mentioned above, we first produced pure, biologically active material by injection of SP6-driven transcripts of appropriate plasmids into X. laevis oocytes. This material secreted by the oocytes in the medium had the same specific activity as natural IL6 in the hybridoma growth factor assay. As it could be labelled at a high specific activity, such IL6 was also used for characterization of the IL6 receptor (Coulie et al., 1987a).

But in order to investigate the many biological functions of IL6, a good source of pure product was necessary. For this purpose we have constructed a plasmid which allows secretion of the hIL6 from yeast cells. This plasmid contains the α-mating factor promoter followed by the α-mating factor signal and pro-sequence, fused to the mature sequence of human IL6. The transformed cells produce between 1 to 5 mg/l of IL6 secreted into the medium. This yeast-produced IL6 has been purified to near homogeneity and has been used in a variety of biological studies as well as for the preparation of a neutralizing rabbit antiserum.

INDUCTION OF IL6 IN VITRO

As mentioned above, Van Damme et al. (1987) have shown that IL1 acts as a natural inducer of IL6 in fibroblasts. We have previously reported on the many similarities in action between TNF and IL1, although these factors each recognize specifically their own receptor (Fiers et al., 1987). Indeed, on a variety of cells, not only fibroblasts, but also cells of epithelial origin, TNF induces IL6, although somewhat more weakly than IL1 (Defilippi et al., 1987). Remarkably, there seems to be a correlation between the sensitivity to the cytotoxic action of TNF and the lack of inducibility of the IL6 gene; this might perhaps indicate that in the transformed, TNF-sensitive cells there is a lack of signalling to the nucleus, such that neither TNF-protecting mechanisms are induced, nor IL6.

INDUCTION OF IL6 IN VIVO

Coulie et al. (1987) have shown that after injection of lipopolysaccharide into mice, a high level of murine IL6 appears in the serum. The concentration reached a maximum level after 2 h, and the peak level was up to thousandfold higher than background. Presumably, this IL6 is mainly produced by monocytes (Aarden et al., 1987), although other contributing compartments, for example the endothelial system, cannot be excluded. The induction of IL6 by bacterial lipopolysaccharides may be the reason why elevated levels of IL6 can be detected after acute infections; for example, high levels of IL6 have been reported in the cerebrospinal fluid of patients with acute infection of the nervous system (Houssiau et al., 1988) and also in the serum of patients with severe burns (Nijsten et al., 1987). It is not clear, however, in such cases to what extent IL6 is directly induced by lipopolysaccharides or by the intermediator IL1.

Undoubtedly, IL6 is part of a complex cytokine regulatory network, and it can also be induced in vivo by endogenous signals. For example, it has been known for a long time that acute phase responses occur upon inflammation, even in the absence of any infection. The induction of the acute phase responses was known to be due to hepatocyte-stimulating factor or HSF, and it was shown that this HSF could be induced by IL1. Of course, it is now well-established that the HSF is identical to IL6 (Gauldie et al., 1987). But also TNF can induce acute phase proteins in vivo (Gresser et al., 1987). As we have seen above, TNF can directly induce IL6 synthesis in appropriate cells. But moreover, TNF also induces IL1 in vivo (Dinarello et al., 1986; Nawroth et al., 1986), and this IL1 may in turn induce a second wave of IL6 induction.

When TNF, either murine or human, is injected in mice, there is a considerable in vivo induction of IL6, albeit the concentrations are much less compared with what can be obtained by injection of lipopolysaccharides (Table).

TNF INDUCES IL6 IN VIVO

LPS (E. coli), hTNF or mTNF in phosphate-buffered saline (PBS; 0.2 ml) was injected i.v. in Balb/c mice (two/group). 2 h later blood was collected (in citrate) by cardiac puncture and plasma prepared.

Treatment		**IL6** (U/ml)
Control (PBS)	1	0
	2	0
mTNF (10 µg)	1	2310
	2	2118
hTNF (30 µg)	1	2840
	2	4928
LPS (10 µg)	1	> 59000
	2	34413

Undoubtedly, this in vivo synthesized IL6 is responsible for the induction of the acute phase proteins. We have observed that murine TNF is much more toxic to mice than human TNF (as the specific activity of the former is threefold higher, we inject threefold less μg murine TNF). The higher toxicity of murine TNF is not observed in the presence of galactosamine, in which condition the mice are equally sensitive to low concentrations of either murine or human TNF. We have shown that there is a strong synergism in lethality between TNF and IL1. Hence, the higher toxicity of the homologous, murine TNF can be explained by a higher induction level of endogenous IL1. Indeed, we have demonstrated that after injection of murine TNF into mice, a much higher, sustained level of IL6 appears in circulation compared with the situation after human TNF treatment. We believe this higher IL6 concentration in the serum is a consequence of phenomena which occur after murine TNF injection (presumably IL1 induction), but is not itself contributory to the enhanced toxicity. Indeed, we have not observed any increase in toxicity by treatment with TNF in combination with murine IL6.

Clinical phase I studies have also been initiated for the treatment of selected cancer patients with recombinant TNF, alone or in combination with IFN-γ. In a collaborative study we have looked at the IL6 concentrations in the serum of the patients treated with TNF by a continuous i.v. infusion for 24 h. Indeed, much enhanced IL6 levels were found in the serum of patients treated with concentrations above 4×10^5 U/m^2 TNF (specific activity 2.2×10^6 U/mg protein). Peak levels were reached about 3 to 6 h after the start of infusion, and there was a crude relationship between dose of TNF administered and IL6 level reached. After reaching a peak level, the IL6 concentration then decreased considerably, despite the continuous infusion of TNF. There was a very considerable variation in the level of IL6 in the different patients, and a possible correlation between this level with clinical parameters is still under investigation. Occasionally, levels of up to 20 ng/ml serum were noted. This IL6 was measured in the hybridoma growth factor assay and was verified as being authentic IL6 by neutralization using monospecific antiserum.

CONCLUDING REMARKS

In the case of inflammation, either localized or systemic, IL6 is released in circulation. IL6 can be synthesized by many cells, both monocytes and macrophages as well as cells of fibroblastic or epithelial origin. The IL6 can be induced by bacterial components, but also by natural triggers such as IL1 or TNF. Both IL1 and TNF can be secreted, but are also known to function locally in a membrane-bound form. We consider IL6 more as the in vivo secondary messenger which tells the whole organism about the ongoing inflammation. IL6 may go to the bone marrow and help (together with IL1 and IL3) in the recruitment and activation of hemopoiesis. IL6 also goes to the various organs of the immune system, where it stimulates, both by growth and by differentiation, various steps in B-cell maturation as well as in the generation of T-lymphocytes. Another very important function of IL6 is its action as an inducer of the acute phase response. Although the physiological function and role of the acute phase proteins is not known, or is only partially known, it is clear that some of these are anti-proteases which may help to limit the damage as a result of the inflammation (Fey and Fuller, 1987).

Clearly, the 26-kDa protein - the orphan without a function (Content et al., 1982) - has come a long way!

ACKNOWLEDGEMENTS

Research in the first author's laboratory has been supported by grants from the "Onderling Overlegde Onderzoeksacties" and IUAP Program (Department of Science Policy), the "Fonds voor Geneeskundig Wetenschappelijk Onderzoek" and the "Algemene Spaar- en Lijfrentekas". B.E. and C.L. thank the IWONL for a fellowship. We are indebted to M. Vandecasteele for editorial assistance.

REFERENCES

Aarden, L.A., De Groot, E.R., Schaap, O.L. and Lansdorp, P.M. (1987). Eur. J. Immunol. 17, 1411-1416.
Billiau, A. (1987). Immunol. Today 8, 84-87.
Content, J., De Wit, L., Pierard, D., Derynck, R., De Clercq, E. and Fiers, W. (1982). Proc. Natl. Acad. Sci. USA 99, 2768-2772.
Content, J., De Wit, L., Poupart, P., Opdenakker, G., Van Damme, J. and Billiau, A. (1985). Eur. J. Biochem. 152, 253-257.
Coulie, P.G., Cayphas, S., Vink, A., Uyttenhove, C. and Van Snick, J. (1987). Eur. J. Immunol. 17, 1217-1220.
Coulie, P.G., Vanhecke, A., Van Damme, J., Cayphas, S., Poupart, P., De Wit, L. and Content, J. (1987a). Eur. J. Immunol. 17, 1435-1440.
Defilippi, P., Poupart, P., Tavernier, J., Fiers, W. and Content, J. (1987). Proc. Natl. Acad. Sci. USA 84, 4557-4561.
Derynck, R., Content, J., De Clercq, E., Volckaert, G., Tavernier, J., Devos, R. and Fiers, W. (1980). Nature (London) 285, 542-547.
Dinarello, C.A., Cannon, J.G., Wolff, S.M., Bernheim, H.A., Beutler, B., Cerami, A., Figari, I.S., Palladino, M.A. and O'Connor, J.V. (1986). J. Exp. Med. 163, 1433-1450.
Fey, G.H. and Fuller, G.M. (1987). Mol. Biol. Med. 4, 323-338.
Fiers, W., Degrave, W., Derynck, R., Devos, R., Gheysen, D., Remaut, E., Stanssens, P., Tavernier, J., Content, J. and De Clercq, E. (1982). In: Primary and Tertiary Structure of Nucleic Acids and Cancer Research (eds M. Miwa, S. Nishimura, A. Rich, D.G. Söll and T. Sugimura) Japan Scientific Societies Press. 227-236.
Fiers, W., Brouckaert, P., Devos, R., Fransen, L., Haegeman, G., Leroux-Roels, G., Marmenout, A., Remaut, E., Suffys, P., Tavernier, J., Van der Heyden, J. and Van Roy, F. (1987). In: Biology of the Interferon System (eds K. Cantell and H. Schellekens) M. Nijhoff. 205-216.
Garman, R.D., Jacobs, K.A., Clark, S.C. and Raulet, D.H. (1987). Proc. Natl. Acad. Sci. USA 84, 7629-7633.
Gauldie, J., Richards, C., Harnish, D., Lansdorp, P. and Baumann, H. (1987). Proc. Natl. Acad. Sci. USA 84, 7251-7255.
Gresser, I., Delers, F., Tran Quangs, N., Marion, S., Engler, R., Maury, C., Soria, C., Soria, J., Fiers, W. and Tavernier, J. (1987). J. Biol. Regul. Homeost. Agents 1, 173-176.
Haegeman, G., Content, J., Volckaert, G., Derynck, R., Tavernier, J. and Fiers, W. (1986). Eur. J. Biochem. 159, 625-632.
Hirano, T., Yasukawa, K., Harada, H., Taga, T., Watanabe, Y., Matsuda, T., Kashiwamura, S., Nakajima, K., Koyama, K., Iwamatsu, A., Tsnunasawa, S., Sakiyama, F., Matsui, H., Takahara, Y., Taniguchi, T. and Kishimoto, T. (1986). Nature (London) 324, 73-76.
Houssiau, F.A., Bukasa, K., Sindic, C.J.M., Van Damme, J. and Van Snick, J. (1988). In press.
Ikebuchi, K., Wong, G.G., Clark, S.C., Ihle, J.N., Hirai, Y. and Ogawa, M. (1987). Proc. Natl. Acad. Sci. USA 84, 9035-9039.
Nawroth, P.P., Bank, I., Handley, D., Cassimeris, J., Chess, L. and Stern, D. (1986). J. Exp. Med. 163, 1363-1375.
Nijsten, M.W.N., De Groot, E.R., Ten Duis, H.J., Klasen, H.J., Hack, C.E. and Aarden, L.A. (1987). Lancet 2, 921.
Poupart, P., Vandenabeele, P., Cayphas, S., Van Snick, J., Haegeman, G., Kruys, V., Fiers, W. and Content, J. (1987). EMBO J. 6, 1219-1224.
Reynolds, F.H., Premkumar, E. and Pitha, P.M. (1975). Proc. Natl. Acad. Sci. USA 72, 4881-4885.
Uyttenhove, C., Coulie, P.G. and Van Snick, J. (1988). J. Exp. Med. In press.
Van Damme, J., Cayphas, S., Opdenakker, G., Billiau, A. and Van Snick, J. (1987). Eur. J. Immunol. 17, 1-7.
Van Snick, J., Cayphas, S., Vink, A., Uyttenhove, C., Coulie, P.G., Rubira, M.R. and Simpson, R.J. (1986). Proc. Natl. Acad. Sci. USA 83, 9679-9683.

Van Snick, J., Vink, A., Cayphas, S. and Uyttenhove, C. (1987). J. Exp. Med. 165, 641-649.
Van Snick, J., Cayphas, S., Szikora, J.P., Renauld, J.C., Van Roost, E., Boon, T. and Simpson, R.J. (1988). Eur. J. Immunol. 18, 193-197.
Weissenbach, J., Zeevi, M., Landau, T. and Revel, M. (1979). Eur. J. Biochem. 98, 1-8.
Weissenbach, J., Chernajovsky, Y., Zeevi, M., Shulman, L., Soreq, H., Nir, U., Wallach, D., Perricaudet, M., Tiollais, P. & Revel, M. (1980). Proc. Natl. Acad. Sci. USA 77, 7152-7156.
Zilberstein, A., Ruggieri, R., Korn, J.H. and Revel, M. (1986). EMBO J. 5, 2529-2537.

Interleukin-6 is the Major Regulator of Acute Phase Protein Synthesis in Rat and Man

J. V. CASTELL, T. ANDUS†, T. GEIGER†, M. GÓMEZ-LECHÓN*, M. DAVID, J. KLAPPROTH, T. HIRANO§, T. KISHIMOTO§, P. C. HEINRICH

Biochemisches Institut and †Medizinische Klinik der Universität, D-7800 Freiburg, F.R.G.
**Centro de Investigación Hospital La Fe, INSALUD, E-46009 Valencia, Spain,*
§Institute for Molecular and Cellular Biology, Division of Immunology, Osaka University, Osaka 565, Japan

ABSTRACT

The regulation of the major acute phase proteins by interleukin-6/hepatocyte-stimulating factor (IL-6/HSF), interleukin-1ß (IL-1ß) and tumor necrosis factor α (TNFα) was studied in rat hepatocyte primary cultures. IL-6 was found to be the most effective inducer of acute phase protein synthesis in vitro and also in vivo. IL-6 was rapidly removed from blood and detected on the surface of hepatocytes. Also in human hepatocyte primary cultures IL-6, when compared to IL-1ß and TNFα, exbihited the strongest capacity to stimulate acute phase protein synthesis.

KEYWORDS

Acute phase proteins : interleukin-1ß : interleukin-6 : hepatocytes : TNFα.

INTRODUCTION

The answer of higher organisms to severe tissue damage caused by burns, physical and chemical traumata, bacterial or parasitic infections is comprised of a series of local and systemic events aimed to restore the altered physiological homeostastis and is called acute phase response (Kushner, 1982; Koj, 1985). The local reaction includes the dilation of blood vesels, alteration in blood flow and clotting, immigration of neutrophils and macrophages, release of lysosomal proteases and cytokines. The systemic reaction is characterized by fever and pain, leukocytosis, and changes in plasma protein composition. Some of the plasma proteins increase during an acute phase response (positive acute phase proteins), while others decrease (negative acute phase proteins). Im man serum levels of C-reactive protein and serum amyloid A increase several hundred-fold, whereas in the rat alpha-2-macroglobulin and alpha-1-acid glycoprotein are the most important positive acute phase proteins. Albumin and transferrin are negative acute phase proteins in both species (Kushner, 1982; Koj, 1985). The underlying mechanisms of acute phase protein regulation in human and animal liver are presently not well understood.

It is known that monocytes and macrophages are attracted and activated at the sites of trauma. Fuller and Ritchie (1982) have observed that LPS-stimulated monocytes synthesize and secrete a hepatocyte-stimulating activity, which they designated hepatocyte-stimulating factor (HSF). Many efforts have been made to identify the HSF.

The two monokines interleukin-1ß (IL-1ß) and tumor necrosis factor alpha (TNFα) have been regarded as the major acute phase mediators present in conditioned media from LPS-stimulated monocytes (Darlington et al., 1986; Perlmutter et al., 1986). Recently, it was found that HSF is functionally and immunologically identical with interleukin-6 (IL-6), also known as BSF-2, IFN-ß2, 26 kDa protein and interleukin HP-1 (Gauldie et al., 1987; Andus et al., 1987a). Here we demonstrate that IL-6/HSF is the most important mediator of acute phase protein synthesis in rat and human hepatocyte primary cultures.

MATERIALS AND METHODS

Chemicals - L-^{35}S/Methionine (>1000 Ci/mmol) and deoxycytidine 5'α-^{32}P/triphosphate (3000 Ci/mmol) were purchased from the Radiochemical Centre (Amersham, UK). Collagenase (>300 units/mg) was from Boehringer (Mannheim, FRG). Protein A-Sepharose CL-4B was obtained from Pharmacia (Freiburg, FRG). Guanidinium thiocyanate was obtained from Fluka (Neu-Ulm, FRG). Antibodies against rat or human plasma proteins were either prepared as described in earlier papers (Geiger et al., 1982; Andus et al., 1983) or purchased from Dakopatts (Hamburg, FRG). Recombinant human IL-6/BSF-2 (5 x 10^6 units/mg protein) was prepared as described (Hirano et al., 1985,1986). Recombinant human IL-1ß (5 x 10^7 units per mg) was from Biogen (Geneva, Switzerland). Recombinant human TNFα (> 1.6 x 10^7 units per mg) was generously supplied by BASF (Ludwigshafen, FRG). Rat albumin cDNA was kindly provided by Dr. A. Alonso (Heidelberg, FRG), rat alpha-1-acid glycoprotein cDNA by Dr. G. Schreiber (Melbourne, Australia), rat cysteine proteinase inhibitor (T-kininogen) by Dr. S. Nakanishi (Kyoto, Japan), ß-fibrinogen cDNA by Dr. A. Mitchell (Parkville, Australia), and the genomic clone of rRNA by Dr. I. Grummt (Würzburg, FRG).

Preparation of hepatocyte primary cultures - Rat hepatocyte primary cultures were prepared as described (Tran-Thi et al., 1985). Human hepatocytes were obtained after perfusion with collagenase of a small surgical biopsy (1.5 g) of a healthy individual. Cell viability was >95%. Hepatocytes (1.5 x 10^5 cells/-well) were seeded on 24-well dishes (Falcon, no. 3047) previously coated with fibronectin (1.5 µg/cm^2) and cultured in Ham's F-12 medium supplemented with 0.2% bovine serum albumin, 10 nM insulin and 2% newborn calf serum. One h later >90% of the cells were attached and medium was changed. After 24 h cells were shifted to Ham's F-12 medium containing 0.2% bovine serum albumin, 10 nM insulin and 10 nM dexamethasone.

Synthesis of acute phase proteins in hepatocytes - After >48 h in culture, rat or human hepatocytes were stimulated with the various cytokines with or without dexamethasone for 20 h. Medium was changed and hepatocytes were labeled for 4 h with 25 µCi of ^{35}S/methionine per ml methionine-free culture medium. The various acute phase proteins were immunoprecipitated from the hepatocyte culture medium, subjected to SDS-PAGE and fluorography as described in previous publications (Geiger et al., 1987; Andus et al., 1987b).

Induction of acute phase protein mRNA by rhIL-6 in vivo - 40 x 10^3 units of rhIL-6 were injected intraperitoneally into male Wistar rats (180-200 g). Animals were sacrificed at various times and total RNA was extracted from livers and hybridized with the specific ^{32}P-labeled cDNA probes (Chirgwin et al., 1979; Feinberg and Vogelstein, 1983).

RESULTS AND DISCUSSION

(A) Regulation of major rat acute phase proteins

As a first approach rat hepatocytes were used as a model system to evaluate the contributions of each of the 3 monokines in respect to the synthesis of acute phase proteins. We studied the dose- and time-dependence of rhIL-1ß, rhIL-6, and rhTNFα on the synthesis of alpha-2-macroglobulin, cysteine proteinase inhibitor, alpha-1-antitrypsin and albumin.

Fig. 1 shows that rhIL-6 (filled circles) strongly stimulated alpha-2-macroglobulin (54-fold) and cysteine proteinase inhibitor (8-fold) at a concentration of

>50 units/ml, but had essentially no effect on alpha-1-antitrypsin synthesis and diminished albumin synthesis by about 60% of controls. Half maximal stimulation of alpha-2-macroglobulin and cysteine proteinase inhibitor synthesis was achieved with about 3 units per ml corresponding to a rhIL-6 concentration of about 30 pM. In contrast, rhIL-1ß (filled triangles) had only a slight effect on alpha-2-macroglobulin (2-3-fold) and a marked effect on albumin synthesis (60% decrease). RhTNFα (filled squares) did not affect the synthesis of any of the 4 acute phase proteins. Since the recombinant mediators may contain trace amounts of lipopolysaccharide (LPS), we incubated hepatocyte primary cultures with LPS in concentrations between 1 pg and 10 µg/ml medium. In this concentration range no effect on the synthesis of acute phase proteins was detected.

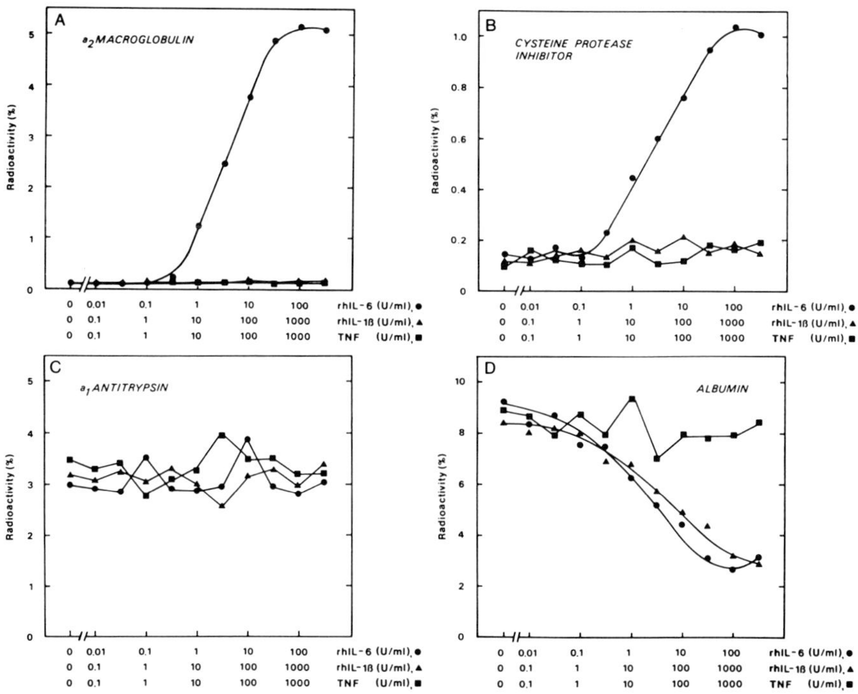

Fig. 1. Dose reponse of regulation of acute-phase proteins by rhIL-6, rhIL-1ß and rhTNFα in rat hepatocyte primary cultures. Rat hepatocyte primary cultures (2.5×10^5 cells/well) were incubated in the presence of 1 µM dexamethasone and the various monokines. After 12 h the cells were labeled with ^{35}S/methionine for 3 h and the 4 acute phase proteins (A-D) were immunoprecipitated from the hepatocyte media and quantitated as described (Andus et al., 1988).

The time course of alpha-2-macroglobulin and cysteine proteinase inhibitor induction revealed an immediate increase after the addition of rhIL-6 (Fig. 2A,B, filled circles). A maximum was observed after 24 h for both proteins. The down-regulation of albumin synthesis by either rhIL-6 (filled circles) or rhIL-1ß (filled triangles) showed a continuous decrease up to 24 h.

In vivo probably all 3 mediators are liberated from monocytes i.e. by LPS, and thus act simultaneously on hepatocytes. Therefore, we incubated the hepatocytes with various combinations of the 3 cytokines (Fig. 3) in order to look for possible interactions. When the induction of alpha-2-macroglobulin (A) and

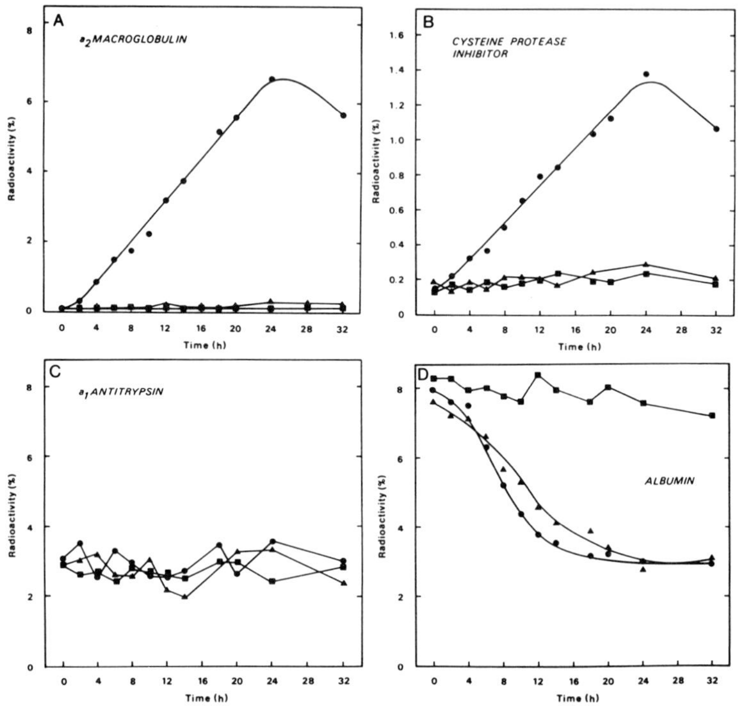

Fig. 2. Time course of acute-phase protein induction by rhIL-6, rhIL1ß and TNFα. Hepatocyte primary cultures (2.5×10^5 cells/well) were incubated in the presence of 1 µM dexamethasone as described in the legend to Fig. 1 with either 100 U/ml of rhIL-6 (●), 500 U/ml rhIL-1ß (▲), or 1000 U/ml of rhTNFα (■). At different times after the addition of the stimulant, the cells were labeled with ^{35}S/methionine for 2 h and the 4 acute phase proteins (A-D) were immunoprecipitated from the hepatocyte media.

cysteine proteinase inhibitor (B) by rhIL-6 was examined in the presence of increasing concentrations of rhIL-1ß, synthesis of the 2 acute phase proteins was strongly impaired at rhIL-1ß concentrations of 10 U/ml (filled circles) and 100 U/ml (filled triangles) and essentially abolished at 1000 U/ml (filled squares) (Fig. 3A,B, left panels). On the other hand, the combination of rhIL-6 and rhIL-1ß resulted in an additive down-regulation of albumin synthesis and alpha-1-antitrypsin synthesis remained unchanged (not shown).

Increasing concentrations of rhTNFα present during the acute phase protein stimulation by rhIL-6 had essentially no influence on the synthesis of alpha-2-macroglobulin (Fig. 3A, right panel). The induction of cysteine proteinase inhibitor synthesis by rhIL-6 was impaired at 1000 U/ml rhTNFα (Fig. 3B, right panel). The combination of rhIL-1ß with rhTNFα did not result in either additive or inhibitory interactions (not shown).

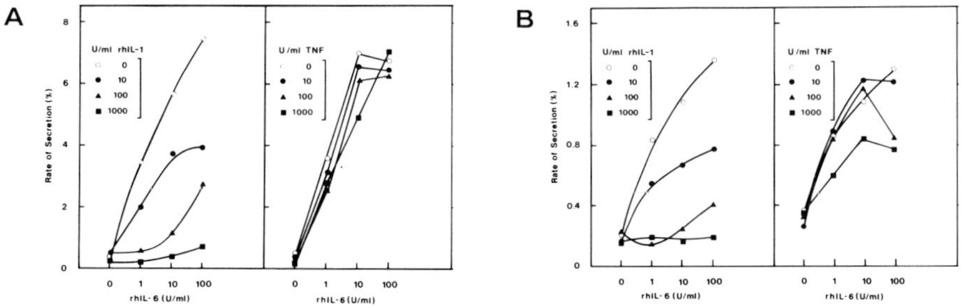

Fig. 3. Dose-response of regulation of acute-phase proteins by combinations of rhIL-6, rhIL-1ß and rhTNFα. Hepatocyte primary cultures (2.5 x 10^5 cells/well) were incubated in the presence of 1 μM dexamethasone and combinations of rhIL-6, rhIL-1ß and rhTNFα. After 18 h the cells were labeled with ^{35}S/methionine for 2 h and alpha-2-macroglobulin (A) and cysteine proteinase inhibitor (B) were immunoprecipitated and quantitated as described in the legend to Fig. 1.

(B) Induction of rat acute phase proteins by interleukin-6 in vivo

The results presented above have shown IL-6 to be the most potent stimulator of acute phase protein synthesis in rat hepatocytes. However, it remained necessary to demonstrate the validity of these observation under in vivo conditions. Therefore, rhIL-6 was intraperitoneally injected into male Wistar rats and changes in the hepatic mRNA levels for alpha-2-macroglobulin, ß-fibrinogen, cysteine proteinase inhibitor, alpha-1-acid glycoprotein and albumin were measured.

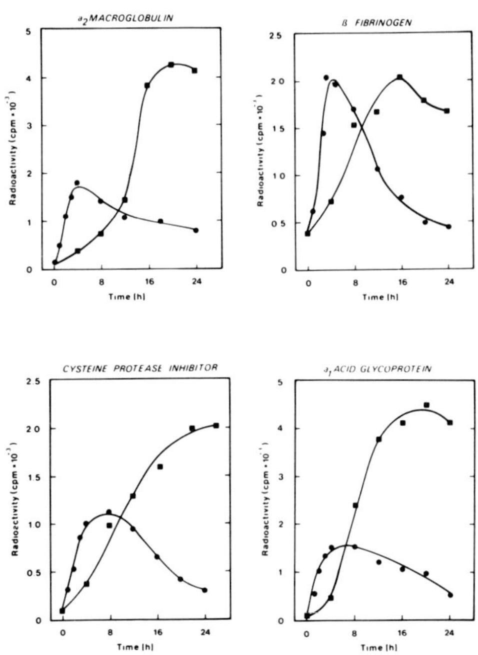

Fig. 4. Comparison of the time courses of induction of acute phase protein mRNAs by rhIL-6 or turpentine. Male Wistar rats (180-220 g body weight) were injected either intraperitoneally with 40 x 10^3 units of rhIL-6 (●) or intramuscularly with 0.8 ml of turpentine (■). At the times indicated in the figure, the animals were sacrificed, the livers excised, total RNA was extracted and analyzed by dot-blot hybridization. The radioactivity of the dots was determined by liquid scintillation counting.

Fig. 4 (closed circles) shows that alpha-2-macroglobulin, ß-fibrinogen, cysteine proteinase inhibitor and alpha-1-acid glycoprotein mRNA levels increase very rapidly after the administration of rhIL-6. On the other hand, albumin mRNA concentrations showed a steady decrease during a period of 24 h. Since the recombinant IL-6 used was expressed in E. coli, possible LPS contamination had to be considered. LPS concentrations in the rhIL-6 and fetal calf serum preparations were determined. As a result of the Limulus amoebocyte assay we had to take into account a maximum LPS contamination of about 0.25 ng per injection. When increasing amounts of LPS were injected in a control experiment, we found no acute phase protein response up to 10 ng of LPS per animal. As an additional control, rhIL-6 was incubated at 95°C for 5 min prior to injection. After this treatment no stimulation of the acute phase protein mRNA levels was observed, although the LPS contamination was still present and active.

When the time course of acute phase protein mRNA induction after rhIL-6 was compared with the one after intramuscular injection of turpentine, it was found that rhIL-6 led to a much more rapid induction of ß-fibrinogen, alpha-2-macroglobulin, cysteine proteinase inhibitor and alpha-1-acid glycoprotein mRNA levels with maxima already at 4 h for ß-fibrinogen, alpha-2-macroglobulin and alpha-1-acid glycoprotein and about 8 h in the case of cysteine proteinase inhibitor (Fig. 4, filled circles). It is obvious from the figure 4 that the maximal acute phase protein mRNA levels after the administration of turpentine (filled squares) are reached much later, i.e. between 16 and 24 h. For albumin only a small difference was observed. The maximal mRNA levels after the administration of turpentine are reached 12-16 h later than after injection of the inflammatory mediator rhIL-6. This delay in acute phase protein response is very likely due to an indirect action of turpentine, where a cascade of reactions including activation of monocytes and macrophages, the formation, secretion and transport of inflammatory mediators from the local abscess to the liver has to proceed, whereas rhIL-6 acts directly on the hepatocytes (Gauldie et al., 1987; Andus et al., 1987a).

(C) Plasma clearance, organ distribution and target cells of rhIL-6 in the rat

The rapid increases as well as the transient mRNA levels of the acute phase proteins found after rhIL-6 injection, compared to the turpentine-induced response could be due to a short half-life of rhIL-6. Therefore, we have investigated the fate of rhIL-6 in the rat.

After intravenous injection of 40,000 units of rhIL-6, blood samples were taken for the determination of the biological activity of rhIL-6 measured by the induction of ß-fibrinogen mRNA in the rat hepatoma cell line Fao. Fig. 5 shows that rhIL-6 activity disappeared very rapidly from the plasma. Furthermore, the

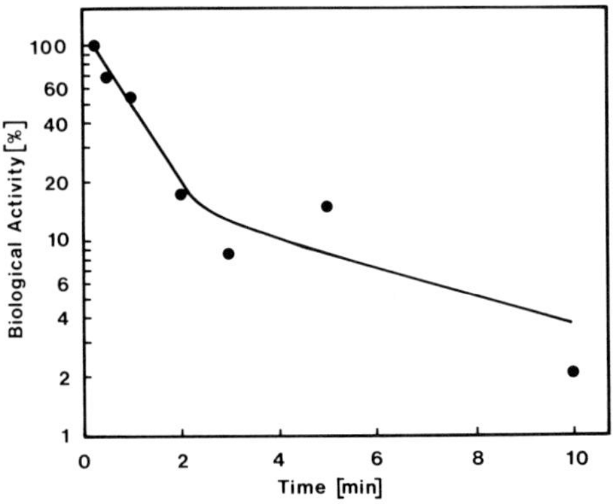

Fig. 5. Clearance of rhIL-6 from rat plasma. 4×10^4 units of rhIL-6 in 0.14 M NaCl/1% fetal calf serum were injected into the tail vein of a male Wistar rat (200 g body weight). At the times indicated in the figure, blood samples of 0.2 ml were taken from the catheterized vena cava inferior and IL-6 activity was determined in the plasma. IL-6 concentrations are expressed as percent of the maximum plasma level at 30 seconds after injection.

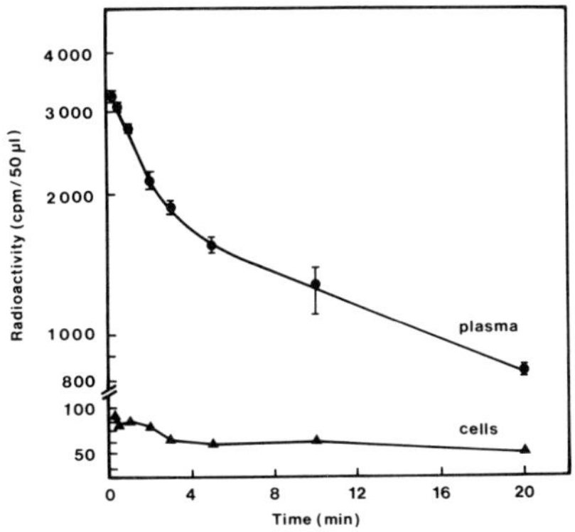

Fig. 6. Disappearance of ^{125}I/rhIL-6 from rat plasma. 1.2 x 10^6 cpm of ^{125}I/rhIL-6 (specific activity 50 kBq per µg) were injected into the tail vein of a male Wistar rat (200 g body weight). At the times indicated, blood samples were taken from the catheterized vena cava inferior. Radioactivity was determined in plasma (●) and in blood cells (▲). Data are expressed as radioactivity per 50 µl of plasma or blood cells, respectively, and represent the average ± S.D. of 4 independent experiments.

plasma half-life of ^{125}I/rhIL6 was studied. Iodination did not lead to a reduction in its biological activity. Fig. 6 shows that the iodinated rhIL-6 disappeared in a biphasic manner. The clearance curve consisted of two exponential components: an initial, fast one, corresponding to an average half-life of about 3 min, whereas the half-life of the second slow component was about 55 min. No ^{125}I/rhIL-6 was bound to blood cells (filled triangles).

The radioactivity measured in plasma corresponded to intact IL-6 with an apparent molecular weight of 21 kDa, as determined by SDS-PAGE under reducing conditions and subsequent to autoradiography (not shown). The ratio of radioactivity in plasma/radioactivity in the IL-6 band in the gel was constant at all time points suggesting that no degradation of ^{125}I/rhIL-6 had occurred 20 min after injection.

Having demonstrated that rhIL-6 is rapidly removed from blood, the question arose, which organs are involved in its clearance. 20 min after intravenous injection of ^{125}I/rhIL-6 liver, kidney, spleen, heart, thymus, lungs, muscle, and small intestine were excised and the radioactivities of the whole organs were determined. Fig. 7 shows clearly that liver is the major target organ for rhIL-6. In 3 independent experiments about 80% of ^{125}I/rhIL-6 that had disappeared from the circulation was found in liver. The radioactive material taken up by the liver was shown by SDS-PAGE to be intact ^{125}I/rhIL-6.

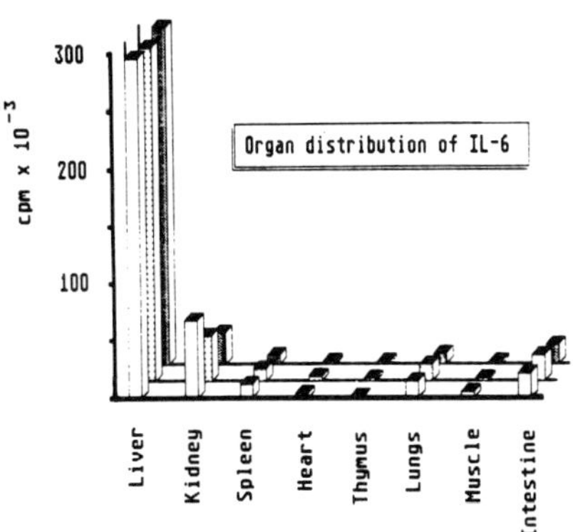

Fig. 7. Organ distribution of ^{125}I/rhIL-6. As described in the legend to Fig. 6, 1.2 x 10^6 cpm of ^{125}I rhIL-6 (specific activity 50 kBq per µg) were intraveneously injected into male Wistar rats. After 20 min, organs were excised and their wet weights and radioactivities were measured. Data are expressed as absolute radioactivity determined in each organ.

To identify the target cells within the liver, we examined liver sections taken 20 min after injection of ^{125}I/rhIL-6 by light microscopy after autoradiography. Autoradiography showed the radioactivity exclusively at the surface of hepatocytes and essentially not on non-parenchymal cells (Fig. 8). No internalization of the radioactively labeled rhIL-6 was observed at this time.

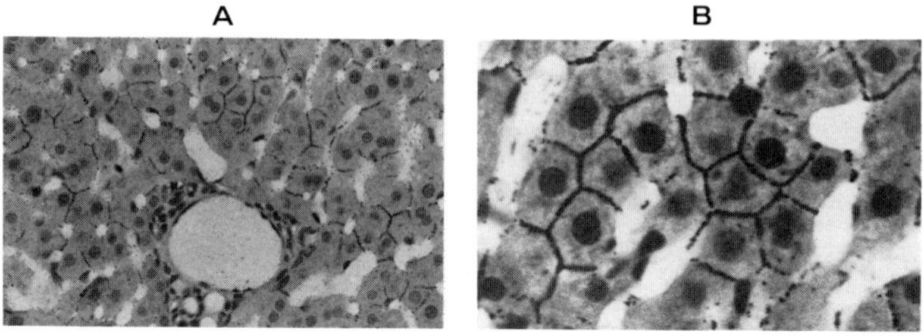

Fig. 8. Distribution of ^{125}I/rhIL-6 in liver. ^{125}I/rhIL-6 (7.5×10^6 cpm, 50 kBq per µg) were injected into the tail vein of male Wistar rats. After 20 min the liver was perfused in situ with 4% glutardialdehyde in 50 mM phosphate (Na/K) buffer, pH 7.4 containing 0.14 M NaCl. After fixation liver pieces were embedded in paraffin, sliced and analyzed by autoradiography and light microscopy. Magnification: A, 600 X; B, 1700 X.

(D) Interleukin-6 is the major regulator of acute phase protein synthesis in human hepatocytes

From the studies presented above, it is evident that (i) IL-6 is preferentially taken up in the liver and bound to the surface of hepatocytes and is (ii) the most important mediator for acute phase protein induction in the rat. Thus far, there has been no direct evidence for IL-6 as an acute phase mediator in human hepatocytes.

Adult human hepatocytes were incubated with 100 units per ml rhIL-6 for 20 h with or without supplementation of 100 nM dexamethasone. This rhIL-6 concentration as well as the time for stimulation was chosen in analogy to experiments, which we had carried out with the human hepatoma cell lines HepG2 and Hep3B2. After labeling hepatocytes with ^{35}S/methionine for 3 h, 12 plasma proteins were immunoprecipitated from the media and analyzed by SDS-PAGE and subsequent fluorography. Essentially for all acute phase proteins the immunoprecipitations led to single radioactively labeled bands. In the cases of fibrinogen and fibronectin the antisera had been raised against the holoproteins. Since fibrinogen is composed of 6 subunits ($\alpha_2\beta_2\gamma_2$) and fibronectin of 2 subunits, the expected polypeptides were detected.

It can be seen in Fig. 9 that the response to rhIL-6 is quite different for the various proteins studied. Serum amyloid A and C-reactive protein are very strongly induced, and a strong stimulation was also found for haptoglobin, alpha-1-antichymotrypsin, and fibrinogen. Only moderate increases were observed for alpha-1-antitrypsin and alpha-1-acid glycoprotein. Alpha-2-macroglobulin, which is no acute phase protein in humans, did not change. In the cases of fibronectin, transferrin and albumin decreases were observed. No newly synthesized serum amyloid P could be detected under our experimental conditions.

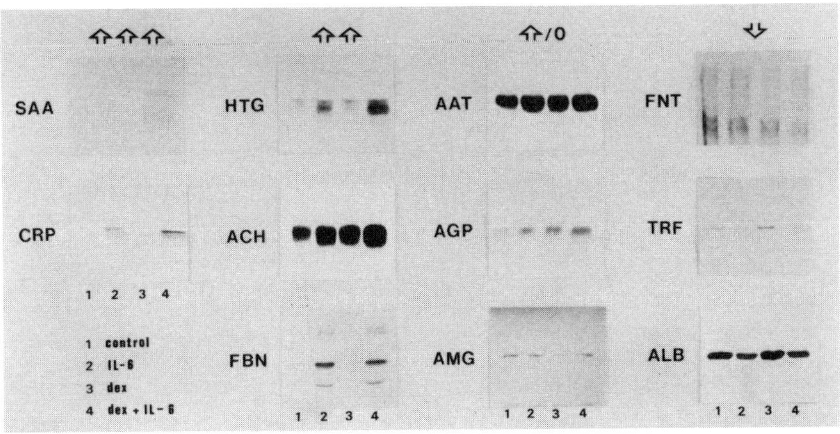

Fig. 9. Induction of acute phase protein synthesis in human hepatocyte primary cultures. Cultured adult human hepatocytes were incubated with 100 U/ml of rhIL-6 (lane 2), 100 nM dexamethasone (lane 3), and 100 U/ml of rhIL-6 plus 100 nM dexamethasone (lane 4) for 20 h. Non-treated hepatocytes were used as a control (lane 1). After a labeling period of 4 h with 25 µCi ^{35}S/methionine per ml. The acute phase proteins were immunoprecipitated with specific antibodies and analyzed by SDS-PAGE and autoradiography. SAA, serum amyloid A; CRP, C-reactive protein; HTG, haptoglobin, ACH, a-1-antichymotrypsin; FBN, fibrinogen; AAT, a-1-antitrypsin; AGP, a-1-acid glycoprotein; AMG, a-2-macroglobulin; FNT, fibronectin; TRF, transferrin; ALB, albumin.

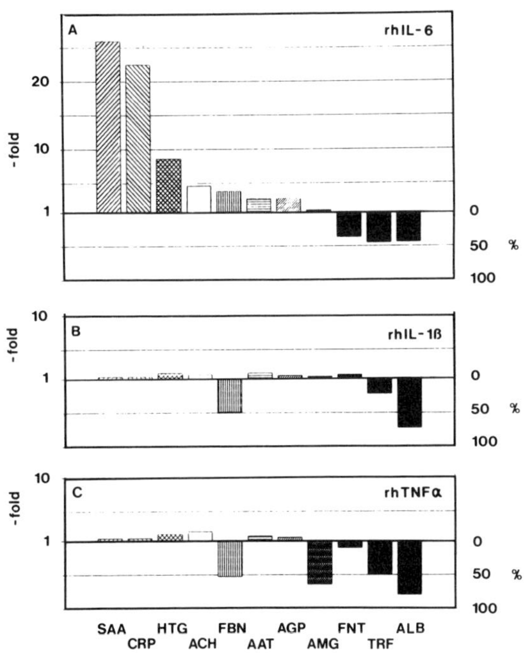

Fig. 10. Acute phase response of human hepatocytes stimulated by rhIL-6, rhIL-1ß and rhTNFa. Human hepatocytes isolated from liver biopsies of healthy donors were serum-free cultured and stimulated with 100 U/ml of rhIL-6 (A), or 300 U/ml of rhIL-1ß (B) or 500 U/ml of rhTNFa (C) for 20 h. After a labeling period of 3 h with ^{35}S/methionine, newly synthesized and secreted proteins were immunoprecipitated and quantified. The abbreviations are the same as those given in the legend to Fig. 9.

Since IL-1 (Dinarello, 1984) and TNFα (Darlington et al., 1986; Perlmutter et al., 1986) are presently considered as important mediators of acute phase protein synthesis in hepatocytes from rodents and hepatoma cell lines, we incubated human hepatocytes in primary culture with rhIL-1ß and rhTNFα. The newly synthesized and secreted proteins were analyzed by immunoprecipitation, their radioactivities were determined and compared to those of IL-6 stimulated hepatocytes. It is shown in Fig. 10A that rhIL-6 stimulated a wide spectrum of acute phase proteins, whereas rhIL-1ß and rhTNFα exhibited only weak stimulatory effects (Fig. 10,B,C). The synthesis of the negative acute phase protein albumin was dramatically decreased (80% inhibition) by rhIL-1ß and rhTNFα. Also, it is remarkable that the levels of the positive acute phase protein fibrinogen, which increased after rhIL-6, decreased in rhIL-1ß and rhTNFα stimulated human hepatocytes. Furthermore, fibronectin and alpha-2-macroglobulin were found to be regulated by only one of the 3 mediators. RhIL-6 impaired fibronectin synthesis and only rhTNFα decreased alpha-2-macroglobulin production.

CONCLUSION

From the results presented in this paper, it is now evident that among the three monokines released by LPS-stimulated human monocytes/macrophages which act on hepatocytes, interleukin-6 is the most important mediator in respect to its capability to regulate acute phase protein synthesis in human liver as well as in the rat (Fig. 11).

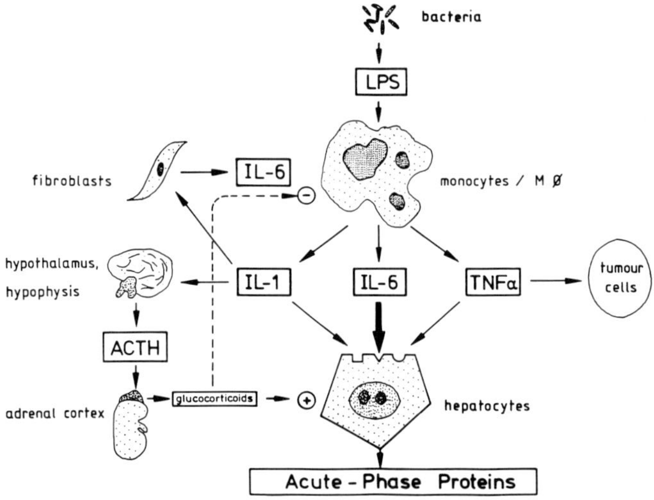

Fig. 11. Schematic representation of acute phase protein regulation in hepatocytes.

ACKNOWLEDGEMENTS

The authors thank Dr. R. Trullenque and Dr. R. Fabra, Servicio de Cirugîa, Hospital General de Valencia, Spain for providing the liver biopsies. J.V.C. is indebted to Consellería de Cultura de Valencia and to INSALUD for facilitating this research. The help of H. Gottschalk in the preparation of this manuscript is greatly acknowledged. This work was supported by grants from the Deutsche Forschungsgemeinschaft, Bonn, SFB 206, Freiburg, and Fondo de Investigaciones Sanitarias de la Seguridad Social, Spain.

REFERENCES

Andus, T., Gross, V., Tran-Thi, T.-A., Schreiber, G., Nagashima, M., and Heinrich, P.C. (1983). Eur. J. Biochem. 133, 561-571.

Andus, T., Geiger, T., Hirano, T., Northoff, H., Ganter, U., Bauer, J., Kishimoto, T., and Heinrich, P.C. (1987a). FEBS Lett. 221, 18-22.

Andus, T., Heinrich, P.C., Bauer, J., Tran-Thi, T.-A., Decker, K., Männel, D., and Northoff, H. (1987b). Eur. J. Immunol. 17, 1193-1197.

Andus, T., Geiger, T., Hirano, T., Kishimoto, T., Tran-Thi, T.-A., Decker, K., and Heinrich, P.C. (1988). Eur. J. Biochem. 173, 287-293.

Chirgwin, J.M., Przybyla, A.E., MacDonald, R..J. and Rutter, W.J. (1979). Biochemistry 18, 5294-5299.

Darlington, G.J., Wilson, D.R., and Lachman, L.B. (1986). J. Cell Biol. 103, 787-793.

Dinarello, C.A. (1984). New England J. Med. 311, 1413-1418.

Feinberg, A.P. and Vogelstein, B. (1983). Anal. Biochem. 132, 6-13.

Fuller, G.M. and Ritchie, D.G. (1982). Ann. N.Y. Acad. Sci. 389, 308-322.

Gauldie, J., Richards, C., Harnish, D., Lansdorp, P., and Baumann, H. (1987). Proc. Natl. Acad. Sci. USA 84, 7251-7255.

Geiger, T., Northemann, W., Schmelzer, E., Gross, V., Gauthier, F., and Heinrich, P.C. (1982). Eur. J. Biochem. 126, 189-195.

Geiger, T., Tran-Thi, T.-A., Decker, K., and Heinrich, P.C. (1987). J. Biol. Chem. 262, 4973-4977.

Hirano, T., Taga, T., Nakano, N., Yasukawa, K., Kashiwamura, S., Shimizu, K., Nakajima, K., Pyun, K.H., and Kishimoto, T. (1985). Proc. Natl. Acad. Sci. USA 82, 5490-5494.

Hirano, T., Yasukawa, K., Harada, H., Taga, T., Watanabe, S., Matsuda, T., Kashiwamura, S., Nakajima, K., Koyama, K., Iwamatsu, A., Tsunasawa, S., Sakiyama, F., Matsui, H., Takahara, Y., Taniguchi, T., and Kishimoto, T. (1986). Nature 324, 73-76.

Koj, A. (1985). Definition and classification of acute-phase proteins. In: The acute-phase response to injury and infection (eds A.H. Gordon and A. Koj) Elsevier, Amsterdam. Vol. 10. 139-232.

Kushner, I. (1982). Ann. N.Y. Acad. Sci. 389, 39-48.

Perlmutter, D.H., Dinarello, C.A., Punsal, P.I., and Colten, H.R. (1986). J. Clin. Invest. 78, 1349-1354.

Tran-Thi, T.-A., Phillips, J., Falk, H., and Decker, K. (1985). Exp. Mol. Pathol. 42, 89-116.

Transmembrane Signalling and Chemical Mediators

The Role of Kinase Activation and Gene Expression in the Action of Interleukin 2

WILLIAM L. FARRAR[1], DOUGLAS K. FERRIS[2], and ANNICK HAREL-BELLAN[1]

[1] *Laboratory of Molecular Immunoregulation, National Cancer Institute—Frederick Cancer Research Facility, Frederick, Maryland 21701–1013*

[2] *Biological Carcinogenesis Development Program, Program Resources Inc., NCI-FCRF, Frederick, Maryland 21701-1013*

ABSTRACT

Interleukin 2 (IL 2) stimulates the activation of several unique kinase systems which interact to decrease negative signals and amplify positive signals to the nucleus. Specific gene transcription is rapidly initiated by IL 2 including, protooncogenes, ornithine decarboxylase, heat shock stress genes and secretory lymphokines.

KEYWORDS

Interleukin 2: Kinases: Phosphoproteins: gene transcription

INTRODUCTION

Signal transduction is a process by which external substances convey "new" information to the cell by transforming the chemical nature of the information into a series of simplified yet amplified chemical "messengers". The first form of information identification occurs at the outer surface of the plasma membrane as a result of the bimolecular interaction between recognition protein (receptor) and the information substance (ligand). The binding of the two molecules causes additional allosteric protein interactions within the transmembrane and proximal cytoplasmic domains of the receptor which then activate "amplifying" systems which create new species of chemical substances which are recognized by internal proteins (enzymes) and thereby affect the physicochemical activity of subcellular proteins. The two most rigorously studied transduction systems of cellular stimuli are the adenylate cyclase (AC) complex (rev. in Gillman, 1984) and phospholipase C activation of phosphatidylinositol (PIP_2) hydrolysis (Michell, 1982). Both systems create unique chemical messengers, in the case of AC cyclic AMP is synthesized from ATP, whereas the hydrolysis of PIP_2 liberates inositol triphosphate (IP_3) and diacylglycerol. Although unique messengers are synthesized by these systems, both sets of chemical "second messengers" result in the activation of protein kinases. In fact, with the possible exception of steroid hormones, all known external-receptor mediated signalling triggers protein phosphorylation.

Long recognized as an exquisitely sensitive means of controlling protein function, protein phosphorylation is a principal biochemical mechanism regulating cellular viability and function. We have examined the ability of IL 2 to stimulate protein phosphorylation in comparison with pharmacological activators of distinct kinase systems. IL 2 also down regulates cyclic AMP accumulation, implying an inhibition of cAMP-dependent kinase activation (Beckner & Farrar, 1986). IL 2 apparently activates a number of distinct kinases which affect phosphorylation of unique substrates (Evans & Farrar, 1987a). For instance, the activation of protein kinase C (PK-C) by phorbol ester or IL 2 leads to the subsequent activation of a Mg^{2+}-dependent serine kinase which phosphorylates the 40S ribosomal S6 protein (Evans & Farrar, 1987b). Such early studies indicate that IL 2 stimulates several unique kinase activities, which are subject to interkinase regulation.

Cell cycle progression is characterized by the expression of genes common to most mammalian cells. We have examined the sequential expression of protooncogenes, ornithine decarboxylase (ODC), IL 2 receptor α (TAC), and a member of the heat shock gene family HSP70. Although many of these genes are modulated by IL 2, potent anti-proliferative signals such as cyclic AMP inhibit the expression of a selected few of these cell progression genes.

RESULTS AND DISCUSSION

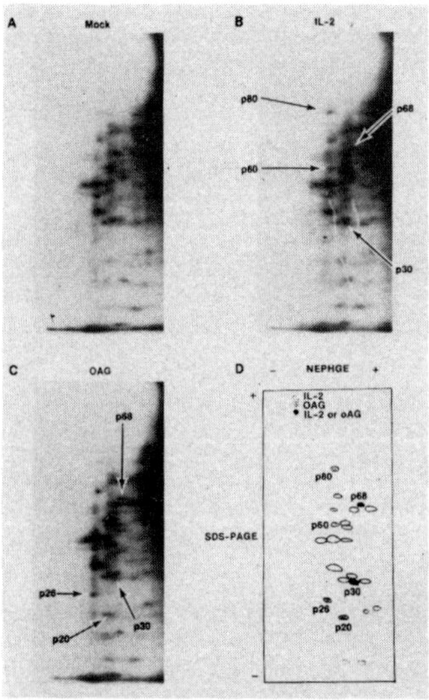

Fig. 1.

IL 2 and Synthetic Diacylglycerol (OAG) Stimulation of Protein Phosphorylation.

CT6 cells were deprived of IL 2 and serum for 18 hrs. prior to $^{32}P\text{-}O\text{-}PO_4$ labelling (Evans & Farrar, 1987a). Labelled cells were stimulated for 10 minutes, 2-D NEPHGE gels are shown.

IL 2 stimulates the rapid phosphorylation of a number of substrates in murine and human T cells. Since some suggestions had been made that IL 2 could stimulate a transient activation of PK-C (Farrar & Anderson, 1985), we tested whether IL 2 and a direct activation of PK-C, with synthetic diacylglycerol (1-oleyl-2-acetylglycerol: OAG), stimulated the phosphorylation of any common substrates in the ^{32}P-phosphate labelled IL 2-dependent murine T cell line CT6. Figure 1 shows 2-D NEPHGE gels comparing IL 2 and OAG stimulation of cellular protein phosphorylation. Panel A is background phosphorylation of unstimulated cells. IL 2 stimulated the rapid phosphorylation (>10 min.) of proteins whose molecular weights corresponded to p30, p60, p68 and p80 Kilodaltons (Fig. 1B). OAG, a direct activator of PK-C, stimulated phosphorylation of p20, p26, p30 and p68 kd proteins (Fig. 1C). The comparison between the physiological ligand and PK-C activator revealed that the stimulated phosphoproteins fell into three categories. First, IL 2 and OAG both stimulated phosphorylation of p68 and p30 proteins. Second, IL 2 stimulated phosphorylation of other proteins not affected by OAG treatment, p80 and p60. Finally, direct activation of PK-C alone by OAG stimulated phosphorylation of unique proteins p26 and p20 (Fig. 1D). Several conclusions can be drawn from these studies (Evans & Farrar, 1987a; Farrar et al., 1986) IL 2 and direct activators of PK-C converge at the phosphorylation of at least two substrates p68 and p30. IL 2, however, is clearly stimulating the phosphorylation of additional substrates p80 and p60 which are not apparently affected by PK-C. The study indicated that IL 2 may in fact, stimulate multiple kinase activities. In order to determine which phosphoproteins may be of critical importance, we examined the effects of a number of growth promoting colony stimulating factors (IL 3, GM-CSF, and G-CSF) for the stimulation of phosphoproteins in myeloid cell lines. A comparative analysis indicated that IL 2, IL 3, and G-CSF all induced phosphorylation of the p68 protein on threonine-serine residues in multiple cell lines (Evans et al., 1987). The high positive correlation of p68 phosphorylation with multiple growth factor stimulation suggested a remarkable conservation of p68 involvement in diverse tissue responses to growth factors. While we have not identified the function of p68, however, we identified the p30 protein as the 40S ribosomal S6 protein (Evans & Farrar, 1987b).

IL 2 and OAG/PMA both stimulated phosphorylation of the 40S ribosomal S6 protein. Shown in Figure 2 is the time-course increase in S6 protein phosphorylation observed _in situ_ following IL 2 treatment of CT6 cells. Stimulation of S6 phosphorylation by PMA or IL 2 was accompanied by increased protein chain initiation suggesting that the level of increased S6 phosphorylation was proportional to increases in the initiation of protein synthesis. Although both IL 2 and PMA stimulated the same phosphorylation pattern, deduced by 2-D tryptic peptide analysis, purified PK-C could not phosphorylate purified S6 protein _in vitro_ in a manner analogous to IL 2 or PMA induced phosphorylation _in situ_. However, another kinase was isolated from CT6 cytosol following IL 2 treatment that had no requirements for Ca^{2+} or phospholipids (as does PK-C), and could phosphorylate S6 _in vitro_. The tryptic phosphopeptide pattern produced from S6 phosphorylated by this kinase _in vitro_ was nearly identical to those obtained from S6 phosphorylated _in situ_ after IL 2 or PMA stimulation. The "S6 kinase" required only Mg^{2+} ions and was insensitive to cyclic AMP-kinase or PK-C inhibitors _in vitro_. These studies suggested the important conclusion that although a specific kinase (such as PK-C) may be directly pharmacologically activated (phorbol esters), other kinases may act as the effector enzyme in the phosphorylation of proteins. Thus, we envision many kinase interactions may occur as a result of IL 2 initiated signal transduction.

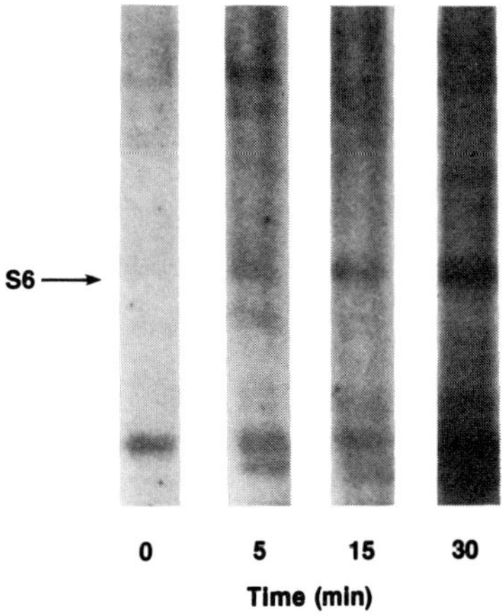

Fig. 2.

IL 2 Stimulation of 40S Ribosomal S6 Protein Phosphorylation.

CT6 cells were prepared as described in Evans and Farrar, 1987a. Cells were stimulated with 1000u rIL 2 (Cetus)/10^7 cells and aliquats removed at indicated time points. S6 protein was prepared as described (Evans & Farrar, 1987b) and run on PAGE.

Kinase system "cross-talk" has also been demonstrated for the signals evoked by IL 2 and PK-C activators and the adenylate cyclase (AC) complex. Activation of AC or elevation of intracellular cyclic AMP by stable analogues inhibits IL 2 driven proliferation of human or mouse T lymphocytes (Beckner & Farrar, 1986, Farrar & Beckner, 1986). Increasing dosages of IL 2, however, mitigates the (ED50) anti-proliferative effects of prostaglandins. IL 2 and a phorbol ester (PMA) were shown to diminish basal cAMP levels in IL 2-dependent murine or human T cells and uncouple PGE_2 stimulation of AC and cAMP accumulation (Beckner & Farrar, 1986). Membrane reconstitution experiments, where purified PK-C was added to CT6 membranes, showed that activation of PK-C was sufficient to inhibit membrane basal AC activity or PGE_2 induced AC activity. These experiments provided new insights that positive and negative signals to the cell, mediated through distinct protein kinase systems, can modulate each other's activities, the balance of which determines the biological response.

Control of gene expression by IL 2 and the anti-growth signal cyclic AMP

IL 2 triggers the transcriptional expression of a number of "consensus" genes common to fibroblasts, myeloid cells and lymphocytes (Cleveland et al., 1987, Harel-Bellan & Farrar, 1987). Specifically, IL 2 modulates the sequential expression of the nuclear protooncogenes c-fos, c-myc, and c-myb. A comparative analysis with serum-stimulated NIH 3T3 fibroblasts and IL 2 treated lymphocytes revealed similar expression of c-fos and c-myc (Cleveland et al., 1987). Other genes such as KC or r-fos were only seen in fibroblasts whereas c-myb was detected in IL 2 stimulated lymphocytes. The regulation of protooncogenes with tyrosine kinase activity (c-abl, c-src, etc.) or those with serine kinase activity (c-raf-1) were unaffected by IL 2 stimulation. Hybridization analyses with cytosolic/membrane protooncogene probes specific for c-fms, neu, c-erbB, c-erbA, C-Ha-ras, v-sis, and N-ras, failed to detect any hybridizing transcripts in CT6 cells. Colony stimulating factor(s) also stimulate c-fos and c-myc expression in factor dependent myeloid cell clones (Harel-Bellan & Farrar, 1987).

In addition to the nuclear protooncogenes, IL 2 stimulates steady state mRNA accumulation and protein synthesis for ornithine decarboxylase, the rate limiting enzyme for polyamine synthesis, and HSP70, a member of the ancient family of stress proteins (Farrar et al., 1988, Ferris et al., 1988). Interestingly, IL 2 modulated over 15-fold the expression of HSP70, a stress protein which characteristically responds to heat shock, metalloproteins, and oxidative stress. The finding that IL 2 modulated the HSP70 gene suggested mammalian cell proliferation utilizes highly conserved pathways which have evolved from primitive microorganismal stress - adaptation responses.

The identification of molecular structures (genes, protein synthesis, etc.) which are amplified by the growth signal (IL 2) has allowed the study of the effects of anti-growth signals. Cyclic AMP is well known for its anti-proliferative effects on T and B-lymphocytes. We have examined the effects of the stable analog 8-Br-cAMP (1mM) on IL 2 stimulated gene expression. Table 1 summarizes our findings of the effects of IL 2, phorbol ester, and cyclic AMP analog on $G_1 \rightarrow S$ phase gene expression in the cytotoxic T cell clones CT6 or CTB6. Cyclic AMP is not a universal inhibitor of gene expression. While c-myc and ODC steady state mRNA levels are reduced by cAMP, mRNA levels for c-fos, c-myb and IL 2 receptor α (TAC) are increased (Farrar et al., 1987, Farrar et al., 1988). Although we found cAMP to stimulate Tac mRNA expression, we found a concomitant inhibition of protein synthesis in the presence of cAMP. The effects of cAMP were seen at independent levels of macromolecular synthesis, both protein synthesis and steady state mRNA levels were affected. Our findings that cAMP can inhibit c-myc expression may be important since recent studies have shown that oligonucleotide "anti-sense" inhibition of c-myc biosynthesis inhibits cellular proliferation in response to plant lectin or IL 2 (Harel-Bellan et al., 1988).

The identification of specific biochemical events and gene expression regulated by IL 2 aids in the development of our understanding of mammalian cell growth. These biochemical and molecular events also serve as fundamental loci at which to examine the effects of potent anti-growth signals. Furthermore, as we identify biochemical signals and genes important in the control of cellular growth, it should become possible to determine their relationships to malignant growth.

Table I
Effects of Exogenous Stimulants on Cell Cycle Genes

mRNA Expression	IL 2	PMA (PKC)	8-Br-cAMP (PK-A)	IL 2 + cAMP
c-fos	+	+	++	+++
c-myc	++++	++	-	-
c-myb	++++	++	++	+++
Tac(p55)	+++	+++	+++	+++
ODC	+++	+++	-	+
HSP70	+++	ND	ND	ND

ND = not done. Data based on relative densitometry and arbitrary assignments. All data was from northern blot analysis (Cleveland et al., 1987, Farrar et al., 1987, Farrar et al., 1988, Ferris et al., 1988)

ACKNOWLEDGEMENTS

The authors would like to thank all past and present collaborators for their contributions. We appreciate the support and encouragement of Drs. Joost J. Oppenheim and Dan Longo and the editorial assistance of Ms. Beth Guyton.

This project has been funded at least in part with Federal funds from the Department of Health and Human Services under contract number N01-CO-74102 with Program Resources, Inc. The content of this publication does not necessarily reflect the views or policies of the Department of Health and Human Services, nor does mention of trade names, commercial products, or organizations imply endorsement by the U.S. Government.

REFERENCES

Beckner, S.K. and Farrar, W.L. (1986) J. Biol. Chem. 261, 3043-3047.
Cleveland, J.L., Rapp, U.R. and Farrar, W.L. (1987) J. Immunol. 138, 3495-3504.
Evans, S.W. and Farrar, W.L. (1987a) J. Cell. Biochem. 34, 47-59.
Evans, S.W. and Farrar, W.L. (1987b) J. Biol. Chem. 262, 4624-4630.
Evans, S.W., Rennick, D., and Farrar, W.L. (1987) Biochem. J. 244, 683-691.
Farrar, W.L. and Anderson, W.B. (1985) Nature 315, 233-235.
Farrar, W.L. and Beckner, S.K. (1986) Transplantation Proc. 5, 25-28.
Farrar, W.L., Cleveland, J., Beckner, S.K., Bonvini, E., and Evans, S.W. (1986) Immunol. Rev. 92, 49-65.
Farrar, W.L., Evans, S.W., Rapp, U.R., and Cleveland, J.L. (1987) J. Immunol. 139, 2075-2080.
Farrar, W.L., Harel-Bellan, A., Cleveland, J.L., and Vinocour, M. J. Immunol., in press.
Ferris, D.K., Harel-Bellan, A., Morimoto, R.I., Welch, W.J., and Farrar W.L. Proc. Natl. Acad. Sci. USA, in press.
Gilman, A.G. (1984) Cell 36, 577-580.
Harel-Bellan, A., Ferris, D.K., Vinocour, M., Holt, J.T., and Farrar, W.L. (1988) J. Immunol. 140, 2431-2435.
Michell, R.H. (1982) Cell Calcium 3, 285-296.

Transmembrane Events in Mast Cell Histamine Release

TERUKO ISHIZAKA

Johns Hopkins University School of Medicine, Subdepartment of Immunology, 5601 Loch Raven Blvd., Baltimore, Maryland USA 21239

ABSTRACT

Bridging of IgE-receptors on mast cells and basophil granulocytes induces an enhancement of phosphatidylinositol (PI) turnover and mobilization of intracellular Ca^{2+}, followed by the activation of protein kinase C. Pretreatment of sensitized mouse bone marrow-derived mast cells (BMMC) with either pertussis toxin (PT) or cholera toxin (CT), which ADP-ribosylates GTP-binding protein Gi or Gs, affected neither the formation of inositol phosphates nor histamine release induced by the bridging of IgE-receptors. In contrast, the treatment of the cells with PT or CT either inhibited or enhanced histamine release induced by IgE-independent stimuli. It was also found that introduction of GTPγS or GTPβS into permeabilized BMMC did not affect the IgE-mediated histamine release. It appears that GTP-binding protein is not involved in the transduction of the triggering signals from IgE-receptors for histamine release.

KEY WORDS

Phospholipase C: inositol trisphosphate: diacylglycerol: GTP-binding protein: pertussis toxin: cholera toxin.

INTRODUCTION

Mast cells and basophils bear receptors specific for IgE and the reaction of cell-bound IgE antibodies with multivalent antigen initiates the release of a variety of inflammatory mediators (Ishizaka, T. 1981). Before the 3rd International Conference on Immunopharmacology in Florence, I discussed the biochemical events involved in the transduction of IgE-mediated triggering signals for mediator release (Ishizaka and White, 1986). In the past three years, remarkable progress has been made in this area and more information became available. Development of sensitive new methods by Tsien et al (1982) to directly measure changes in the concentration of intracellular Ca^{2+} such as Quin-2 or Fura-2, made it possible for us to analyze initial movement of intracellular Ca^{2+} upon antigen stimulation. Furthermore, possible role of other biochemical processes, such as PI turnover, protein kinase C and guanyl nucleotide (GTP)-binding proteins in the mediator release have been explored. In this presentation, I would like to briefly summarize the progress made in the past three years on the biochemical processes involved in mediator release from mast cells.

Mobilization of intracellular calcium:

After Quin-2 became available, we examined mobilization of intracellular free calcium upon antigen stimulation using rat peritoneal mast cells (White et al, 1983). Purified rat mast cells sensitized with IgE antibody were first loaded with Quin-2 and challenged with antigen in the presence of Ca^{2+}. The concentration of intracellular free calcium rapidly increased, reaching maximum within 10 sec. When the same cells were challenged with antigen in the presence of EGTA, a small but significant increase in intracellular free calcium was observed. Since influx of Ca^{2+} can be excluded in the presence of EGTA, this increase appears to be due to the release of calcium from intracellular stores. In rat mast cells, a comparable amount of histamine was released when they were challenged with antigen in the presence or absence of EGTA. The results suggest that Ca^{2+} released from intracellular pools was sufficient for inducing a maximum histamine release from rat mast cells.

Similar experiments were repeated using cultured human basophils and IL-3 dependent mouse mast cell line PT-18 cells. Antigen challenge of sensitized mouse mast cells in the presence of Ca^{2+} resulted in a rapid increase in intracellular Ca^{2+}. In the presence of EGTA, a reduced, but significant Quin-2 signal was observed. In both PT-18 cells and human basophils however, presence of EGTA during the antigen challenge greatly reduced not only Quin-2 signal but also histamine release. The results suggested that Ca^{2+} influx was required to achieve maximum histamine release from human basophils and IL-3 dependent mouse mast cells. These results indicate that requirement of Ca^{2+}-influx for mediator release is different depending on the mast cells derived from different sources.

Another important information obtained through the experiments with Quin-2 was that the mobilization of intracellular Ca^{2+} was an earliest biochemical change detected following the bridging of IgE receptors. In our previous studies on rat mast cells and cultured human basophils, we had shown a transient increase in the phospholipid methylation and cAMP rise after the receptor bridging (Ishizaka and Ishizaka, 1984). However, mobilization of intracellular Ca^{2+} preceded the increase in phospholipid methylation and ^{45}Ca uptake, in all of rat mast cells, mouse mast cells and cultured human basophils.

The role of phosphatidylinositol turnover:

Recently, the role of phosphatidylinositol (PI) turnover in signal transduction was studied in many types of cells, and the results suggested an essential role of PI turnover in mobilization of intracellular Ca^{2+} (Streb et al, 1983). In the mast cell and basophil systems, the reaction of cell-bound IgE antibodies with multivalent antigen induced the activation of phospholipase C and resulted in the hydrolysis of inositol phospholipids. When bone marrow-derived mouse mast cells (BMMC) sensitized with IgE antibodies were challenged with specific antigen, phosphatidylinositol 4,5-bisphosphate was hydrolyzed and generated inositol 1,4, 5-trisphosphate (IP3), inositol 1,4-bisphosphate (IP2) and inositol 1 monophosphate (IP) (Fig. 1) (Saito et al, 1987). As shown in the figure, stimulation of the cells with thrombin also resulted in the generation of IP3, IP2 and IP, but kinetics of the generation of phosphatidylinositol breakdown products were different depending on the stimulus.

The stimulation of sensitized BMMC with either antigen or thrombin also generated an accumulation of 1,2-diacylglycerol (DAG). As shown in Fig. 2, kinetics of the generation of DAG paralleled the kinetics of histamine release in both antigen-induced and thrombin-induces systems (Saito et al, 1987). These results suggest that stimulation of PI turnover and generation of IP3 and DAG may play an important role in transduction of the triggering signals for mediator release.

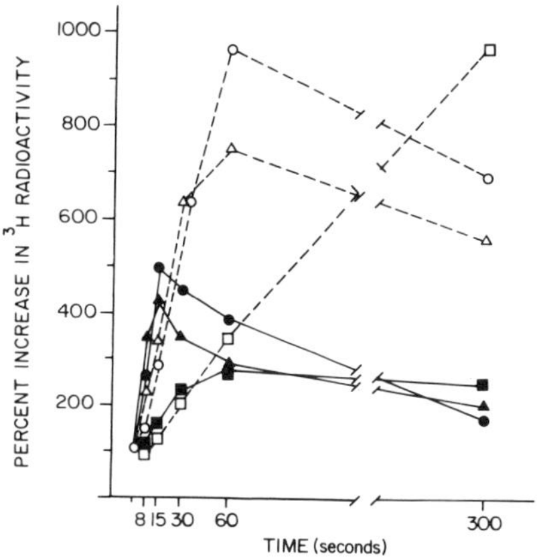

Fig. 1. Kinetics of generation of IP3 (Δ), IP2 (o) and IP (□) by DNP-HSA or by thrombin (▲,●,■,), in BMMC sensitized with anti-DNP-IgE antibodies.

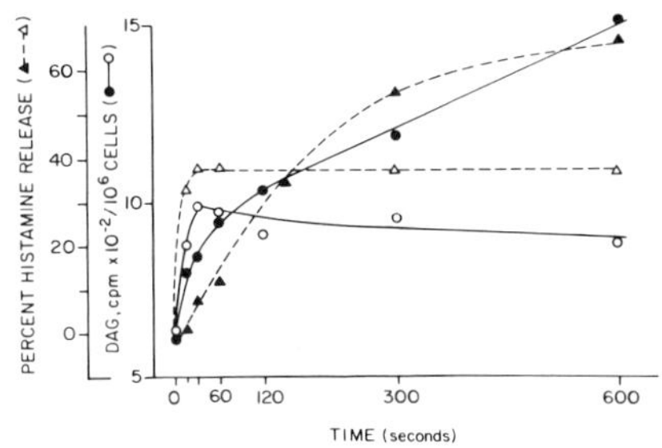

Fig. 2. Kinetics of generation of DAG (●——●) and histamine release (▲——▲) by DNP-HSA, or by thrombin (o----o, Δ----Δ), from BMMC sensitized with anti-DNP IgE-antibodies.

Activation of protein kinase C:

Since the bridging of IgE on mast cells induces the accumulation of DAG, one can expect that protein kinase C may be activated by antigen challenge. As previously reported (White et al, 1985), stimulation of sensitized mouse mast cells with antigen resulted in a rapid increase in C-kinase activity associated with plasma membrane which reached maximum by 30 sec, then gradually decreased to control levels. The protein kinase C activity remaining in the cytosol slightly diminished over the same period. It was also found that an increase in C-kinase activity precedes histamine release.

Recently, similar results were obtained in human basophils by Warner and MacGlashan (1988). Stimulation of purified human peripheral blood basophils with an optimal concentration of anti-IgE resulted in a rapid increase in membrane associated C-kinase which reached a maximum 1 min after the stimulation, and then declined slowly over the next 30 min. White and Metzger (1988) also showed translocation of C-kinase from cytosol to membrane fraction upon stimulation of sensitized RBL cells with PMA or antigen. In their experiments, however, they demonstrated that RBL cells depleted of C-kinase failed to respond to PMA or Ca^{2+}-ionophore for degranulation, but responded to antigen for a significant degranulation. The results suggest that the activation of C-kinase may not be essential for antigen-induced mediator release.

Possible role of GTP-binding proteins in mediator release:

Another new topic in the field is the possible role of GTP-binding proteins in mediator release. It has been established that receptors for various hormones link to one of the two GTP-binding proteins, Gs or Gi, which mediates either the activation (Gs) or inhibition (Gi) of adenylate cyclase. Pertussis toxin (PT) induces the ADP-ribosylation of α subunit of Gi (Giα) (Katada and Ui, 1982), while cholera toxin ADP-ribosylates Gsα (Gill and Meren, 1978, Cassel and Pfeuffer, 1978). Accumulated evidence suggests that GTP-binding proteins are involved in the signal transduction in various types of cells. In view of these observations, we studied possible participation of GTP-binding proteins in the mediator release from mast cells, in collaboration with Drs. Ui and Okajima in Japan and Dr. Sha'afi, University of Connecticut (Saito et al, 1987, 1988).

It was demonstrated that IgE-mediated histamine release from rat mast cells, bone marrow-derived mouse mast cells (BMMC), cultured human basophils and human peripheral blood basophils was not affected by pretreatment of the cells with highly purified pertussis toxin. In contrast, the pretreatment with PT inhibited compound 48/80-induced histamine release from rat mast cells, thrombin-induced histamine release from BMMC, and F-Met-Leu-Phe-induced or C5a-induced histamine release from human basophils in a dose-dependent manner (Saito et al, 1987). The treatment of sensitized BMMC with PT resulted in the inhibition of thrombin-induced histamine release, but did not affect the antigen-induced IgE-mediated histamine release even when more than 97% of α subunit of Gi (41 Kd) had been ADP-ribosylated by the pretreatment. Furthermore, analysis of the mechanisms for the inhibition of thrombin-induced histamine release by the PT-treatment indicated that the treatment neither affected thrombin-induced generation of IP3, IP2, IP and 1,2-diacylglycerol (DAG) nor thrombin-induced Quin-2 signal. It was also found that the PT treatment affected neither the antigen-induced nor thrombin-induced arachidonic acid release. The results suggested that the inhibition of histamine release induced by IgE-independent stimuli is due to the effect of PT on the later stages of histamine release, distal to the mobilization of intracellular Ca^{2+}.

In the next series of experiments, we studied the effect of cholera toxin (CT) which induces ADP-ribosylation of α subunit of stimulatory GTP-binding protein Gs, using BMMC as a model system. It was found that preincubation of BMMC with cholera toxin (CT) resulted in the parallel increase in intracellular cAMP and an enhancement of histamine release by thrombin, but failed to show any effect on antigen-induced histamine release, even when more than 90% of α subunit (43 Kd and 48 Kd) of Gs had been ADP-ribosylated by the pretreatment (Saito et al, 1988).

These results suggest that neither PT-sensitive GTP-binding protein Gi, nor CT-sensitive Gs plays an essential role in the transduction of IgE-mediated triggering signals for histamine release. However, these results do not exclude the possibility that some novel GTP-binding protein other than Gi or Gs may be involved in the IgE-mediated histamine release. Indeed, possible participation of GTP-binding protein in histamine release from mast cells was first demonstrated by Gomperts (1983). He had shown that introduction of a non-hydrolyzable GTP analogue, such as GTPγS, into permeabilized rat mast cells caused histamine release in response to the addition of extracellular Ca^{2+}. Furthermore, Fernandez et al (1984), demonstrated that introduction of GTPγS into the cytosol of rat mast cells by patch pipette technique induced Ca^{2+}-independent degranulation. Based on these observations, we explored possible involvement of a novel GTP-binding protein in the IgE-mediated histamine release from mast cells.

Effect of GTPγS and GDPβS on IgE-mediated histamine release:

Following the method described by Gomperts with slight modifications, we established the conditions for permeation of rat mast cells and BMMC using ATP. When various concentrations of GTPγS were introduced into the permeabilized rat mast cells or BMMC, these cells released histamine in response to the addition of extracellular Ca^{2+}. Using these permeabilized rat mast cells and BMMC, we analyzed possible linkage between IgE-mediated histamine release and GTPγS-induced histamine release.

In the experiments shown in Fig.3, sensitized BMMC were permeabilized, and various concentration of GTPγS was introduced into aliquots of the cells. After the cells were resealed with Mg^{2+}, one set of the cells were challenged

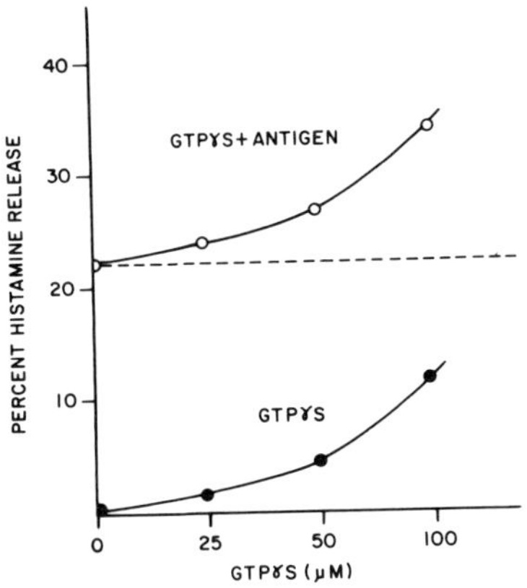

Fig. 3. Various concentrations of GTPγS were introduced into 2 sets of permeabilized BMMC sensitized with anti-DNP IgE antibodies. After the cells were resealed with Mg^{2+}, one set of the cells were challenged with a suboptimal concentration of DNP_{12}-HSA in the Tyrode solution containing 1.6 mM Ca^{2+}. Other set of cells were resuspended in the same Tyrode solution and both sets were incubated at 37°C for 10 min for histamine release.

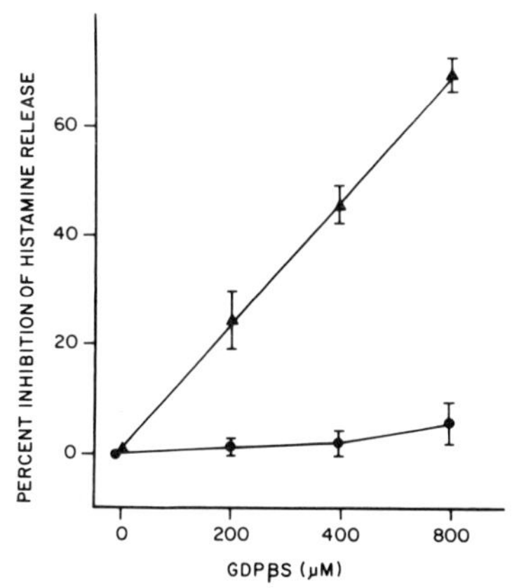

Fig. 4. Various concentrations of GDPβS were introduced into two sets of BMMC sensitized with anti-DNP IgE antibody. To one set of cells, 100 M of GTβγS was introduced together with GDPβS. Resealed cells were resuspended in Tyrode solution containing 1.6 mM Ca^{2+} and histamine release was measured. Another set of cells containing GDPβS were challenged with an optimal concentration of DNP-HSA for histamine release.

with a suboptimal concentration of antigen in Tyrode solution containing 1.6 mM Ca^{2+}. Another set of cells were resuspended in the same Tyrode solution. The percentage of histamine released by antigen challenge from the GTPγS-containing cells corresponded to the sum of that induced by GTPγS alone and histamine release from control cells. The results indicate that the GTPγS does not have synergistic effect on antigen-induced histamine release, suggesting that antigen-induced histamine release and GTPγS-induced histamine release may go through independent pathways.

In order to test this hypothesis, a GDP analogue, GDPβS was introduced into permeabilized cells and the effect of GDPβS on IgE-mediated histamine release was examined. As shown in Fig. 4, introduction of various concentrations of GTPβS did not affect the antigen-induced histamine release. As expected, introduction of GTPβS together with GTPγS into permeabilized cells resulted in the inhibition of GTPγS-induced histamine release in a dose-dependent fashion.

Another striking difference in the GTPγS-induced and IgE-mediated histamine release was observed in the sensitivity of the responses to intracellular cAMP level. As demonstrated by Gomperts (1983) in rat mast cells, an increase in intracellular cAMP by preincubation of BMMC with IBMX or Forskolin, did not

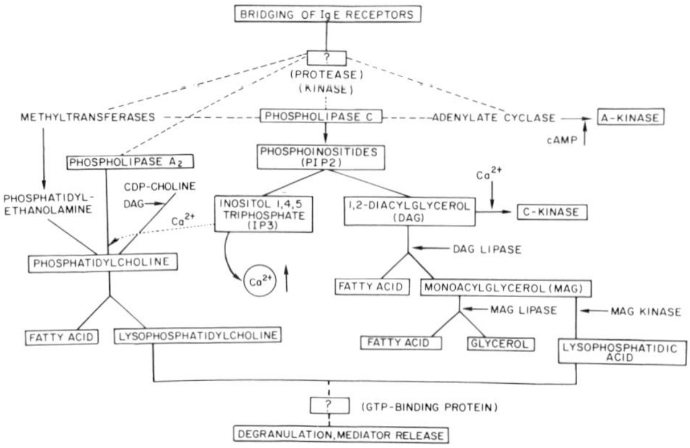

Fig. 5. Enzymes activated by bridging of IgE receptors on mast cells and basophils.

affect GTPγS-induced histamine release. The same treatment resulted in the inhibition of antigen-induced histamine release and PI turnover in a dose-dependent manner. Thus it appears that GTPγS-induced histamine release and IgE-mediated histamine release go through distinct pathways. The results support the concept that GTP-binding protein does not play a crucial role in the transduction of IgE receptor-mediated triggering signals for mediator release from mast cells.

Enzymes activated by receptor bridging:

Bridging of IgE receptors activates a variety of membrane-associated enzymes, such as a putative serine protease (Ishizaka and Ishizaka, 1984), phospholipase C (PLC) (Kennerly *et al*, 1979; Beaven *et al*, 1984; Mush and Siegel, 1986), phospholipase A_2 (PLA_2), methyltransferases (Ishizaka *et al*, 1980), and adenylate cyclase (Fig. 5). Stimulation of PI turnover results in an accumulation of DAG in the plasma membrane and the release of IP3 into cytoplasm. IP3 triggers mobilization of intracellular Ca^{2+}, and DAG in turn activates protein kinase C. IgE-mediated activation of PLA_2 (Garcia-Gil and Siraganian, 1986), and cAMP-dependent protein kinase (Holgate *et al*, 1978) had been demonstrated. An increase in intracellular Ca^{2+} and DAG further facilitates the activation of phospholipase A_2 and diacylglycerol lipase, respectively, and in turn induces the release of free arachidonic acid (AA) and lysophospholipids, monoacylglycerol (MAG) and lysophosphatidic acid. Since all of these products are membrane-active fusogens, they may cause the fusion of granular membrane and degranulation. However, many fundamental questions remain to be answered. First of all, we do not know yet how triggering signal is transmitted from IgE receptors to the enzymes. We have no evidence for possible association of IgE receptors with protein kinase or coupling of the receptors to GTP-binding protein. Neither the sequence of the activation of various enzymes nor obligatory process for the mediator release is clearly understood, because none of the inhibitors available at the moment is strictly specific for one enzyme.

At present, a general consensus is that the activation of PLC and PLA_2 may play a central role in the cascade of IgE-dependent mediator release. Since the activation of PLC would result in mobilization of intracellular Ca^{2+}, activation of C-kinase and formation of fusogens (c.f. Fig. 5), possible role of PLC in the mediated release has been emphasized. However, our recent experiments on the effect of a phospholipase inhibitor (ONO-RS-082, ONO Pharmaceutical Co., Japan), may suggest an important role of PLA_2 in IgE-mediated histamine release from BMMC. Preincubation of sensitized BMMC with various concentrations of the inhibitor resulted in a dose-dependent inhibition of antigen-induced histamine release and arachidonate release but did not affect the hydrolysis of inositol phospholipids. On the other hand, the inhibitor had much less inhibitory effect on IgE-mediated histamine release from human basophils. It is possible that crucial enzymes for IgE-dependent mediator release may differ, depending on mast cells/basophils of different species and/or different stages of maturation.

ACKNOWLEDGEMENT

I would like to express my gratitude to Drs. K. Ishizaka, H. Saito and T. Nakamura, The Johns Hopkins University, Baltimore, Md., Dr. M. Ui, University of Tokyo; Dr. F. Okajima, Gumma University, Japan, Dr. R. I. Sha'afi and Mr. T. F. P. Molski, University of Connecticut, Farmington, CN., for their collaboration and Mrs. Chiew G. L. Ko for her excellent technical assistance.

This work was supported by research grant AI-10060 from the U.S.H.H.S. and the research grant from Hyde and Watson Foundation. This paper is publication No. 726 from the O'Neill Laboratories, the Good Samaritan Hospital, Baltimore, Md.

REFERENCES

Beaven, M. A., Moore, J.P., Smith, G.A., Hesketh, R.T. and Metcalfe, J.C. (1984). J. Biol. Chem. 259, 7137-7142.
Cassel, D. and Pfeuffer, T. (1978). Proc. Natl. Acad. Sci. USA 75, 2669-2683
Fernandez, J. M., Neher, E. and Gomperts, B.D. (1984). Nature 313, 543-545.
Garcia-Gil, L. M. and Siraganian, R.P. (1986). J. Immunol. 136,359-363.
Gill, D. M. and Meren, R. (1978). Proc. Natl. Acad. Sci. USA 74, 3050-3054.
Gomperts, B. D. (1983). Nature 306, 64-66.
Holgate, S. T., Lewis, R.A. and Austen, K.F. (1980). J. Immunol. 124, 2093-2099.
Ishizaka, T. (1981). J. Allergy and Clin. Immunol. 67, 90-96.
Ishizaka, T., Hirata, F., Ishizaka, K. and Axelrod, J. (1980). Proc. Natl. Acad. Sci. USA 77, 1903-1907.
Ishizaka, T. and Ishizaka, K. (1984). Prog. Allergy 34, 188-235.
Ishizaka, T. and White, J.R. (1986). Advances in Immunopharmacology, ed.by Chedid, L. Hadolen Pergamon Press 201-209.
Katada, T. and Ui, M. (1982). J. Biol. Chem. 257, 7210-7216.
Kennerly, D. A., Sullivan, T.J. and Parker, C.W. (1979). J. Immunol. 122, 152-159.
Mush, M. W. and Siegel, M .I. (1986). Biochem. 234, 205-212.
Saito, H., Okajima, F., Molski, T.F.P., Sha'afi, R.I., Ui, M. and Ishizaka, T. (1987). J. Immunol. 138, 3927-3934.
Saito, H., Okajima, F.,m Molski, T.F.P., Sha'afi, R.I., Ui, M. and Ishizaka, T. (1988). Proc. Natl. Acad. Sci. USA 85, 3504-3508.
Streb, H., Irvine, R.F., Berrige, M.J. and Schulz, I. (1983). Nature 306, 67-68.
Tsien, R. Y., Pozzan, T. and Rink, J.J. (1982). J. Cell. Biol. 94, 325-334.
Warner, J. A. and MacGlashan, D.W. (1988). FASEB J. 2, A1226 (Abstract).
White, J. R., Ishizaka, T., Ishizaka, K. and Sha'afi, R.I. (1983). Proc. Natl. Acad. Sci. USA 81, 3978-3982.
White, J. R., Pluznik, D.H., Ishizaka, K. and Ishizaka, T. (1985). Proc. Natl. Acad. Sci. USA 82, 8193-8197.
White, K. N. and Metzger, H. (1988). FASEB J. 2, A1235 (Abstract.

An Approach to the Mode of Action of Lipocortins

BERNARD ROTHHUT, CHRISTINE COMÉRA
and FRANÇOISE RUSSO-MARIE

*Unité de Pharmacologie Cellulaire, INSERM UA 285, Institut Pasteur,
25 rue du Dr. Roux, 75724 Paris Cédex 15, France*

Abstract

Lipocortins are a family of proteins whose major function is to inhibit phospholipase A2, a key enzyme involved in the production of inflammatory mediators such as prostaglandins, leukotrienes and paf-acether. The mechanism of action of anti-inflammatory steroids is in part attributed to the synthesis and/or release of lipocortins. These proteins are thought to be regulated by phosphorylation involving tyrosine kinases such as the EGF receptor and the retrovirally coded protein kinase $pp60^{src}$, as well as the serine/threonine protein kinase C. Recently lipocortins were identified as members of a new family of calcium-dependent / phospholipid binding proteins including other proteins found in the literature under the names calelectrin, endonexin, calpactin, chromobindin, synhibin, calcimedin, and annexin. The comparison of available amino acid sequences showed that all these proteins contain a conserved consensus sequence of 17 amino acids. Recent kinetic studies revealed a substrate concentration-dependent inhibition of the enzyme by lipocortin involving a calcium-dependent binding to the phospholipid rather than an enzyme-inhibitor interaction. Whatever the mechanism of inhibition, these proteins are able to exert an anti-inflammatory effect in an animal model, but it is not yet known whether they can reproduce all the effects induced by anti-inflammatory steroids.

Key words

Glucocorticosteroids / lipocortin / phospholipase A2 / Ca^{2+} and phospholipid-binding protein anti-inflammatory effect.

Introduction

A simplified inflammatory reaction can be described as a stimulus-response coupling event occuring on the cell membrane leading to activation of phospholipase A2, a key enzyme involved in the formation of pro-inflammatory mediators such as prostaglandins, leukotrienes and paf-acether. In inflammatory cells, the signal-induced activation of phospholipase A2 releases mediators able to reactivate other cells.

Glucocorticosteroids are the most widely used anti-inflammatory agents and studies of their mechanism of action led to the discovery of lipocortins. These hormones cross the plasma membrane and act inside the cells by binding to a specific receptor. The complex (hormone-receptor) interacts with the cellular DNA, inducing transcription into mRNA and traduction into specific proteins. These proteins are in part responsible for the anti-inflammatory effect induced by steroids (Russo-Marie et al, 1979). The studies on these induced proteins led to the discovery and the purification of a family of proteins named lipocortins.

Several groups described this phenomenon. Hirata et al (1980) described in rabbit neutrophils, a steroid-induced protein they named "lipomodulin". Blackwell et al (1980) demonstrated the same mechanism in rat macrophages and gave the name of "macrocortin". In our laboratory we worked on rat renomedullary interstitial cells in culture and proposed the name "renocortin" for the steroid-induced factor (Cloix et al, 1983). All these proteins were identified by their biochemical properties (molecular weights of 40 kDa cleaved into smaller fragments of 30 and 15 kDa), biological activities, (inhibition of soluble phospholipases A2 in an *in vitro* assay), and biological regulation (phosphorylation by protein kinases) (Hirata, 1981). The use of monoclonal antibodies against the different proteins, led to the finding that all these factors were immunologically related (Rothhut et al, 1983) and therefore the common name of "lipocortin" was adopted (proteins induced by corticoids and modulating phospholipids) ((Di Rosa et al, 1984).

Lipocortins are constitutive proteins

Lipocortins were first described as steroid-induced and -released proteins inhibiting phospholipase A2. All the groups had initially reported the lipocortins in the supernatants of treated cells or in the peritoneal fluid. The demonstration and the finding of intracellular forms of lipocortins (Rothhut et al, 1984) without steroid treatment, raised new questions on the mode of action of the hormones. Using a monoclonal antibody against rat lipocortin, we could find immunoprecipitated proteins inside control cells, demonstrating the existence of endogenous forms of lipocortins. One possibility could be that the steroids induce "de novo" protein synthesis which is released out of the cell and possess a very high specific activity for inhibiting phospholipase A2.

Purification, regulation and sequence of lipocortins

Recently Biogen cloned and sequenced lipocortin I (Wallner et al , 1986)) and a different protein they named lipocortin II (Huang et al, 1986) Both proteins exhibit similar biochemical properties : they possess anti-phospholipase A2 activities. By peptide mapping, amino acid sequence and immunological analyses, they identified lipocortin I (or p35) as the substrate of the EGF receptor tyrosine kinase from A431 cells (Blake-Pepinsky and Sinclair, 1986). In a similar way, they demonstrated that lipocortin II (or p36) was the substrate for the retrovirally encoded tyrosine kinase pp60^{src} (Huang et al, 1986; Kristensen et al, 1986). These two proteins have 50% sequence homology, are coded by two different genes and only the mRNA level of lipocortin I was increased after glucocorticoid treatment. At the same time other groups working on calpactins, (cytoskeletal proteins interacting with actin in a calcium-dependent manner), published amino acid sequences (Glenney, 1986). By comparing the different amino acid sequences it became clear that lipocortin I and II are respectively identical to calpactin II and I. In addition other calcium binding proteins which bind to biomembranes have sequence homology with lipocortin I and II (Geisow et al, 1986). It became obvious that there exists a family of proteins sharing the following properties : they bind reversibly to biological membranes in a calcium-dependent manner, they inhibit phospholipases A2 and they all contain a highly conserved consensus sequence of 17 amino acids (Geisow, 1986). In the literature the following different names for this new family of proteins are found : calelectrin (Walker, 1982), endonexin (Südhof et al, 1984), p68/p70 (Owens et al, 1984), protein I and II (Gerke and Weber, 1984), synexin (Creutz et al, 1978), chromobindin (Creutz et alwa, 1983), calcimedin (Moore, 1986), annexin (Geisow et al, 1987). For simplicity and convenience, these proteins will be referred to as lipocortins.

Mode of action of lipocortins

We have investigated the purification of the lipocortins from human mononuclear cells. Based on calcium dependent binding to biological membranes we were able to purify six proteins having lipocortin-like activities (Rothhut et al , 1987; Coméra et al, submitted). Among these proteins we characterized and identified a 32 kDa lipocortin, using immunological and biological criteria. With respect to lipocortin, the pure protein inhibited soluble phospholipases A2 in a dose-dependent manner but only when low concentrations of negatively charged phospholipids were used as a substrate. This suggested a substrate concentration-dependent inhibition of the enzyme by lipocortin, involving a calcium-dependent binding to the phospholipid rather than an enzyme-inhibitor interaction. (Davidson et al, 1987; Aarsman et al, 1987). Another alternative could be a dissociation of the inactive enzyme-inhibitor complex in the presence of an excess of phospholipids (Aarsman et al, 1987). We can not conclude whether one mechanism or the other is involved, or both.

Pharmacological aspects

The first demonstration of a pharmacological effect of purified lipocortin I has recently been published by Cirino et al, 1987).
In our laboratory, Errasfa and Russo-Marie (manuscript in preparation) developed an animal model (a polyacrylamide gel induced granuloma in mice) to test the anti-inflammatory effects of a 36 kDa lipocortin purified from mice lungs (Errasfa and Russo-Marie, 1988). As dexamethasone, an intravenous injection of the protein inhibited the production of prostaglandins, leukotrienes as well as cell migration to the inflammatory site.
Another pharmacological approach was also developed in our laboratory by Maridonneau-Parini and coworkers. In ovalbumin-sensitized guinea-pigs, aerosolization of lipocortin (32 kDa protein, Rothhut et al, 1987) before antigen challenge, almost totally abolished the allergic bronchospasm. These results suggest that the therapeutic effect of glucocorticosteroids administered by aerosol in asthmatic diseases may be mimicked -even more rapidly- by lipocortin.

Conclusion

These different results raise several questions concerning the role of the different proteins of the lipocortin family and the regulation of their synthesis and activity by glucocorticosteroids. Up to now only lipocortin I has been described to be induced by steroids. Lipocortins main fonction is to inhibit the activity of phospholipase A2 by a mechanism involving calcium-dependent binding to the phospholipidic substrate. Are these proteins able to modulate other membrane interacting proteins? (phospholipase C, protein kinase C ...). These proteins reproduce in part the anti-inflammatory effect of the glucocorticosteroids. Are they responsible for all the effects of the hormones? The answers to these questions will lead to the development of a new class of anti-inflammatory and anti-allergic drugs.

Acknowledgments

We thank Dr. Isabelle Maridonneau-Parini and Mourad Errasfa for their pharmacological contributions.

References

Aarsman, A.J., Mynbeek, G., Van Den Bosch, H., Rothhut, B., Prieur, B., Coméra, C., Jordan, L. and Russo-Marie, F. (1987). FEBS Lett. 219, 176-180.

Blackwell, G.J., Carnuccio, R., Di Rosa, M., Flower, R.J., Parente, L. and Persico, P. (1980). Nature 287, 147-149.

Blake-Pepinsky, R. and Sinclair, L.K. (1986). Nature 321, 81-84.

Cirino, G., Flower, R.J., Browning, J.L., Sinclair, L.K. and Pepinsky, R.B. (1987). Nature 328, 270-272.

Cloix, J-F., Colard, O., Rothhut, B. and Russo-Marie, F. (1983). Br. J. Pharmacol.79, 312-321.

Coméra, C., Rothhut, B. and Russo-Marie, F. (1988). Submitted.

Creutz, C.E., Pazoles, C.J. and Pollard, H.B. (1978). J. Biol. Chem. 253, 2858-2866.

Creutz, C.E., Dowling, L.G., Sando, J.J., Villar-Palasi, C., Whipple, J.H. and Zaks, W.J. : (1983). J. Biol. Chem. 258, 14664-14674.

Davidson, F.F., Dennis, E.D., Powell, M.P. and Glenney, J.R. (1987). J. Biol. Chem. 262, 1698-1705.

Di Rosa, M., Flower, R.J., Hirata, F., Parente, L. and Russo-Marie, F. (1984). Prostaglandins 28, 441-444.

Errasfa, M. and Russo-Marie, F. (1988). Biochem. Biophys. Res. Commun. 153, 1271-1275.

Geisow, M.J., Fritsche, U., Hexham, J.M., Dash, B. and Johnson, T. (1986). Nature 320, 636-638.

Geisow, M.J. (1986). FEBS Lett. 203, 99-103.

Geisow, M.J., Walker, J.H., Boustead, C. and Taylor, W. (1987). Bioscience Reports 7, 289-298.

Gerke, V. and Weber, K. (1984). EMBO J. 3, 227-233.

Glenney, J.R. Jr. (1986). Proc. Natl. Acad. Sci. USA 83, 4258-4262.

Hirata, F., Schiffmann, D., Venkatasubramanian, K., Salomon, D. and Axelrod, J. (1980) . Proc. Natl. Acad. Sci. USA 77, 2533-2536.

Hirata, F. (1981). J. Biol. Chem. 256, 7730-7733.

Huang, K.S., Wallner, B.P., Mattaliano, R.J., Browning, J.L., et al. (1986). Cell 46, 191-199.

Kristensen, T., Saris, C.J.M., Hunter, T., Hicks, L.J., Noonan, D.J., Glenney, J.R. and Tack, B. (1986). Biochemistry 25, 4497-4503.

Moore, P.B. (1986). Biochem. J. 238, 49-54.

Owens, R.J., Gallagher, C.J. and Crumpton, M.J. (1984). EMBO J. 3, 945-952.

Rothhut, B., Russo-Marie, F., Wood, J., Di Rosa, M. and Flower, R.J. (1983). Biochem. Biophys. Res. Commun. 117, 878-884.

Rothhut, B., Russo-Marie, F., Cousin, M. and Lando, D. (1984). In Proceedings of the 9th IUPHAR Congress of Pharmacology, P. Turner, W. Paton, J.F. Mitchell (eds), The Macmillan Press ltd, London, 43-46.

Rothhut, B., Coméra, C., Prieur, B., Errasfa, M., Minassian, G. and Russo-Marie, F. (1987). FEBS Lett. 219, 169-175.

Russo-Marie, F., Paing, M. and Duval, D. (1979). J. Biol. Chem. 254 8498-8504.

Südhof, T.C., Ebbecke, M., Walker, J.H., Fritsche, U. and Boustead, C. (1984). Biochemistry 23, 1103-1109.

Walker, J.H. (1982). J. Neurochem., 39, 815-823.

Wallner, B.P., Mattaliano, R.J., Hession, C., et al. (1986). Nature 320, 77-80.

Protein Kinase C and Signal Transduction in T Lymphocytes

N. BERRY and K. ASE

Department of Biochemistry, Kobe University School of Medicine, Chuo-ku, Kobe 650, Japan

ABSTRACT

Protein Kinase C (PKC), is involved in the signal transduction of a variety of stimulatory agents which activate human T lymphocyte proliferation. In this study, the role of PKC in T cell activation has been investigated in the light of two developments in this field. Firstly, recent reports have shown that PKC exists as several structurally and biochemically distinct subspecies. Immunocytochemical analysis of a pure T lymphocyte population with polyclonal antisera specific for these subspecies revealed that T lymphocytes express the PKC subspecies encoded by α, βI and βII, but not by γ cDNA sequences. Secondly, it has been shown that contamination of a T lymphocyte population by even a low percentage of macrophages can markedly affect the response to stimulatory agents. Examination of interleukin-2 receptor (IL-2R), expression and proliferation in a pure T lymphocyte population in response to PHA-M, TPA and OAG show that elevation of the intracellular calcium concentration synergises with PKC activation to cause IL-2R expression. TPA also elicits an additional stimulatory effect, similar to that of macrophages, which results in T cell proliferation. The implications of these results and the direction of future work are discussed.

KEYWORDS

Human T lymphocyte: protein kinase C: proliferation: interleukin 2 receptor.

INTRODUCTION

The Protein kinase C (PKC) enzyme, ubiquitous in the tissues of all species tested, is physiologically activated by the receptor-mediated hydrolysis of inositol phospholipids, which generates two intracellular signals. One of these is inositol-1,4,5-trisphosphate (IP3), which mediates the elevation of intracellular calcium concentration ($[Ca]_i$), and the other is diacylglycerol, which activates PKC. As this signal transduction pathway is initiated by a variety of external stimuli, such as hormones, growth factors and neurotransmitters, PKC is thought to be involved in the activation of a range of cellular responses, including proliferation, differentiation and the secretion of several biologically active substances (For reviews see Nishizuka, 1984; 1986).

There is considerable evidence that PKC is involved in the activation of proliferation of human T lymphocytes. Physiological activation of T lymphocytes is via the T cell receptor (Ti/T3 complex), (Acuto and Reinherz, 1985), as a result of which the T cell receptor is phosphorylated and down-regulated, the interleukin-2 receptor (IL2-R), is expressed and interleukin-2 (IL-2) is secreted. The IL-2 then acts on IL2-R in an autocrine fashion resulting in proliferation (Reinherz et al, 1982; Meuer et al, 1984).

Activation of T lymphocyte proliferation, in vitro, by monoclonal antibodies to the Ti/T3 complex, or by binding of IL-2 to IL-2R, resulting in proliferation, causes hydrolysis of inositol phospholipids and elevation of $[Ca]_i$ (Imboden and Stobo, 1985; Bonvini et al, 1987). Moreover, activation by monoclonal antibodies to the Ti/T3 complex, by lectins and by IL-2 causes an apparent translocation of PKC to the cell membrane, which is an indication of PKC activation (Farrar and Ruscetti, 1986). Thus, activation of T lymphocyte proliferation via the Ti/T3 complex or by binding of IL-2 to IL-2R results in the hydrolysis of inositol phosholipids and, consequently, PKC activation.

The intracellular mechanisms triggered by the inositol phospholipid signal transduction pathway can be mimicked by using calcium ionophores to raise $[Ca]_i$ and either phorbol esters, for which PKC is believed to be the cell surface receptor (Castagna et al., 1982), or diacylglycerol analogues to activate PKC. Activation of the signal transduction pathway in this way results in phosphorylation and down-regulation of the Ti/T3 complex, IL-2R expression, IL-2 secretion and proliferation (Cantrell et al, 1985; Truneh et al, 1985; Kaibuchi et al, 1985; Manger et al, 1987). Whether PKC is wholly responsible for all of these T lymphocyte responses is not clear but the application of two recent developments in this field to signal transduction in T lymphocytes may provide more information to elucidate the mechanism of activation.

The first development is that molecular cloning of PKC purified from brain tissue of several mammalian species revealed that, rather than the existence of one PKC molecule, there are at least seven structural subspecies of PKC (see Ono et al, 1987; 1988; Coussens et al, 1987; Kubo et al, 1987). Three of these subspecies, which correspond to the cDNA sequences α, βI, βII and γ have been resolved by column chromatography. These purified subspecies display different activation requirements and possibly different phosphorylation specificities and are differentially localised in a number of tissues and cell types (Sekiguchi et al, 1987; 1988; Ido et al, 1987; Shearman et al, 1987; Saito et al, 1988). It is possible, therefore, that the activation of a certain PKC subspecies might be responsible for a particular cell response.

The second development is in the preparation of pure T lymphocyte populations. Experiments have previously been carried out either on established clonal cell lines or on normal T lymphocytes separated from tissues and blood. The former, because of their transformed nature, may not represent accurately signal transduction in normal cells and the latter, because macrophages were eliminated by their adherence to plastic, were contaminated with 2-5% of these cells. Recent experiments, however, using pure T lymphocyte populations prepared by elimination of contaminating cells by monoclonal antibodies and fluorescent activated cell sorting or complement mediated lysis, have shown that the presence of a low number of macrophages can markedly affect the T lymphocyte response (Linch et al, 1987).

We have begun to investigate the role of PKC in T lymphocyte proliferation in the light of these developments, firstly by determining the PKC subspecies expressed in a pure T lymphocyte population and then by examining the response of a pure T cell population to activation by the lectin phytohaemagglutinin-M (PHA-M), the phorbol ester phorbol-12-myristate-13-acetate (TPA) and the diacylglycerol analogue oleoyl acetyl glycerol (OAG).

MATERIALS AND METHODS

Preparation of a Pure T Lymphocyte Population

Peripheral venous blood was obtained from healthy volunteers and depleted of erythrocytes by mixing with 0.75 volumes of 1% (w/v) dextran in normal saline and incubating at room temperature for 45 min. Mononucleocytes were then separated by centrifugation of the plasma over Ficoll-Hypaque (Nycomed, Norway). These were depleted of B lymphocytes and macrophages, firstly, by passage through a nylon wool column, as described by Dixon and Uyemura (1987), except that all procedures were carried out at room temperature, and secondly by incubation in plastic culture dishes at 2 x 10^7 cells/20ml RPMI 1640 (Gibco), containing 20mM HEPES and 10% autologous serum/dish, for 30 min at room temperature. At this point "semi-pure" T lymphocytes were set aside so that a comparison of the proliferative response of semi-pure and pure T cells could be made. Finally, the T lymphocyte preparation was treated with 'T Cell Lymphokwik' (One Lambda Inc., CA), at 1 x 10^7 cells/0.8 ml reagent. This reagent contains the appropriate antibodies to eliminate contaminating B lymphocytes, macrophages, granulocytes and pre-activated T lymphocytes by complement mediated lysis.

Immunocytochemical Staining

T lymphocytes were stained with polyclonal antisera raised against synthetic oligopeptide sequences specific for each of the PKC subspecies encoded by α, βI, βII, and γ rat cDNA (Ase et al, 1988). Cytocentrifuge preparations of para-formaldehyde fixed, permeabilised T cells were incubated with the appropriate antiserum, diluted in 0.1M Tris/HCl at pH 7.6, containing 4% normal human serum, overnight at 4°C. The immunostaining procedure was completed using an anti-rabbit immunoglobulin streptavidin/biotin-peroxidase immunostaining kit (Biogenex, CA), according to the manufacturers instructions, except that incubation with biotinylated antiserum and streptavidin was at 4°C for 2 hrs and 1 hr respectively. A colour reaction was developed using 3,3'diaminobenzidine.

For staining of the antigens CD3, CD4, CD8, HLA-DR and IL-2R, the monoclonal antibodies CD3NU-T3, CD4NU-TH/1, CD8NUTs/c, HLA-DR Ia1 and CD25 TAC respectively, (donated by J Minowada, Fujisaka Cell Center) were used. Cytocentrifuge preparations of acetone fixed T lymphocytes were incubated with the appropriate antibody, diluted to 10 μg/ml in 0.1M Tris/HCl at pH 7.6, for 1 hr at room temperature. The staining procedure was completed using an anti-mouse immunoglobulin streptavidin/biotin-peroxidase staining kit (Biogenex, CA), according to the manufacturers instructions and employing 3,3' diaminobenzidine as substrate for the colour reaction.

Dehydrated, mounted slides were photographed using a Nikon Optiphot microscope-camera system using Fuji Minicopy 32 ASA film.

(^{3}H) Thymidine Proliferation Assay.

T lymphocytes, in RPMI 1640, containing 20mM HEPES and 10% autologous serum, were plated out into 96-well flat-bottomed plates at 10^5 cells/well and incubated with the appropriate stimuli at 37° C in a humidified atmosphere of 5% CO_2 for 72 hrs. For the final 6 hr of incubation the cells were pulsed with (^{3}H) thymidine (0.5 uCi/well; 2.0 Ci/mM sp. activity, NEN Research Products). Incorporated radioactivity was quantitated by scintillation spectrometry. Stock solutions of phorbol-12-myristate-13 acetate (TPA; Chemsyn Science Lab., Kansas) and oleoyl acetyl glycerol (OAG; Nacalai Tesque inc., Kyoto) were made in dimethyl sulphoxide (DMSO). They were diluted into cell culture medium to give a final concentration of 0.05% DMSO. Phytohaemagglutinin M (PHA-M) was obtained from EY Laboratories Inc.).

RESULTS

Composition of the T Lymphocyte Preparations.

T lymphocytes, purified by the procedure described in Materials and Methods, were immunocytochemically stained with monoclonal antibodies to the CD3, CD4 and CD8 antigens, all expressed by T lymphocytes, and to the HLA-DR antigen expressed by macrophages and by activated T lymphocytes. The "semi-pure" T lymphocyte preparation (see Materials and Methods) was composed of approximately 95% CD3 antigen positive cells and between 5-10% HLA-DR antigen positive cells, presumably because of the presence of approximately 5% macrophages and a variable number of preactivated T lymphocytes. In the "pure" T lymphocyte preparation there were >99% positive CD3 antigen positive cells and 0% HLA-DR positive cells. Both the semi-pure and pure T lymphocyte preparations were composed of approximately 60% CD4 antigen positive cells and 40% CD8 antigen positive cells.

Determination of the Expression of PKC Subspecies by Purified T Lymphocytes

Pure T lymphocyte populations were immunocytochemically stained with polyclonal antisera specific for each of the PKC subspecies encoded by α, βI, βII and γ rat cDNA. These antisera were used at a dilution, which, when preadsorbed by the appropriate peptides, resulted in no immunostaining. A positive staining reaction was observed with each of the antisera to α, βI and βII but not with the antiserum to γ (FIG 1). A similar staining distribution, albeit of different intensities, of pre- dominantly cytoplasmic staining, with some membrane localisation in the more intensely staining cells, was noted with all three PKC subspecies. Staining of the subspecies was also heterogeneous in intensity throughout the T cell population, ranging from negative to strongly positive. A comparison of the staining obtained with the antisera to the PKC subspecies and that obtained with the antibodies to CD4 and to CD8 showed that the heterogenous staining was not due to differential staining of the CD4/CD8 antigen positive T lymphocyte subpopulations.

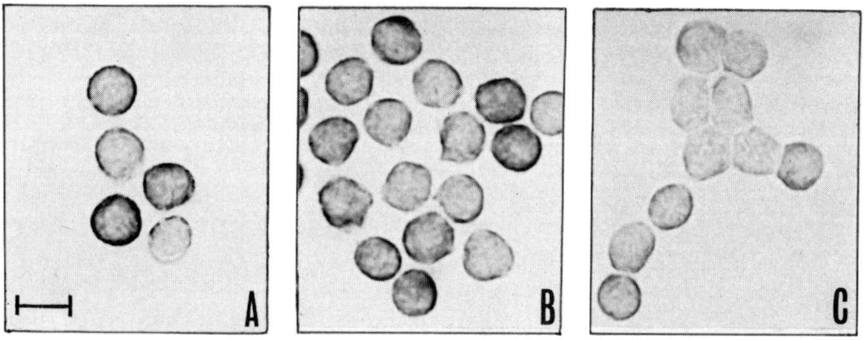

FIG 1 Immunocytochemical staining of a pure T cell population, prepared as described in Materials and Methods, with polyclonal antisera specific for the PKC subspecies encoded by α(A), βI(B) and βII(C) cDNA. Staining in all three cases is predominantly cytoplasmic, with some membrane localisation in the more intensely staining cells, and heterogenous in intensity throughout the T cell population.
Photograph taken using a x100 objective and oil immersion. Bar = 20 μm.

An Examination of the Response of Semi-Pure and Pure T Lymphocyte Preparations to Activation by PHA-M, TPA and OAG.

A comparison was made of the proliferative response, assessed by (^{3}H) thymidine uptake, of semi-pure and pure T lymphocytes to activation by PHA-M, TPA and OAG (FIG 2). Semi-pure T lymphocytes showed a proliferative response to PHA-M, a slight proliferative response to TPA and no response to OAG, whilst pure T lymphocytes did not respond to any of these stimulants alone. A combination of PHA-M and TPA had a synergistic effect on the proliferation of both semi-pure and pure T lymphocytes, although the response of the former population was markedly higher. A combination of PHA-M with OAG also had a synergistic effect on the response of semi-pure T lymphocytes, but not on that of pure T lymphocytes.

The induction of Tac antigen expression, as an indication of IL2-R expression, in response to these reagents was examined by immunocytochemical staining with a monoclonal antibody directed against the Tac antigen. Both TPA and OAG, in combination with PHA-M induced the pure T lymphocytes to express the Tac antigen although the percentage of cells expressing the antigen was higher when activated with TPA and PHA-M (65%) than with OAG and PHA-M (32%).

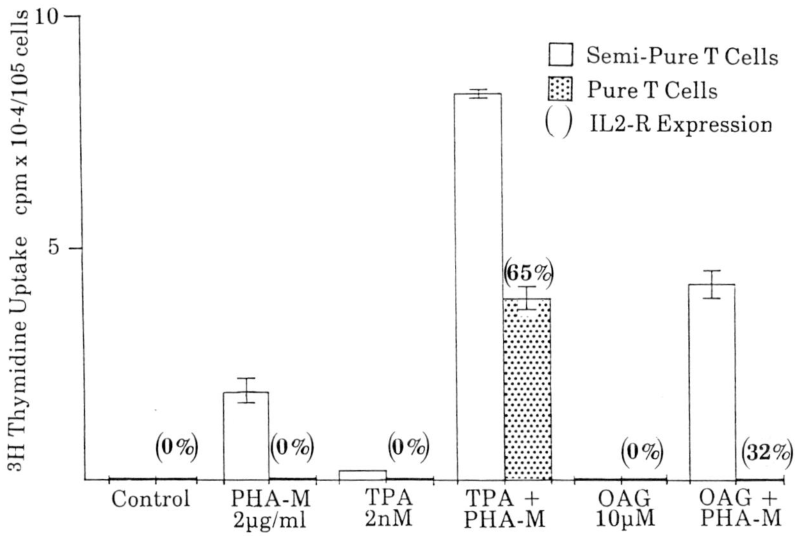

FIG 2 A comparison of the response of semi-pure and pure T lymphocyte preparations to stimulation by PHA-M, TPA and OAG. Pure T lymphocytes were plated out at 10^5 cells/well of a 96-well plate and incubated with the appropriate stimulants at the concentrations shown for 72 hr. (^{3}H) Thymidine was added for the final 6 hr of incubation. The data shown is the mean of triplicate wells. For IL-2R expression, cells from triplicate wells were pooled, cytocentrifuged and stained with a monoclonal antibody directed against the TAC antigen.

DISCUSSION

The role of PKC in the activation of T lymphocyte proliferation was investigated in this study, firstly, by determining the subspecies of PKC expressed by these cells and then by examining their response to reagents which raise $[Ca]_i$ and which activate PKC.

Immunocytochemical staining showed that a pure T lymphocyte population, which was composed of >99% T lymphocytes and 0% macrophages or preactivated T lymphocytes, expressed α, βI and βII but not γ PKC subspecies. These results confirm the data obtained by the isolation of PKC subspecies from a pure T lymphocyte population by hydroxyapatite column chromatography, where two peaks of PKC activity were obtained whose elution profile and whose biochemical characteristics correlated closely to rat brain PKC subspecies type II (βI & βII) and type III (α) (Shearman et al, manuscript in preparation).

The distribution of all three PKC subspecies was predominantly cytoplasmic, with some membrane localisation in intensely staining cells. A cytoplasmic distribution of PKC has also been observed in other resting or unactivated cell types, including lymphocyte cell lines and human neutrophils (Girard et al, 1987; Deli et al, 1987). There was no difference, at the resolution of light microscopy, in the intracellular distribution of the different subspecies. The intensity of staining of all three subspecies was heterogenous in the T lymphocyte population. This was apparently not due to differential staining of the CD4/CD8 T cell subsets but may be responsible for the normal distribution of IL2-R expression and proliferation shown by activated T lymphocytes (Cantrell and Smith, 1984).

The co-expression of multiple subspecies of PKC in resting human T lymphocytes observed in this study has also been noted in cloned T cell lines (Huang et al, 1987; Sawamura et al, manuscript in preparation) and may be an important factor in T cell activation. Of particular significance is the finding that type II (βI & βII) PKC isolated from human T lymphocytes is activated, in vitro, by phosphatidylserine and diolein in the absence of calcium, whilst activation of type III (α) PKC requires micromolar concentrations of calcium. It is possible that reagents which have different effects on intracellular calcium levels (see Linch et al, 1987), may differentially activate PKC subspecies and, consequently, elicit specific cell responses.

A comparison of the activation of pure T lymphocytes and semi-pure T lymphocytes (containing approximately 5% macrophages and 5-10% preactivated T lymphocytes) showed that the presence of even a low percentage of macrophages or preactivated T lymphocytes significantly alters the proliferative response to PHA-M, OAG and TPA, as previously reported by others (Davis and Lipsky, 1985; Katzen et al, 1987). Pure T lymphocytes proliferate only when activated by a combination of PHA-M and TPA. PHA-M is thought to activate T lymphocytes via the Ti/T3 complex by the hydrolysis of inositol phopholipids, thereby raising [Ca]i and activating PKC, although it should be noted that these experiments were carried out on semi-pure T cell populations (see Linch et al, 1987; Farrar and Ruscetti, 1986). The phorbol ester, TPA, directly activates PKC (Castagna et al, 1982). It appears that the effect of TPA partially replaces that of macrophages (or, possibly, preactivated T cells) because semi-pure T lymphocytes are capable of responding to PHA-M alone. This effect, however, cannot be attributed simply to the activation of PKC because a combination of PHA-M with OAG, a diacylglycerol analogue, and, therefore, an activator of PKC, does not induce T lymphocyte proliferation.

The reason for the different effects of TPA and OAG is not understood. It is possible that TPA initiates another signal transduction mechanism as well as activating PKC. Alternatively, there is considerable evidence that the duration and extent of activation of PKC by TPA is greater than by OAG, presumably because it integrates into the cell membrane and is stable for several hours (Farrar and Ruscetti, 1986; Manger et al, 1987). It is possible that, by either of these mechanisms, TPA activates a different range of PKC suspecies than OAG.

The response of pure T cells to PHA-M, TPA and OAG was also examined by analysis of Tac antigen expression, as an indication of IL-2R expression. A combination of either TPA or OAG with PHA-M induced Tac expression, showing that, along with the stimulatory effect of PHA-M (presumably $[Ca]_i$ elevation), PKC activation induced Tac antigen expression. Evidence that PKC activation results in IL2-R expression has been previously reported (see Farrar and Ruscetti, 1987). Whether the Tac antigen is expressed as part of the low or high affinity IL2-R (see Teshigawara et al, 1987), is presently under investigation.

In conclusion, elevation of the $[Ca]_i$ elicited by PHA-M synergises with PKC activation to cause IL-2R expression. TPA induces an additional stimulatory effect, similar to that of macrophages, which results in T lymphocyte proliferation. The basis of these activation mechanisms is not understood but it is possible, as T lymphocytes co-express α, βI and βII PKC subspecies, that differential activation of the subspecies may be responsible. This possibility is the focus of our future investigations into the role of PKC in the activation of proliferation of T lymphocytes.

ACKNOWLEDGMENTS

The authors would like to thank Prof. J. Minowada for donation of the anti- T lymphocyte monoclonal antibodies. The research in the Department of Biochemistry, Kobe University School of Medicine was supported in part by research grants from the Scientific Research Fund of the Ministry of Education, Science and Culture, Japan; Muscular Dystrophy Association; Yamanouchi Foundation for Research on Metabolic Disorders; Mercke Sharp & Dohme Research Laboratories; Biotechnology Laboratories of Takeda Chemical Industries, Ajinomoto Central Research Laboratories, Meiji Institute of Health Sciences, and New Lead Research Laboratories of Sankyo Company. N.B. is a recipient of a research fellowship from the Yamada Science Foundation.

REFERENCES

Acuto, O. and Reinherz, E.L. (1985). New Eng. J. Med. 312, 1100-1111.
Ase, K., Saito, N., Shearman, M.S., Kikkawa, U., Ono, Y., Igarashi, K., Tanaka, C. and Nishizuka, Y. (1988). J. Neuroscience In Press.
Bonvini, E., Ruscetti, F.W., Ponzoni, M., Hoffman, T. and Farrar, W.L. (1987) J. Biol.Chem. 262, 4160-4164.
Cantrell, D.A. and Smith, K.A. (1984). Science 224, 1312-1316.
Cantrell, D.A., Davies, A.A. and Crumpton, M.J. (1985). Proc. Natl. Acad. Sci. 82, 8158-8162.
Castagna, M., Takai, Y., Kaibuchi, K., Sano, K., Kikkawa, U. and Nishizuka, Y. (1982). J. Biol. Chem. 257, 7847-7851.
Coussens, L., Rhee, L., Parker, P. and Ullrich, A. (1987). DNA 6, 389-394.
Davis, L. and Lipsky, P.E. (1985). J. Imm. 135, 2946-2952.
Deli, E., Kiss, Z., Wilson. E., Lambeth, J.D. and Kuo J.F. (1987). FEBS Lett. 221, 365-369.
Dixon, J.F.P. and Uyemura, K (1987). Immunol. Invest. 16, 189-200.
Farrar, W.L. and Ruscetti, F.W. (1986) . J. Imm. 136, 1266-1273.
Girard, P.G., Stevens, V.L., Blackshear. P.J., Merrill, A.H., Wood, J.G. and Kuo, J.F. (1987) Cancer Res. 47, 2892-2898.
Huang, F.L., Yoshida, Y., Nakabayashi, H., Knopf. J.L., Scott-Young III, W. and Huang, K-P. (1987). Biochem. Biophys. Res. Comm. 149, 946-952.
Ido, M., Sekiguchi, K., Kikkawa, U. and Nishizuka, Y. (1987). FEBS Lett 219, 215-218.
Imboden, J.B. and Stobo, J.D. (1985). J. Exp. Med. 161, 446-456.
Kaibuchi, K., Takai, Y. and Nishizuka, Y. (1985), J. Biol. Chem. 260, 1366-1369
Katzen, D., Chu, E., Terhost, C., Leung, D.Y., Gesner, M., Miller, R.A. and Geha, R.S. (1985). J. Imm. 135, 1840-1845.
Kubo, K., Ohno, S. and Suzuki, K. (1987) FEBS Lett 223, 138-142.
Linch, D.C., Wallace, D.L. and O'Flynn, K. (1987) Imm. Rev. 95, 137-159.
Manger, B., Weiss, A., Imboden, J., Laing, T. and Stobo, J.D. (1987). J. Imm. 139, 2755-2760.

Meuer, S.C., Hussey, R.E., Cantrell, D.A., Hodgdon, J.C., Schlossman, S.F., Smith, K.A. and Reinherz, E.L. (1984). Proc. Natl. Acad. Sci. (USA) 81, 1509-1513.

Nishizuka, Y. (1984). Nature 308, 693-698.

Nishizuka, Y. (1986). Science 233, 305-312.

Ono, Y., Fujii, T., Ogita, K., Kikkawa, U., Igarashi, K. and Nishizuka, Y. (1987). FEBS Lett. 226, 125-128.

Ono, Y., Fujii, T., Ogita, K., Kikkawa, U., Igarashi, K. and Nishizuka, Y. (1988). J. Biol. Chem. In Press.

Saito, N., Kikkawa, U., Nishizuka, Y. and Tanaka, C. (1988). J. Neurosci. 8, 369-383

Sekiguchi, K., Tsukuda, M., Ogita, K., Kikkawa, U. and Nishizuka, Y. (1987). Biochem. Biophys. Res. Comm. 145, 797-802.

Sekiguchi, K., Tsukuda, M., Ase, K., Kikkawa, U. and Nishizuka, Y. (1988). J. Biochem. In Press.

Shearman, M.S., Naor, Z., Kikkawa, U. and Nishizuka, Y. (1987). Biochem. Biophys Res. Comm. 147, 911-919.

Teshigawara, K., Wang, H-H., Kato, K. and Smith, K.A. (1987). J. Exp. Med. 165, 223-238.

Truneh, A., Albert, F., Golstein, P. and Schmitt-Verhulst, A-M. (1985). Nature 313, 318-320.

Reinherz, E.L., Meuer, S., Fitzgerald, K.A., Hussey, R.E., Levine, H. and Schlossman, S.F. (1982). Cell 30, 735-743.

Regulation of Human Eosinophil Phenotype

M. E. ROTHENBERG and K. F. AUSTEN

Department of Medicine, Harvard Medical School, and the Department of Rheumatology and Immunology, Brigham and Women's Hospital, Boston, MA 02115, USA

ABSTRACT

Human mature eosinophils have been cultured for up to 2 weeks by coculture with endothelial cells, or by culture in enriched medium supplemented with interleukin 3, interleukin 5, granulocyte/macrophage colony-stimulating factor, or the serum of a patient with the idiopathic hypereosinophilic syndrome. Compared to the freshly isolated eosinophils, the cultured eosinophils underwent phenotypic changes characterized by enhanced calcium ionophore-induced leukotriene C_4 generation, enhanced cytotoxicity for antibody-coated larvae of Schistosoma mansoni and hypodensity as defined by sedimentation analysis. These findings and an integrated view of the regulation of eosinophil postmitotic phenotype are presented.

KEYWORDS

Eosinophils: Cytokines: Interleukins: Endothelium: Parasites.

INTRODUCTION

Over the past decade, there has been a rapid increase in our knowledge of eosinophils. It has become clear that activated eosinophils release potent inflammatory mediators, that eosinophils exist as heterogeneous subpopulations of cells with different phenotypes, and that the tissue microenvironments in which these cells reside play an important role in regulating their function and phenotype. This review will focus on our current understanding of the role of eosinophils in allergic diseases and their regulation by the tissue microenvironment in which they reside.

FUNCTION OF EOSINOPHILS

Both human (Vadas et al., 1979) and rat (Ramalho-Pinto et al., 1978) eosinophils are potent killers of opsonized helminthic parasites such as the larvae of Schistosoma mansoni. Human eosinophils possess receptors for complement fragments (Anwar and Kay, 1977; Ottesen et al., 1977), and for the F_c portions of IgG (Anwar and Kay, 1977; Ottesen et al., 1977), IgM (DeSimone et al., 1982a), and IgE (Capron et al., 1981) and are thought to utilize these receptors for recognition of opsonized targets. There are three very basically charged proteins (designated as major basic protein, eosinophil cationic protein, and eosinophil peroxidase) present in the granule of the human eosinophil which are believed to be the principal cytotoxic factors produced by this effector cell. In electron microscopic studies, eosinophils have been shown to kill schistosomula larvae by discharging their granule content onto the surface of the worm (Caulfield et al., 1985). Major basic protein, which accounts for ~55% of the weight of the human eosinophil granule, is toxic to parasites such as the larvae of Schistosoma mansoni (Butterworth et al., 1979) and Trichinella spiralis (Wassom and Gleich, 1979), as well as the protozoan parasite Trypanosoma cruzi (Kierszenbaum et al., 1981). In addition to its cytotoxicity for parasites, guinea pig major basic protein can also damage tracheal epithelium in culture (Frigas et al., 1980). This protein has been found in the toxic range in the sputa of patients with asthma (Frigas et al., 1981) and in the tears of patients with vernal conjunctivitis (Udell et al., 1981). It has also been detected by immunofluorescence in the damaged respiratory epithelium of patients with asthma (Filley et al., 1982). Major basic protein may be further involved in allergic disease by causing histamine release from basophils and mast cells (O'Donnell et al., 1983). Human eosinophil cationic protein is also a potent toxin for schistosomula; in a comparative study it appears to be ~10-fold more cytotoxic than major basic protein (Ackerman et al., 1985). Human eosinophil cationic protein damages targets by inserting voltage-insensitive, ion-nonselective transmembrane channels (Young et al., 1986). Finally, eosinophil peroxidase, in the presence of halide and hydrogen peroxide, generates hypohalous acid, which kills a variety of targets such as schistosomula (Jong et al., 1981) and mycobacteria (Klebanoff and Shepard, 1984). At low concentrations this protein can induce noncytolytic exocytosis of histamine from mast cells, whereas at high concentrations the protein lyses the mast cells (Henderson et al., 1980). This enzyme is distinguished from neutrophil myeloperoxidase on the basis of spectral differences (Archer et al., 1965) and its ability to preferentially oxidize bromide (Weiss et al., 1987).

The human eosinophil also generates lipid mediators de novo. After eosinophil stimulation, arachidonic acid is liberated from membrane-bound phospholipids by the action of phospholipases. This free arachidonic acid is oxidatively metabolized via the 5-lipoxygenase pathway to the cysteinyl leukotrienes C_4, D_4, and E_4 (formerly collectively known as slow reacting substance of anaphylaxis) (Lewis and Austen, 1984). The cysteinyl leukotrienes induce vasopermeability and bronchoconstriction in normal donors (Weiss et al., 1982) and patients with asthma (Adelroth et al., 1986). They also stimulate in vitro mucus secretion from airway tissue explants (Marom et al., 1982), but without evidence of stereospecificity as would be expected for a receptor-mediated response (Coles et al., 1983). The eosinophil is the chief peripheral blood source of cysteinyl leukotrienes. In contrast to the neutrophil, which generates selectively leukotriene B_4, the human eosinophil generates large amounts of leukotriene C_4, but not leukotriene B_4, in response to activation with calcium ionophore (Owen et al., 1987a) or IgG-coated beads (Shaw et al., 1985). Free arachidonic acid can also be metabolized by the 15-lipoxygenase pathway of these cells to form lipoxins (Henderson et al., 1984) which function as immune regulators in vitro (Samuelsson et al., 1987). The eosinophil also generates substantial amounts of 1-alkyl-2-acetylglyceryl-3-phosphorylcholine (also known as platelet-activating factor) (Lee et al., 1984), a potent chemotactic and chemokinetic factor for eosinophils (Wardlow et al., 1986). It has been postulated that the generation of platelet-activating factor is a mechanism by which eosinophils can amplify the influx of other eosinophils into sites of inflammation.

HETEROGENEITY OF EOSINOPHILS

The isolation of eosinophils from patients with eosinophilia-associated diseases such as helminthic infections (DeSimone et al., 1982b), bronchial asthma (Fukuda et al., 1985), and the idiopathic hypereosinophilic syndrome

(DeSimone et al., 1982b; Winqvist et al., 1982; Prin et al., 1983, 1984) has led to the identification of heterogeneous populations of eosinophils. A portion of the eosinophils isolated from these patients have lower-than-normal mean sedimentation density properties (designated hypodense eosinophils) (Table). Hypodense eosinophils are activated cells compared to normodense eosinophils from healthy donors in that hypodense eosinophils exhibit an increase in the following functional parameters: resting oxygen and glucose consumption (Winqvist et al., 1982; Prin et al., 1983, 1984), deoxyglucose uptake (Winqvist et al., 1982), N-formyl-L-methionyl-L-leucyl-L-phenylalanine-stimulated superoxide generation (Prin et al., 1984), chemotaxis to platelet-activating factor (Wardlow et al., 1986), antibody-mediated cytotoxicity for helminths (Prin et al., 1983), and leukotriene C_4 generation in response to stimulation with calcium ionophore (Kajita et al., 1985) or IgG-coated beads (Shaw et al., 1985). In addition, the hypodense population of eosinophils possesses more low affinity receptors for IgE which can participate in antibody-dependent killing of parasites (Capron et al., 1981). This increased number of IgE receptors has important implications in the clinical setting of elevated IgE because it indicates that, in addition to the mast cell, the eosinophil can be a pivotal cell in IgE-mediated allergic diseases. We recently found that hypodense eosinophils from a patient with the idiopathic hypereosinophilic syndrome have prolonged in vitro survival compared to normodense eosinophils from the same patient or from healthy donors (Owen et al., 1988). Furthermore, the small fraction of normodense eosinophils from this patient were functionally activated as compared to normodense cell populations isolated from healthy donors (Table). The findings of hypodense eosinophils in the pleural exudates of some patients with peripheral blood eosinophilia (Winqvist et al., 1982) and pulmonary infiltrative eosinophilia (Prin et al., 1984), even though the eosinophils present in their blood are predominantly normodense, suggest that hypodense eosinophils may represent the phenotype of eosinophils that exists in tissue.

REGULATION OF EOSINOPHIL PHENOTYPE

Eosinophils are thought to remain in the bloodstream for 6-12 hours before they enter connective tissues where they survive for at least several days (Spry, 1971). Although we often think of the eosinophil as a peripheral blood leukocyte, ~300 times more eosinophils exist in tissues than in the circulation (Rytomma, 1960). Eosinophils tend to reside in areas exposed to the external environment, such as the skin, the mucosa of the bronchi and gastrointestinal tract, and in the connective tissue immediately under the epithelial layer. The first indication that the microenvironment in which eosinophils reside might be important in regulating their phenotype was the finding that eosinophils could be maintined in vitro for at least 14 days when cultured in the presence of living endothelial cells or their conditioned medium (Rothenberg et al., 1987); they could also be maintained in enriched medium supplemented with only 10^{-11} M granulocyte/macrophage colony-stimulating factor (Owen et al., 1987b), interleukin 3 (Rothenberg et al., 1988a) or interleukin 5 (Rothenberg et al., 1988b,c). During the first 7 days of culture in the presence of any of these three cytokines or in the presence of endothelial cells, the eosinophils underwent a change in their sedimentation characteristics such that they were converted from normodense cells to hypodense cells. These eosinophils exhibited an augmented capacity for killing antibody-coated larvae of Schistosoma mansoni, and generated more leukotriene C_4 when activated with calcium ionophore than freshly isolated eosinophils. Upon short-term exposure to these cytokines, the cells responded with the same increases in function and with an increase in their uptake of deoxyglucose (Rothenberg et al., 1988c) but did not undergo an appreciable change in their density sedimentation properties (Table). These postmitotic changes in the human eosinophil were induced in vitro by those same three cytokines (interleukin 3, interleukin 5, and granulocyte/macrophage colony-stimulating factor) that caused progenitor cells to proliferate and differentiate along an eosinophil lineage (Clark and Kamen, 1987).

These effects were not induced by interleukin 1, interleukin 2, interleukin 4, tumor necrosis factor, platelet-derived growth factor, or fibroblast-growth factor (Rothenberg et al., 1988a).

CHARACTERISTICS OF DIFFERENT SUBPOPULATIONS OF HUMAN EOSINOPHILS[a]

	Resting Normodense[b]	Activated Normodense[c]	Hypodense[d]
Density	High	High	Low
Receptors			
Complement	+	ND	+++
IgG	+	ND	+++
IgE	-	ND	+++
In Vitro Survival			
No cytokine	-	-	+
Cytokine	+++	+++	+++
Function			
Antibody-dependent cytotoxicity	+	+++	+++
Ionophore-induced LTC_4 generation	+	+++	+++
Chemotaxis to PAF[e]	+	ND	+++
Superoxide generation	+	ND	+++
Oxygen/Glucose Consumption	+	ND	+++
Hexose Transport	+	+++	+++

a The relative expression of each parameter is indicated by: -, negligible; +, moderate; +++, high; ND, not determined.

b Normodense eosinophils isolated from the peripheral blood of healthy reference donors.

c Normodense eosinophils isolated from a patient with the idiopathic hypereosinophilic syndrome, or after a 60-minute treatment of eosinophils from healthy donors with interleukin 3, interleukin 5, or granulocyte/macrophage colony-stimulating factor.

d Hypodense eosinophils isolated from patients with hypereosinophilia.

e PAF, platelet-activating factor.

These findings suggest that the local microenvironment regulates the activation of normodense eosinophils and their conversion to the hypodense phenotype (Figure). They also suggest that the activation of normodense eosinophils is an acute event, while the acquisition of the hypodense phenotype requires prolonged cytokine exposure. In a patient with the idiopathic hypereosinophilic syndrome, we found that activation of eosinophils in vivo can occur before normodense eosinophils have acquired the hypodense phenotype (Owen et al., 1988). Because we observed that specific cytokines induce resting normodense eosinophils to become activated cells that eventually become hypodense cells, we examined the serum of this patient for the presence of an activity that would influence eosinophils from healthy donors. Indeed, this serum caused a dose-dependent increase in the in vitro viability of normodense eosinophils from healthy donors and converted them to activated hypodense cells (Owen et al., 1988). Although the cytokine(s) present in the serum of this patient has not yet been identified, this finding suggests that the hypereosinophilic state may develop due to the excess production of cytokines that are usually confined in the microenvironment.

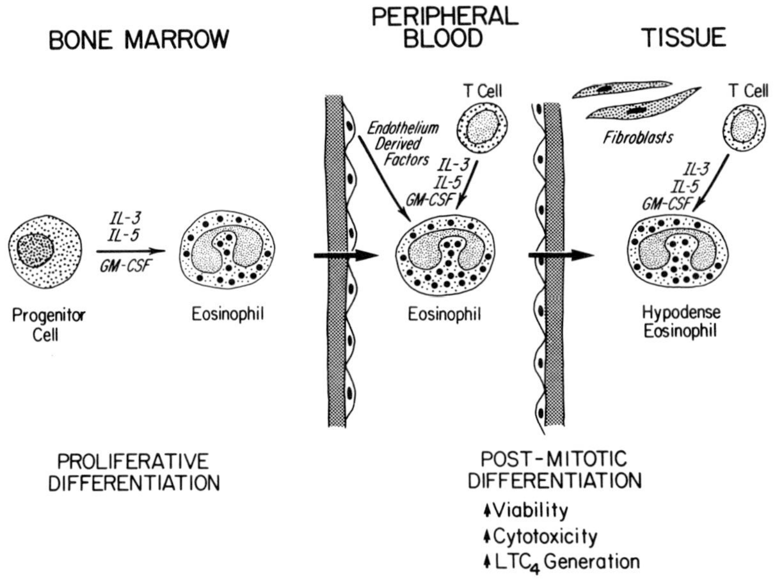

Eosinophil differentiation scheme--Interleukin 3 (IL-3), interleukin 5 (IL-5), and/or granulocyte/macrophage colony-stimulating factor (GM-CSF) regulate the proliferation and differentiation of human bone marrow progenitor cells into eosinophils. Most eosinophils in the peripheral blood are normodense in healthy states. When these mature eosinophils are acutely exposed to IL-3, IL-5, GM-CSF, or cytokines made by endothelial cells, they become functionally activated. After prolonged exposure to these cytokines in the peripheral blood or tissue, the activated normodense eosinophils are converted to activated hypodense cells. In the tissue, these same cytokines can be produced by local T lymphocytes and/or connective tissue cells.

FUTURE CONSIDERATIONS

There has been a rapid increase in our understanding of the function and regulation of mature eosinophils. The eosinophil appears to be important in defense against certain parasitic infections by mediating antibody-dependent cellular cytotoxicity for helminths. When activated, the eosinophil releases large amounts of preformed granule cationic proteins and newly generated lipid mediators which possess potent and diverse pro-inflammatory capabilities. Eosinophils exist as heterogeneous subpopulations of cells whose viability, phenotype, and function appear to be regulated by their microenvironment. It is likely that the cytokines produced by constitutive and infiltrative cells regulate the activation and phenotype of tissue-localized eosinophils. The cellular sources of eosinophil-directed cytokines include T-lymphocytes which are known to produce interleukin 3, interleukin 5, and granulocyte/macrophage colony-stimulating factor, and fibroblasts and endothelial cells which are also known to produce granulocyte/macrophage colony-stimulating factor. Distinct murine T-lymphocyte subsets have been identified based on their production of cytokines (Mosmann et al., 1986; Cherwinski et al., 1987). One such subset (designated TH2) preferentially produces both interleukin 4 (which promotes both IgE biosynthesis by B cells and also mast cell growth) and interleukin 5; the other subset (TH1) preferentially elaborates interleukin 2 and γ-interferon. It will be important to determine if distinct T cell subsets exist in humans which are responsible for preferentially elaborating the cytokines which play a role in allergic inflammation and parasitic infection (e.g., interleukins 3, 4, and 5). Furthermore, the excess production of these cytokines (that might occur in the idiopathic hypereosinophilic syndrome) may involve a common pathogenetic mechanism since some of the hematopoetic cytokines are related in genetic structure (Tanabe et al., 1987). Defining the postmitotic phenotypes of eosinophils (Table) present in the various tissues of patients with allergic diseases will have important implications in the development of pharmacologic therapy directed against the products elaborated in increased amounts by these cells. Future therapy may also be directed at modulating the production of cytokines produced by T-lymphocytes, endothelial cells, and/or fibroblasts which regulate the functional state of mature cells with inflammatory potential.

REFERENCES

Ackerman, S.J., Gleich, G.J., Loegering, D.A., Richardson, B.A. and Butterworth, A.E. (1985). Am. J. Trop. Med. Hyg. 34, 735-745.
Adelroth, E., Morris, M.M., Hargreave, F.E. and O'Byrne, P.M. (1986). N. Engl. J. Med. 315, 480-484.
Anwar, A.R.E. and Kay, A.B. (1977). J. Immunol. 119, 976-982.
Archer, G.T., Air, G., Jackas, M. and Morell, D.B. (1965). Biochim. Biophys. Acta 99, 96-101.
Butterworth, A.E., Wassom, D.L., Gleich, G.J., Loegering, D.A. and David, J.R. (1979). J. Immunol. 122, 221-229.
Capron, M., Capron, A., Dessaint, J.-P., Torpier, G., Johansson, S.G.O. and Prin, L. (1981). J. Immunol. 126, 2087-2092.
Caulfield, J.P., Lenzi, H.L., Elsas, P. and Dessein, A.J. (1985). Am. J. Pathol. 120, 380-390.
Clark, S.C. and Kamen, R. (1987). Science 236, 1229-1237.
Cherwinski, H.M., Schumacher, J.H., Brown, K.D. and Mosmann, T.R. (1987). J. Exp. Med. 166, 1229-1244.
Coles, S.J., Neill, K.H., Reid, L.M., Austen, K.F., Nii, Y., Corey, E.J. and Lewis, R.A. (1983). Prostaglandins 25, 155-170.
DeSimone, C., Donelli, G., Meli, D., Molinari, A., Rosati, F. and Sorice, F. (1982a). Immunobiology 162, 116-127.
DeSimone, C., Donelli, G., Meli, D., Rosati, F. and Sorice, F. (1982b). Clin. Exp. Immunol. 48, 249-255.
Filley, W.V., Ackerrman, S.J. and Gleich, G.J. (1982) Lancet 2, 11-16.
Frigas, E., Loegering, D.A. and Gleich, G.J. (1980). Lab. Invest. 42, 35-43.
Frigas, E., Loegering, D.A., Solley, G.O., Farrow, G.M. and Gleich, G.J. (1981) Mayo Clin. Proc. 56, 345-353.
Fukuda, T., Dunnette, S.L., Reed, C.E., Ackerman, S.J., Peters, M.S. and Gleich, G.J. (1985). Am. Rev. Respir. Dis. 132, 981-985.
Henderson, W.R., Chi, E.Y. and Klebanoff, S.J. (1980). J. Exp. Med. 152, 265-279.
Henderson, W.R., Harley, J.B. and Fauci, A.S. (1984). Immunology 51, 679-686.
Jong, E.C., Mahmoud, A.A.F. and Klebanoff, S.J. (1981). J. Immunol. 126, 468-471.
Kajita, T., Yui, Y., Mita, H., Taniguchi, N., Sato, H., Mishima, T. and Shida, T. (1985). Int. Archs. Allergy Appl. Immunol. 78, 406-410.
Kierszenbaum, F., Ackerman, S.J. and Gleich, G.J. (1981). Am. J. Trop. Med. Hyg. 30, 775-779.
Klebanoff, S.J. and Shepard, C.C. (1984). Infect. Immun. 44, 534-536.

Lee, T., Lenihan, D.J., Malone, B., Roddy, L.L. and Wasserman, S.I, (1984). J. Biol. Chem. 259, 5526-5530.
Lewis, R.A. and Austen, K.F. (1984). J. Clin. Invest. 73, 889-897.
Marom, Z., Shelhamer, J.H., Bach, M.K., Morton, D.R. and Kaliner, M. (1982). Am. Rev. Respir. Dis. 126, 449-451.
Mosmann, T.R., Cherwinski, H., Bond, M.W., Giedlin, M.A. and Coffman, R.L. (1986). J. Immunol. 136, 2348-2357.
O'Donnell, M.C., Ackerman, S.J., Gleich, G.J. and Thomas L.L. (1983). J. Exp. Med. 157, 1981-1991.
Ottesen, E.A., Stanley, A.M., Gelfand, J.A., Gadek, J.E., Frank, M.M., Nash, T. E. and Cheever, A.W. (1977). Am. J. Trop. Med. Hyg. 26, 134-141.
Owen, W.F., Jr., Soberman, R.J., Yoshimoto, T., Sheffer, A.L., Lewis, R.A. and Austen, K.F. (1987a). J. Immunol. 138, 532-538.
Owen, W.F., Jr., Rothenberg, M.E., Silberstein, D.S., Gasson, J.C., Stevens, R. L., Austen, K.F. and Soberman, R.J. (1987b). J. Exp. Med. 166, 129-141.
Owen, W.F., Rothenberg, M.E., Soberman, R.J., Sheffer, A.L., Stevens, R.L. and and Austen, K.F. (1988). Clin. Res. 36, 615a.
Prin, L., Capron, M., Tonnel, A.-B., Bletry, O. and Capron, A. (1983). Int. Archs. Allergy Appl. Immunol. 72, 336-346.
Prin, L., Charon, J., Capron, M., Gassot, P., Taelman, H., Tonnel, A.-B. and Capron, A. (1984). Clin. Exp. Immunol. 57, 735-742.
Ramalho-Pinto, F.J., McLaren, D.J. and Smithers, S.R. (1978). J. Exp. Med. 147, 147-156.
Rothenberg, M.E., Owen, W.F., Jr., Silberstein, D.S., Soberman, R.J., Austen, K.F. and Stevens, R.L. (1987). Science 237, 645-647.
Rothenberg, M.E., Owen, W.F., Jr., Silberstein, D.S., Woods, J., Soberman, R.J. Austen, K.F. and Stevens, R.L. (1988a). J. Clin. Invest., in press.
Rothenberg, M.E., Owen, W.F., Soberman, R.J., Austen, K.F. and Stevens, R.L. (1988b). FASEB 2, A1598.
Rothenberg, M.E., Pomerantz, J.L., Owen, W.F., Jr., Avraham, S., Soberman, R.J. Austen, K.F. and Stevens, R.L. (1988c). J. Biol. Chem., in press.
Rytomma, T. (1960). Acta Pathol. Microbiol. Scand. 50 (suppl.), 1-118.
Samuelsson, B., Dahlén, S.-E., Lindgren, J.-A., Rouzer, C.A. and Serhan, C.N. (1987). Science 237, 1171-1176.
Shaw, R.J., Walsh, G.M., Cromwell, D., Moqbel, R., Spry, C.J. and Kay, A.B. (1985). Nature (London) 316, 150-152.
Spry, C.J.F. (1971). Cell. Tissue Kinet. 4, 351-364.
Tanabe, T., Konishi, M., Mizuta, T., Noma, T. and Honjo, T. (1987). J. Biol. Chem. 262, 16580-16584.
Udell, I.J., Gleich, G.J., Allansmith, M.R., Ackerman, S.J. and Abelson, M.B. (1981). Am. J. Ophthalmol. 92, 824-828.
Vadas, M.A., David, J.R., Butterworth, A., Pisani, N.T. and Biongok, T. (1979). J. Immunol. 122, 1228-1236.
Wassom, D.L. and Gleich, G.J. (1979). Am. J. Trop. Med. Hyg. 28, 860-863.
Wardlow, A.J., Moqbel, R., Cromwell, O. and Kay, A.B. (1986). J. Clin. Invest. 78, 1701-1706.
Weiss, J.W., Drazen J.M., Coles, N., McFadden, E.R., Jr., Weller, P.F., Corey, E.J., Lewis, R.A. and Austen, K.F. (1982). Science 216, 196-198.
Weiss, S.J., Test, S.T., Eckmann, C.M., Roos, D. and Regiani, S. (1987). Science 234, 200-203.
Winqvist, I., Olofsson, T., Olsson, I., Persson, A.-M. and Hallberg, T. (1982). Immunology 47, 531-539.
Young, J.D., Peterson, C.G., Venge, P. and Cohn, Z.A. (1986). Nature (London) 321, 613-616.

Workshop Sessions

Bacteria and Natural Products as Immunomodulators (II)

M. A. PARANT* and H. TAKADA**

*Institut Biomédical des Cordeliers, 15 rue de l'Ecole de Médecine, 75270 Paris 06, France

**Osaka University Faculty of Dentistry, Dept. Oral Microbiology, 1–8 Yamadaoka, Suita, Osaka 565, Japan

RU 41740 (K. PNEUMONIAE GLYCOPROTEIN) ENHANCES RESISTANCE TO EXPERIMENTAL CANDIDIASIS AND STIMULATES PHAGOCYTIC FUNCTIONS
P. Smets*, M.F. Salles*, M. ROMMAIN*, R. ZALISZ*, and M. GUENOUNOU**
* Laboratoires Cassenne, C.R.I. Roussel Uclaf, Osny, France; ** UER de Médecine Paris Ouest, Garches, France

IN VIVO RESTORATION OF NEUTROPHIL MIGRATION BY RU 41740 (BIOSTIM) INTRAVENOUSLY OR ORALLY ADMINISTERED, USING A SKIN SUCTION BLISTER MODEL IN HAIRLESS RATS
M. Rommain, C. Brossard, R. Zalisz, and P. Smets
Laboratoires Cassenne, C.R.I. Roussel Uclaf, Osny, France

EFFECT OF RU 41740 ON AUTOLOGOUS HAEMOPOIETIC RECONSTITUTION IN IMMUNOSUPPRESSED MICE
F. Rezzoug*, J.L. Touraine*, and P. Smets**
* Hôpital Edouard Herriot, 69437 Lyon 03, France

INDUCTION OF INTERLEUKIN 1 (IL-1) ACTIVITY IN SERUM FOLLOWING ORAL ADMINISTRATION OF RU 41740, A BACTERIAL IMMUNOMODULATOR
S. Perin*, F. Vacheron **, R. Zalisz***, P. Smets ***, and M. Guenounou**
* Université Pasir Sud, Chatenay-Malabry 92296, France; ** UER de Médecine Paris Ouest, Garches, France; ***Laboratoires Cassenne, C.R.I. Roussel Uclaf Osny, France

GRANULOMA FORMING AND CYTOKINE INDUCING ACTIVITIES OF MYCOLIC ACID-CONTAINING GLYCOLIPIDS FROM *NOCARDIA RUBRA*
S. Oka, Y. Natsuhara , Y. Kato, K. Kaneda, and I. Yano
Osaka City University Medical School, Osaka; Osaka Research Institute of Sawai Pharmaceutical Co, Osaka; Tokyo Medical and Dental University, School of Medicine, Tokyo, Japan

EFFECT OF THE GANGLIOSIDE GM_1P ON IMMUNE SURVEILLANCE OF ^{60}Co-IRRADIATED MICE
E. Tubaro, L. Belogi, C. Croce, and G. Cavallo
Wellcome Italia S.p.A. Research Laboratories, Rome, Italy

In this workshop, which is the second one of this Conference concerned with natural immunomodulators, 6 presentations were delivered. None of them was dealing with a novel product. Experimental studies have been pursued on the immunopharmacological properties of Biostim, a compound currently used in human therapy, with another bacterial preparation from *Nocardia rubra*, and also with a calcium-mediated metastable form of a monoasialoganglioside GM-1. The amount of new information on bacterial extracts remained limited since elucidation of their mode of cellular action is speculative unless purification and characterization of the active part(s) be achieved.

Dr Smets opened the session with a summary on the development and therapeutic properties of Biostim. This extract containing glycoprotein from *Klebsiella pneumoniae* has been reported to reduce infectious episodes in patients prone to recurrent infections. He then described the effect of Biostim on the survival rate of mice infected with *Candida albicans* organisms. The stimulating effect of the product on polymorphonuclear cells was assessed by its priming effect on the oxidative metabolism of mouse peritoneal cells or human blood cells stimulated with zymosan.

In the second paper on Biostim presented by Dr Zalisz, the polymorphonuclear cell migration was evaluated *in vivo*. A skin succion blister model was adapted in hairless rats and the restoration of cell migration induced with Biostim was determined after treatment with an anti-inflammatory drug. In this model, Biostim was shown to be active either by the intravenous or by the oral route in restoring neutrophil migration capacity.

Another aspect of the immunopotentiating properties of Biostim was reported by Dr Rezzoug. The study deals with hemopoietic reconstitution in a classical mouse model after sublethal irradiation. Pretreatment with Biostim induced an increase in the number of CFU-S in the spleen and in bone marrow cell cultures. This kind of investigation is being pursued at the level of mediators.

Dr Guenounou was presenting new data concerned with IL-1 production *in vivo* in mice and in Rhesus monkeys. IL-1 activity was determined by LAF activity in sera after gel filtration in animals given Biostim by the oral route during 3 to 4 days. An IL-1 activity was detectable in the serum of animals at day 4 and 5 after the beginning of Biostim administration. This activity was found only in low molecular fractions. Additional information regarding the presence of radiolabeled material in the blood of monkeys after oral doses of Biostim did not appear conclusive since the radioactive material found in animals was not characterized as the intact product.

After four presentations concerned with Biostim, the discussion started at the point of LPS content in this bacterial extract and its possible role in immunopharmacological properties. The authors answered accurately that the effect of Biostim by the oral route excluded that it was due to LPS content, and they noted that stimulating activities were obtained with purified fractions not containing LPS. Dr MacVittie who did not deliver an oral presentation but had described in her poster hemopoietic effects of Biostim, was asked to give her opinion since she demonstrated that only a minimal stimulation was obtained after oral treatment. Obviously, differences in the experimental models did not allow to draw any conclusion.

Dr Oka is working with mycolic acid-containing glycolipids extracted from *Nocardia rubra* to establish structure-activity relationships. Several glycolipids were isolated by TLC and administered intravenously in the form of a water/oil/water emulsion. One week after a single injection of glucose mycolate, granuloma formation was important in the mouse lung. By contrast, fructose mycolate or arabinose mycolate did not cause significant granuloma formation. Thus, a specific structure of carbohydrate moiety seemed essential for granuloma formation activities as it was found to play an important role in immune responses. Moreover, IL-1 and CSF activities were detected in lung cultures only when obtained from mice treated with the granulomagenic glycolipids.The role of these mediators is being considered to clarify the mechanism of granuloma formation. The author also reported that a strong priming effect on LPS-induced

TNF production was observed with glucose mycolate as well as with trehalose dimycolate but not with other glycolipids.

The last communication of the workshop was given by Dr Tubano. This work dealt with immunostimulating activity of the ganglioside GM_1P. This substance has been shown to increase mouse T- and B-lymphocyte blastogenesis, natural killer (NK) activity *in vivo*, and to prime animals for IL2 production in cell cultures. Moreover, a direct evidence for increased expression of IL-2 receptors was provided by immunofluorescence and FACS analysis of spleen cells from treated mice. This substance was also used to stimulate resistance to *Candida* infection in mice sensitized by gamma-irradiation. Regarding the mortality rate of animals receiving a lethal dose of irradiation, a significant protection was reported in pre-treated animals. A rapid recovery in blood neutrophil and bone marrow cells indicated a positive effect on stem cells.

In summary, all these studies showed a great interest for animal models demonstrating an increased resistance. It might important to compare side effects and to look for inflammatory reactions in the various experimental models. A special effort is still required to determine conditions for a therapeutic effect. The discussion left the participants with the feeling that a lot of research has yet to be done to define mechanisms of action of natural immunoregulatory products. It seemed also imperative to progressively consider more precise molecular and biochemical targets for manipulation of the immune system.

Bacteria and Natural Products as Immunomodulators (III)

T. TOKUNAGA* and S. TSUNG-TANG**

*National Institute of Health, Tokyo, Japan

**Dept. Immunology, Cancer Institute, CAMS, Zuoanmen Wai Panjiyao, Beijing, China

The research area on immunomodulators from bacteria and natural products is relatively large, and, therefore, this workshop was the third one in the three serially organized workshops on the modulators. In this session, 8 oral presentations and 6 posters were delivered. These 14 papers dealt with 6 immunomodulators, namely, PSK, OK432, MY-1, Cholera toxin and Vitamin A. Table I classified the number of papers for the each agent.

Table I. Immunomodulators Appeared in 14 Presentations in the Workshop

Immunomodulator	Oral	Poster	Total
PSK	5	3	8
OK432	1	2	3
MY-1	1	0	1
Cholera toxin	1	0	1
Vitamin A	0	1	1

According to the remarkable technological progress in the recent years, many immunomodulators have been developed and produced by gene-engineering or chemical synthesis. For instance, 7 kinds of recombinant interleukine, from IL-1 to IL-7, are shown in this International Symposia. It seems likely that the complete cytokine networks could be reconstituted <u>in vitro</u> by the cytokines produced already or in the future by gene technology. On the other hand, an essential part of bacterial lipopolysaccharide for macrophage activation, for instance, was chemically synthesized. Instead of natural products, such chemically synthesized agents may play more important roles as immunomodulators in the future. One of the chairpersons (Tokunaga) thinks that the line of study on the agents with known structures which are produced by gene technology or chemical synthesis is correct from the historical standpoint, however, it seems not easy to accomplish in the near future. At present, therefore, there is a consensus of opinion that studies on natural products as immunomodulators for medical use possess significan and important meanings. At the same time, it should be mentioned for developing natural immunomodulators that studies on mechanism of action on the candidate agents are especially necessary and important.

PSK (Krestin) is a protein-bound polysaccharide isolated and has been used broadly for treatment of various cancers for these several years in Japan.

The route of administration of this drug is oral, and its side effect has been reported to be very small. However, the mechanism responsible for its clinical benefits is not well understood yet. In this workshop, various aspects of mode of action of PSK were discussed in the 8 papers.

Drs. Kamisato and Nowakowski (N.Y., USA) reported their findings on morphological and metabolic alterations produced by PSK in macrophages. Their previous studies using mouse peritoneal macrophage cultures showed that PSK (100 μg/ml) induced marked morphological changes (spreading and elongation) and altered protein and DNA synthesis. The rate of protein synthesis, measured by ^{35}S-methionine incorporation, increased 20-fold after 4 days in the presence of PSK; DNA synthesis was induced in macrophage cultures after 3 days in the presence of PSK and reached maximum level after 5 days. Fibroblasts could not be detected until day 7 of culture, and were removed efficiently (90-95%) by trypsin. The possibility of lymphocytes contributing to the observed levels of DNA synthesis was evaluated in cell mixing experiments: freshly collected peritoneal cells were separated into adherent and non-adherent populations; cultures containing each of these populations alone or mixed at a 1:1 ratio were incubated with or without PSK, and incorporation of ^{3}H-TdR was measured on day 4. The results indicated that in their system PSK induced DNA synthesis only in cultures of adherent macrophage. In order to determine accurately changes induced by PSK in morphology and cell number, suspension cultures of macrophages were established in Teflon vials. Addition of PSK resulted in the appearance of multinucleated giant cells (up to 75% on day 11). The direct effects of PSK on macrophages may represent in part the mechanism of the therapeutic action of this glycan _in vivo_. It is interesting to notice that macrophage activation usually accompanies DNA synthesis inhibition, however, in their system, DNA synthesis started after 3 days of incubation, resulting in forming giant cells without cell division.

PSK activates cytotoxic lymphocytes that act on autologous fresh tumor cells and cultured tumor cell lines in human. These facts were reported by Drs. Uchida and Kakitsubata (Kyoto, Japan). According to them, _in vitro_ exposure to PSK of blood and tumor-associated lymphocytes resulted in an augmentation and induction of NK cell activity in previously reactive and nonreactive cases, respectively. In addition, the PSK-treated lymphocytes were able to kill tumor cells that were freshly isolated from the same patients. The induction or enhancement of NK and autotumor killing activity of PSK was time- and dose-dependent, and it was seen at PSK concentrations equivalent to those obtained in blood of PSK-treated cancer patients. The PSK effect appeared to be independent of interferon and interleukin 2 induction. PSK showed no direct cytotoxic effects in these systems. They mentioned that the anti-tumor activity of PSK may be in part mediated through activation of NK and autotumor killing systems.

It seems interesting to know the effect of PSK against microbial infection. The research group of Drs. Sakagami, Harada, Konno, Sato, Osawa, Fujimaki, Komatsu (Tokyo, Japan) reported previously that PSK stimulated production of differentiation-inducing factor (DIF) from macrophages, and activated the function of polymorphonuclear cells (PMN). Based on these observations, they investigated here possible antimicrobial activity of PSK. Mice were given intraperitoneally (ip) single infections of PSK (0.8-80 mg/kg) and 48 hr later _E. coli_ (1 MLD) were challenged ip. DIF activity was assayed with NBT reagent, using U-937 human monoblastic cell line as target cells. Superoxide generation was assayed by luminol-dependent chemiluminescence (LDCL). Pretreatment with PSK protected the mice from the lethal effect of _E. coli_ infection. Ip administration of PSK resulted in a transient induction of DIF with a peak at 1-2 hr after PSK. The rapid decay of DIF activity was followed by PMN accumulation and superoxide generation by peritoneal exudate cells. Time-dependent changes of these two phenomena were almost superimposed with each other; the both activities reached to the peaks after 24 to 48 hr, and thereafter declined.

They suggested a possible association of PSK-induced antimicrobial activity and PMN induction/activation. This is a new information on PSK action, and it is desirable to compare the DIF-inducing ability of PSK with those of other control agents.

Very interestingly, it was reported that PSK is also effective against human immunodeficiency virus (HIV) infection in vitro. This finding was reported by Drs. Yamamoto, Tochikura and Nakashima (Yamaguchi, Japan). They used either a novel infection system using human T-cell lymphotropic virus type I (HTLV-I)-carrying MT-4 cells or a coculture system using MOLT-4 cells and its virus-producing cells MOLT-4/HIV which induces multinucleated giant cells very efficiently. PSK almost completely blocked the cytopathic effect such as giant cell formation and HIV-specific antigen expression both in MT-4 cells and MOLT-4 cells at a concentration of 0.4 and 0.3 mg/ml, respectively. Moreover, PSK inhibited reverse transcriptase in a non-competitive fashion in vitro. It is unknown yet, however, whether these effects are specific for HIV or HIV-infected cells. Further investigations are expected.

Dr. Mickey (North Carolina, USA) reported the effects of combination of PSK with anti-tumor chemotherapeutic drugs against rat prostate adenocarcinoma. The purpose of his study was to determine whether PSK enhanced the effects of conventional therapy in this rat model. Solid tumors were initiated by injecting $1x10^6$ vial tumor cells (MAT LyLu) subcutaneously into Copenhagen rats. This tumor metastasizes to lung and lymph nodes and is lethal to the untreated host in 30 days. All therapy started on day 7 after tumors were palpable. The conventional agents cyclophosphamide (20 mg/kg/wk), cisplatin (3 mg/kg/wk), 5-fluorouracil (50 mg/kg/wk) and PSK (200 mg/kg/48 hrs) were given singly. PSK was also combined with each of the conventional agents and therapy continued for various times. Changes in metastatic progression and changes in growth rates of the tumor at the injected sites were monitered. PSK therapy alone did not change tumor growth characteristics. Each of the conventional agents was effective in increasing the tumor doubling times but none could decrease the metastatic capabilities. Combination therapy with PSK and any of the conventional agents increased tumor doubling times and group mean survival times and decreased mestatic rates. The beneficial effects of combination therapy with PSK were time-dependent but not drug-dependent. In combination therapy, when tumor progression decreases PSK enhances host NK cells and affects the metastatic cell subpopulation. He thinks this may have clinical significance.

Soluble suppressor factor (SSF) released from Con-A induced suppressor cells or cells of monocyte like cell line U-937 was described previously by Dr. Toge, et al. In this workshop, Drs. Toge, Yamaguchi, Kameda, Yanagawa and Hattori (Hiroshima, Japan) reported that PSK abrogated SSF-mediated suppression by blocking of binding sites for SSF on lymphocyte surface. Namely, the suppression of normal lymphocyte proliferative response to PHA by SSF from either Con-A induced suppressor cells or U-937 cells was significantly abrogated by PSK. The release of SSF, however, was not blocked by treatment of U-937 cells with PSK. Moreover, the suppression of lymphocyte proliferative response to PHA by SSF was completely blocked by the pretreatment of effector lymphocytes with PSK. PSK competed with wheat germ agglutinin (WGA) which recognized the same receptor as SSF, in binding on lymphocyte surface. Serum from cancer patients, as well as N-acetyl-D-glucosamin (NAG) also competed with WGA, while immunosuppressive acidic protein did not. Neither PSK nor serum competed with anti-CD4 monoclonal antibody. Thus, PSK may abrogate SSF mediated suppression by specific blocking of the binding sites for SSF on the surface of effector lymphocytes.

The effects of PSK was influenced strongly by its route of injection. Drs. Ryoyama and Ryoyama (Kanazawa, Japan) reported previously that the sera of adult mice given PSK inhibited tumor growth, but the growth inhibition activity of serum was greatly affected by injection routes of PSK. Here, they reported by a poster that C57BL/6 mice were given single s.c. or f.p. injection of PSK (125 mg/kg) on Day-7 and i.p. injection of sheep red blood cells (SRBC; 10^6 or 10^8) on Day 0. After 4 days, one group of the mice was devoted to a humoral response and the other mice were given f.p. injection of SRBC (10^8) to see 24 hr DTH response. Mitogenic response against Con A, PHA and LPS of splenic and thymic cells which received s.c. or f.p. injection of PSK 7 days before were almost the same as those of normal mice. Splenic humoral immune response against SRBC were augmented by s.c. injection of PSK. However, f.p. injection of PSK significantly inhibited the humoral response. Meanwhile, DTH response against SRBC were not significanly influenced by PSK. They conclude that injection routes of PSK selectively modify humoral immune response.

Drs. Nakagami, Ikeda, Lin, Ito, Kimoto and Oka (Tokyo, Japan) reported previously that serum immunosuppressive substance (IS) which is a glycoprotein obtained from the ascitic fluids of advanced cancer patients is found to be higher than patients with benign tumors or normal persons. They reported here by a poster the serum IS levels in tumor bearing rats and the patients with urogentital tumor. Bladder carcinoma BC-47 was transplanted subcutaneously in the back of AC1 rats, and the serum levels of IS, tumor growth rates and survival rates were measured. PSK was administered orally for 14 time after tumor inoculation, and serum IS was measured by single radial immunodiffusion method using anti-IS antiserum. Serum IS increased with tumor growth, but PSK administration inhibited the increase in the serum IS levels, and the suppression of tumor growth and prolongation of survival time were observed. Clinically, serum IS levels increased with advance of the disease, and the mean IS level in the group given PSK was lower than that of non PSK group. They think that the IS is a useful parameter for predicting tumor growth and the therapeutic effect of immunomodulators such as PSK.

OK-432 is a streptococcal preparation that is called Picibanil, and used broadly also in Japan. In this workshop, 3 papers dealt with OK-432, one orally and two by posters. Drs. Moriya, Nunomura, Nanjo, Kataoka, Saito, Sugawara, Yoshida and Ishida (Tokyo and Sendai, Japan) analyzed the effector cells induced by OK-432. BALB/c-+/+ mice implanted ip with syngeneic fibrosarcoma BAMC-1 were cured by 5 every other day injections(ip) of OK-432 starting day2 after tumor implantation. In the case of BALB/c-nu/nu mice, however, the number of tumor cells decreased transiently until day8, then rapidly increased finally causing death of the host. When peritoneal exudate cells (PEC) of +/+ mice treated as above were transferred into peritoneal cavity of nu/nu mice treated similarly as +/+ mice on or after day7 of tumor implantation, more than 85% of the recipients survived. The effector cells in the PEC were nylon wool column nonadherent, and had surface markers as $Thy1^+$, $L3T4^+$, $Lyt2^-$, $AsGM1^-$, LAA^+ cells. They conclude that induction of $L3T4^+$ cells at tumor site may be essential for tumor eradication by OK-432 in this system.

Drs. Toge, Kuroi, Sawamura, Kuninobu and Hattori studied the action mechanism of OK-432 from the standpoint of the reduction of suppressor cell activity of human peripheral blood lymphocytes. Suppressor cells were induced in normal lymphocytes by serum from advanced cancer patients as well as Concanavalin-A (Con-A). Their activities were significantly reduced when they were generated _in vitro_ by Con-A or cancer serum in the presence of OK-432, however, the reduction was not observed when OK-432 was added in the effector phase. $CD4^+$ cells were found to act as inducer cells in the generation of suppressor cells and the increase of $CD4^+2H4^+$ cells (suppressor inducer T cells) by the stimulation with cancer serum or Con-A was observed. The increase of suppressor inducer T cells was inhibited by the presence of OK-432. They suggest that OK-432 may interfere with the induction of suppressor cells through the inhibition of suppressor inducer T cells.

Drs. Nanjo, Moriya, Hashimoto, Kamijo, Kataoka, Saito, Sugawara, Yoshida and Ishida (Tokyo and Sendai, Japan) studied antitumor effect of OK-432. OK-432 could cure BALB/c mice bearing BAMC-1 ascites tumor, when the agent was injected i.p. every other days for five times. Although a single i.p. injection of either OK-432 or a lymphokine (interferon or IL-2) showed only the minimum antitumor effect, the combined administration of both induced stronger therapeutic effects. Furthermore, the sequence of administration of both agents is critical to induce curative effects. The injection of OK-432 on day 2 followed by either interferon or IL-2 on day 4 or day 6 was effective while injections of either lymphokines on day 2 followed by OK-432 on day 4 showed no therapeutic effect. They think that these may warrant further investigation on therapeutic protocols with the combined use of OK-432 and lymphokines.

A fraction extracted from BCG and designated MY-1, which was composed of 70% DNA and 28% RNA, was previously reported to have strong antitumor activities against various syngeneic mouse and guinea pig tumors and to have no direct cytotoxicity to the tumor cells. To clarify the mechanism of its antitumor activity, Kuramoto, Shimada and Tokunaga (Tokyo, Japan) studied the role of NK cells induced by MY-1. When EL4 tumor cells were inoculated together with MY-1 into C57BL/6 mice, the tumor growth was markedly suppressed. This tumor suppression was abrogated by pretreatment of the mice with anti-asialo GM1 antibody. MY-1 showed no such activity in NK-deficient beige mice, but the activity was restored by transfer of untreated C57BL/6 spleen cells, but not by those pretreated with anti-asialo GM1 and complement. Intralesional injection of MY-1 into Meth A tumor of BALB/c mice regressed the tumore and augmented NK activity of cells in the tumor-draining lymph nodes, but not in the remote lymph nodes. Morphologically, it was also observed that MY-1 induced an infiltration of asialo GM1-positive, NK-like cells at the injection site. These results indicate that NK cells activated by MY-1 play an important role in the antitumor activity of MY-1, at least in mice.

Drs. Hussain, Himeno, Tokuda, Asano and Nomoto (Fukuoka, Japan) reported immunomodulative effect of chorela toxin (CT) in mice, C3H/He mice were injected 2 μg of CT at various intervals before assay (Day-21 to Day 0). Thymocytes markedly decreased in number and phenotypes in such cells were clearly shifted from "cortical type" to "medullary type" in Day-2 and Day-4 treated groups. Spleen T cells increased relatively, especially in Lyt-1 and Lyt-2 fractions, while surface IgM positive B cells rather decreased. Natural killer activity or <u>in vivo</u> and <u>in vitro</u> cytotoxic T cell activity were markedly suppressed in early stages after CT treatment but completely recovered within 21 days. Mixed lymphocyte reaction (MLR) was profoundly suppressed in all of the groups. Furthermore, EL-4 tumor of C57BL/6 origin grew progressively and killed the host mice when such tumor cells were inoculated on Day 0. On the contrary, marked augmentation of plaque forming cells (PFC) and delayed type hypersensitivity (DTH) to SRBC was seen in all the treated mice. Taken together, CT appears to have an immunomodulative effects suppressing class-I restricted immune response like cytotoxic T cell activity, and augmenting class-II restricted immune response like helper T activity and DTH.

Vitamin A as an immunomodulator was reported by a poster by Drs. Kashida, Totsuka and Takeyama (Saitama, Japan). They investigated the antitumor effect of vitamin A (retinyl palmitate) by using the doubly grafted tumor system. BALB/c mice were inoculated intradermally with Meth A fibrosarcoma cells ($1x10^6$ cells) on the right inguinal region on day 0, and later on the left ($3x10^6$ cells) on day 13. Intratumoral (i.t.) administration of Vitamin A (33.3 mg/kg/day, day 4-8) into the primary tumor completely prevented growth of the secondary tumor. Without primary inoculation, Vitamin A (s.c. day 4-8) had no effect. Also, Vitamin A showed no effect on the growth of Ehrlich tumors implanted in place of the secondary Meth A. Other parenteral routes (i.v., i.p., and s.c.) were also effective, but required higher doses.

The immune spleen cells taken from the cured mice completely prevented growth of Meth A tumors, when measured by Winn assay. Administration of anti-thymocyte serum abrogated the Vitamin A action. They concluded that Vitamin A enhances tumor immunity by acting directly on the tumor cells and/or immunocytes interacting with the tumor cells.

Glucans and Immunomodifiers (I)

J. K. CZOP* and G. CHIHARA**
*Harvard Medical School, Boston, Massachusetts, USA
**National Cancer Center Research Institute, Tsukiji, Tokyo, Japan

In this workshop, 14 presentations were given, each of which provided further evidence for the pharmacologic activity of fungal and yeast β-glucans in rapidly augmenting numerous biologic responses that are associated with nonimmune host defense.

Eight of the presentations dealt with lentinan, a β-glucan consituent of an edible mushroom, Lentinus edodes (Berk.) Sing., which was first isolated and appreciated for its anti-tumor activity by Dr. Chihara and coworkers (Cancer Res. 30:2776, 1970) nearly 20 years ago. Controlled clinical trials with lentinan have been ongoing in Japan for the past 5 years and the results obtained thus far indicate that lentinan is efficacious as a therapeautic adjuvant. Lentinan has several features which make its usage more acceptable than other adjuvant materials, namely that it is noninfectious and relatively nonimmunogenic. In light of its potentially beneficial effects, lentinan exhibits no side effects that could conceivably be detrimental to an already compromised host.

Two of the presentations dealt with the glucans derived from Saccharomyces cerevisiae, which have been demonstrated by Dr. Di Luzio and coworkers (Trends Pharmacol. Sci. 4:344, 1983) to be active in augmenting host defense mechanisms against a variety of biologic insults. Yeast glucan is a β-glucan similar in structure to lentinan and appears to initiate a cascade of interactions that can be envisioned to convert the glucan-treated animal into an arsenal of defense. The administration of glucan to laboratory animals protects them from a variety of highly lethal microorganisms, promotes tumor regression, and increases survival against sublethal and lethal doses of irradiation. Like lentinin, it is noninfectious and poorly immunogenic.

Four of the presentations dealt with additional β-glucans of fungal origin: sonifilan, sizofiran, Sclerotinia sclerotiorum glucan (SSG), and grifolan. Using a mouse tumor model, Dr. Inomata and coworkers showed that radiation therapy in conjunction with the administration of sonifilan is more effective in inhibiting tumor growth than either treatment alone. Examination of tumor filtrates from irradiated animals receiving sonifilan revealed subsets of T-lymphocytes and a high proportion of macrophages, the latter of which were not present in tumor filtrates from animals treated with radiation alone.

Drs. Tsuchiya and Kumagai showed that a variety of biologic responses are stimulated by the fungal anti-tumor glucan, sizofiran. The treatment of mice with sizofiran augmented proliferation of their thymocytes and spleen cells cultured with mitogens and/or cytokines, increased production of IL-1 by their peritoneal macrophages cultured with LPS, increased production of IL-2 and IL-3 by spleen cells cultured with con A, and increased the levels of colony-stimulating activity (CSA) in serum. Studies on the levels of CSA in serum, and in culture supernatants of two types of cells isolated from SSG-treated mice, namely cells from spleens and from Peyer's patches, were presented by Dr. Suzuki and coworkers. Unlike all other studies presented in this symposium, SSG was given orally rather than by injection, and was shown to increase serum levels of CSA and to induce synthesis of CSA by cultures of the two types of isolated lymphoid cells.

Dr. Adachi and coworkers examined the the effects of chemical modification of grifolan, a β-1,3 glucan with 1,6 branches in several in vitro assays, such as activation of the alternative complement pathway, and carbon clearance and lysosomal enzyme release by peritoneal macrophages obtained from grifolan-treated and untreated mice. They showed that carboxymethylation of hydroxyl groups and carboxylation of side branches resulted in the loss of activity in some of their assays, suggesting that different portions of native grifolan were responsible for each of its many effects.

Dr. Chihara opened the oral part of the symposium by presenting an overview of his work with lentinan, most of which focused on the tumor-inhibitory effects of this fungal β-glucan in mice. A major feature of lentinan is that it is highly effective in suppressing allogeneic, syngeneic, and autochthonous tumors in vivo, but lentinan is not cytotoxic against tumor cells in tissue culture systems. Thus, its tumor inhibitory capacity appears to involve the participation of many types of cells and their bioreactive products. The tumor suppressive effects of lentinan are accompanied by vascular dilation and hemorrhage, which can be measured in the outer ears of mice. Drs. Maeda and Watanabe showed that the capacity of lentinan to induce tumor suppression and vascular dilation and hemorrhage was decreased by the treatment of lentinan with DMSO, urea, and NaOH; removal of these chemical agents from lentinan preparations caused a return of both biologic responses. These data suggested that the sparingly soluble nature of lentinan contributes to at least some of its functional activity.

Dr. Jeannin and coworkers presented data on the effects of lentinan in a rat model of colon cancer metastastes. Multiple i.p. injections of lentinan over a 10 day period induced the disappearance of metastastes and significantly increased survival. Drs. Taguchi and Kaneko presented results of a 4-year followup of phase III randomized control clinical trials with lentinan. In combination with the neoplastic drug Tegaful, lentinan prolonged the lifespan of patients with advanced and recurrent stomach and colorectal cancer. The efficacy of lentinan as a therapeutic adjuvant was most promising for patients with breast cancer.

Dr. Yamanishi and coworkers presented data on natural killer cell activities before and after administration of lentinan to normal controls and to patients with gastric cancer. Flow cytometric analysis with monoclonal antibodies revealed that in cancer patients, lentinan-induced increased numbers of both leu 11 and leu 7 positive cells, whereas in normal controls, it significantly increased the numbers of leu 11, but not leu 7, positive cells. Dr. Akiyama and coworkers presented studies of the combined effects of lentinan and monoclonal 17-1A antibody against human colorectal carcinoma cells. In vitro studies showed that peritoneal macrophages from lentinan-treated normal and nude mice exhibited enhanced antibody-dependent cytotoxicity by a mechanism involving increased expression of Fc-IgG receptors. In vivo studies showed that lentinan administration increased the tumor regressive effects of monoclonal 17-1A.

Additional studies of lentinan and macrophage activities were presented by Dr. Abel and coworkers. In response to i.p. injection of lentinan to tumor-bearing mice, the number of macrophages in peritoneal lavages was increased and reached a maximal value 5 days after injection. Cell increase was accompanied by increases in cell pinocytosis, as assessed by the uptake of FITC-dextran and horseradish peroxidase, and cell phagocytosis of latex beads.

The two presentations with yeast glucans were markedly different from each other. Dr. Landauer and coworkers presented data on the effects of soluble yeast glucans and the behavior of mice. Using a computerized monitor of animal activity, they showed that IV injection of soluble glucan induced a dose-dependent decrease in ambulation and rearing, that is, the mice became more lethargic. Dr. Janusz and coworkers presented work on human monocyte β-glucan receptors which initiate phagocytosis of unopsonized particulate activators of the alternative complement pathway, such as zymosan particles, glucan particles, and Candida albicans. Using acid-solubilized yeast glucan particles as starting material, they isolated a soluble heptaglucoside that functionally impaired monocyte ingestion of zymosan particles. Analysis of function, composition, and mass of smaller yeast-derived oligoglucosides revealed that the heptaglucoside was the smallest functional unit ligand recognized by monocyte β-glucan receptors. Dr. Czop concluded the oral part of the symposium by presenting additional data from studies of the monocyte β-glucan receptors which suggested that the yeast heptaglucoside interacts with only one of several β-glucan receptors present on mononuclear phagocytes.

Glucans and Immunomodifiers (II)

K. NOEL MASIHI* and SHIGEO SUZUKI**

*Robert Koch Institute, Federal Health Office, Berlin, F.R.G.

**Tohoku College of Pharmacy, Sendai, Japan

Glucans are potent immunomodulators of natural origin possessing a broad spectrum of host defense-stimulating activities. Purification and elucidation of precise chemical structures of glucans from various sources have led to an extensive study of the structure-activity relationships of this unique class of immunomodulators. Intense interest in the practical application of glucans was amply reflected in the experimental as well as clinical studies reported at this workshop. Eight papers representing the recent advances in this field were selected. Additionally, two papers dealing with N-acetyl chitohexaose and a conjugate of bakers' yeast mannan and mitomycin C have been included in this workshop, because these saccharides have been shown to be relating materials to fungal cell wall components as well as glucans. The following eight papers were actually presented at the workshop and were discussed in detail.

Therapeutic use of glucan in radiation-injured mice: survival-enhancing and hemopoietic effects.
M.L.Patchen, T.J.MacVittie, I.Brook and T.Elliott

Effector mechanism of antitumor effect at a distant site in the "double grafted tumor system" of PSK, a protein-bound polysaccharide preparation.
T.Ebina, K.Ishikawa and H.Kohya

Antitumor effect of N-acetylchitohexaose against syngeneic mouse tumors.
T.Matsumoto, K.Tsukada, A.Tokoro, S.Suzuki and M.Suzuki

Inhibition of mitomycin C-induced sister chromatid exchanges in mice bone marrow cells by a protein-bound polysaccharide, PSK.
J.Hasegawa, M.Hosokawa and H.Kobayashi

Antitumor effect of mannan-mitomycin C conjugate (WNM-MMC) against mouse MH134 hepatoma.
S.Suzuki, K.Aizawa, T.Matsumoto, K.Tsukada and M.Suzuki

Serum glycoproteins and HLA types as a prognostic marker and individualization of treatment for gastric cancer.

K.Ogoshi, T.Mitomi, Y.Kondoh and K.Iwata

The effect of preoperative intratumoral PSK injection in gastric cancer patients and the localization of PSK.

H.Tomochika, A.Gouchi, K.Ensako, F.Hamada, S.Fuchimoto and K.Orita

AM3 (an oral BRM) enhances the spontaneous bone-marrow recovery in breast cancer patients undergoing short-term adjuvant radio-chemotherapy.

D.E.Levy, I.Rosetti, B.Dosoretz, P.M.Marquez, G.Sada and V.G.Villarrubia

Dr. Patchen and colleagues have previously shown that the administration of glucan isolated from Saccharomyces cerevisiae prior to irradiation can enhance the survival of mice. In an extension of this work, Dr. Patchen reported that glucan can also enhance survival when administered therapeutically after irradiation. Endogenous hemopoietic spleen colony-forming units and bone marrow granulocyte-macrophage colony-forming cell numbers were significantly increased in glucan-treated animals. This indicates accelerated hemopoietic stem cell regeneration in irradiated mice treated with glucan. Synergistic activity with an antibiotic, pefloxacin, was observed in glucan-treated mice and enhanced survival was obtained.

PSK, also known as Krestin, is a protein-bound beta glucan isolated from mycelia of Coriolus versicolor. Dr. Ebina described the effect of PSK in a "double grafted tumor system" in which BALB/c mice are intradermally injected into the right and left flanks at the same time with Meth-A tumor cells. PSK exerted antitumor effect on both the sites even when it was injected only in the right flank tumor on day 3. Intratumoral administration of PSK induced polymorphonuclear and macrophage infiltration in the tumor and generated Lyt-1 positive cells in the regional lymph nodes and spleen. Tumor infiltrating lymphocytes from PSK-treated animals, but not controls, could inhibit the growth of Meth-A cells in the Winn assay.

Dr. Matsumoto studied the antitumor activity of N-acetylchitohexaose (NACOS-6) in C57BL/6 mice using Lewis lung carcinoma. Lung metastasis could be inhibited by intravenous administration of NACOS-6. Interestingly, significant activity of NACOS-6 could be observed even in resected mice.

Dr. Hasegawa observed that sister chromatid exchanges in the bone marrow cells of mice treated with antitumor drug mitomycin C were considerably increased when compared with untreated controls. Simultaneous treatment with PSK reduced the frequency of sister chromatid exchanges in a dose dependent manner. This suggests that PSK can inhibit the mutagenic activity of mitomycin C.

Dr. Suzuki, co-chairman of this workshop, presented an interesting approach to increase the activity of antitumor agents. The mannan of Saccharomyces cerevisiae was conjugated to mitomycin C. The conjugate in saline was administered intravenously 1-5 times on days 7-15 after the subcutaneous implantation of MH134 hepatoma cells. All schedules employed in this study were effective but the administration of 1 mg/kg/day of the conjugate for 3-5 days conferred a marked antitumor effect. This novel conjugate of mannan and mitomycin C appears promising and warrants further studies.

Dr. Ogoshi investigated the levels of pre-operative serum glycoproteins and carcinoembryonic antigen in gastric cancer patients. HLA antigens were determined after patients had undergone gastrectomy and post-operative adjuvant chemotherapy. Poor survival was observed in patients with abnormal levels of carcinoembryogenic antigen and glycoproteins and association with HLA-A11 or B-60. A group of patients received, in addition to the chemotherapy, also immunomodulators like PSK and OK-432. Immunochemotherapy conferred better survival rates than chemotherapy alone in patients having HLA-A2 and normal levels of carcinoembryogenic antigen and glycoproteins.

Dr. Tomochika performed pre-operative endoscopic intratumoral injection of PSK in gastric cancer patients and investigated the distribution of PSK by immunohistological techniques. PSK was taken up by macrophages and an increase in the OKT 4 positive cells was induced in the peripheral blood and regional lymph nodes. Anti-PSK antibody positive cells were detected in tumor tissues and regional lymph nodes. These observations suggest that pre-operative intratumoral injection of PSK can be useful in improving the post-operative prognosis in gastric cancer patients.

AM3 is a protein complexed beta 1-6 polyglycan and is obtained from cell wall of Candida utilis. Unlike most other glucans, AM3 is fully active by the oral route. Dr. Levy reported on a double blind clinical trial with breast cancer patients who had undergone radiotherapy and 3 cycles of chemotherapy. Twenty of the 40 patients received a 3g/day dose of AM3 daily by the oral route. Several hematologic parameters prior to 4th chemotherapy cycle were compared with the baseline values. A significant number of patients who were only on chemotherapy developed mild-moderate bone marrow hypoplasia which was reflected in the numbers of white blood cells and platelets. Except in 2 of 19 patients, AM3 accelerated the spontaneous bone-marrow recovery in breast cancer patients undergoing radio-chemotherapy.

A number of interesting observations have emerged from the presentations and discussion of glucans and immunomodifiers. The therapeutic efficacy of glucan after irradiation, in particular when used in combination with antibiotics, suggests an interesting modality for eventual treatment of radiation sickness in early phases. Agents like PSK can exert antitumor activity even at locations which are distant from the original intratumoral injection site. The capacity to reduce mutagenic effect of cytotoxic drugs is noteworthy. The conjugation of mannans with drugs like mitomycin C produces agents capable of potent antitumor action. A similar approach can be used for development of new immunomodulator-drug combinations for infectious diseases including AIDS. The low toxicity of glucans has certainly contributed to its application in clinical situations. The results of newer clinical studies reported are encouraging. In summary, the various experimental and clinical presentations at this workshop have extended previous observations and indicated directions for future investigations.

Synthetic Immunomodifiers (I)

I. AZUMA* and G. RENOUX**
*Institute of Immunological Science, Hokkaido University, Sapporo, Japan
**Centre Hospitalo-Universitaire Bretonneau, Tours, France

1) Influence of Immuthiol on Pituitary Hormone Levels in Man
G. Renoux, E. Lemaire, M. Renoux, P. Lecomte, and J.-C. Besnard

2) The Biological Activities of Two Human Main Metabolites of Ubenimex
F. Abe, H. Kuramochi, K. Takahashi, M. Ishizuka and T. Takeuchi

3) Inhibition of Experimental Allergic Encephalomyelitis by MS-6044, a Novel Immunomodulating Agent
O. Mizuno, M. Kumakura, A. Matsubara and I. Yamamoto

4) Specific Suppressive Effect of a New Anti-Rheumatic Drug, Bucillamine, on Mitogen-Induced Mouse Spleen Cell Proliferation
S. Mita and K. Matsunaga

5) The New Effects of Lobenzarit Disodium (CCA) on the Immunological Dysfunction in MRL/l Mice
K. Nakamura, J. Abe, Y. Takeda, T. Nakano and Y. Sugawara

6) The Generation of Neutrophils by Dihydroheptaprenol, a Synthetic Polyprenol Derivative, in Experimental Animals
K. Tsukidate, K. Kitoh, A. Suganuma, Y. Sugihara, K. Katsu and I. Azuma

7) Effect of TOK-8801, a Novel Immunomodulating Agent, on the DTH Reactions and Immunologically Induced Arthritis in Mice and Rats
K. Shibata, T. Kobayashi, M. Fujiwara, N. Takayanage, K. Matsunari, K. Nitta and I. Yamamoto

8) L-BCDF and Autoimmunity in MRL/lpr Mice-Suppression by a Novel Immunomodulator, SM-8849
F. Nishikaku and Y. Koga

9) Augmentation of Host Mediated Antitumor Activities by a New Synthetic BRM, RS-0481
A. Hishinuma, T. Kobayashi and T. Nishimura

10) Adjuvant Activity of a Synthetic Nonapeptide of Human Interleukin 1β
L. Nencioni, L. Villa, P. Bossu, A. Tagliabue and D. Boraschi

Dr. Renoux reported the influence of diethyldithiocarbamate (Imuthiol®) on pituitary hormone levels in man. No changes were found in blood samples evaluated at 30 or 60 min, during imuthiol administration. Within 24 hr post administration, imuthiol (10 mg/kg) have no influence on HGH, IGF1, LH, and PRO levels. Furthermore, a woman asking for termination of pregnancy, voluntered with the i.v. administration of 10 mg/kg imuthiol: PRO levels remained at 1600 U/ml during the time of observation, and no trouble on pregnancy was observed. In contrast, imuthiol has induced a mean 2/3 reduction in TSH levels ($P<0.001$ to controls), as early as 2 hr post administration (180 min after the start of treatment), which decrease remained as such as at 24 hr. Above data suggest that, in contrast with thymosin, the recruiting and activating capacities of imuthiol are not associated with increased production of the hormones involved in protein synthesis and growth. The data suggest also that imuthiol does not interfere with the release of these hormones. Of interest is the strong influence of imuthiol on TSH release: an analysis of the finding shows that low levels (around 0.5 mU/l) were not significantly modified, whereas levels higher than 2.0 mU/l were markedly diminished. This might be a consequence of the increase in brain dopomine content induced by imuthiol (a β-dopamine hydroxilase inhibitor), as dopamine inhibits TSH.

Dr. Abe reported the biological activities of two of the main human metabolites of ubenimex, (-)-N-[2S, 3R)-3-amino-2-hydroxy-4-(4'-hydroxy) phenylbutyryl]-L-leucine (OH-ubenimex) and (2S, 3R)-3-amino-2-hydroxy-4-phenylbutyric acid [(2S, 3R)-AHPA]. The degree of inhibition of aminopeptidase (APase) on mouse-peritoneal resident macrophages and the growth of IMC carcinoma in mice by OH-ubenimex were similar to ubenimex. In contrast, the inhibition of mouse spleen cell APase activities in vitro, blastogeneses of mouse T and B cells in vitro, delayed cutaneous hypersensitivities in mice, and the growth of C1498 in vivo and HeLaS3 cells in vitro was weaker than ubenimex. (2S, 3R)-AHPA slightly inhibited only the macrophage APase activities and had practically no effect on the other activities.

Dr. Mizuno described the effects of 5-(4-phenyl-1,3-butadienyl)-1,2-dithiol-3-thione (MS-6044), a novel synthetic compound on various immune responses. MS-6044 enhanced in vitro anti-SRBC PFC and Con A- and LPS-induced proliferative responses of murine splenocytes. Oral administration of this compound resulted in the augmentation of the primary PFC response to SRBC in ICR mice. MS-6044 showed no or slightly inhibitory effect on carrageenin-induced rat paw edema and adjuvant arthritis. However, this compound not only reduced the clinical signs especially in relapsing phases of experimental allergic encephalomyelitis induced in Lewis rats by immunization with an emulsion of guinea pig spinal cord in complete Freund's adjuvant, but also rescued most of the immunized animals from death when administered orally at a dose as low as 0.3 mg/kg daily from day 8 after the immunization. These results suggest that MS-6044 may have an immunomodulating activity and that it may be a possible therapeutic agent for the human autoimmune diseases such as multiple sclerosis.

Dr. Mita reported the effect of bucillamine on Con A-induced mouse spleen cell proliferation in compare with D-penicillamine (D-pen) which showed an inhibitory effect in the presence of copper. Bucillamine (0.1 mM) reduced DNA synthesis of mouse spleen cells to 20% of that of the control culture, whereas D-pen did not reduce the DNA synthesis significantly at the concentration of 0.1 mM. D-pen showed an inhibitory effect only in the presence of copper. The inhibitory effect of bucillamine was not affected by catalase which reduced the inhibitory effect of D-pen plus copper. SA981, an intramolecular disulfide derivative of bucillamine, also showed the same degree of inhibition as bucillamine. These results indicate that the bucillamine has a specific inhibitory effect on mouse spleen cells and this effect is not observed with D-pen and is not mediated by the production of hydrogen peroxide.

Dr. Nakamura reported the new effects of lobenzarit disodium (CCA; disodium 4-chloro-2,2'-iminodibenzoate) on the immunological disorders developed with age in MRL/l mice. Mice were given CCA orally 5 days a week at doses of 5 or 10 mg/kg from 6 to 21 weeks of age. CCA significantly retarded the lymphadenopathy observed in these mice. The analysis by flow cytometry indicated that CCA prevented the decrease of $Thy1^+$ and $L3Ta^+Lyt2^+$ cells in thymus, and the increase of $Thy1^+B220^+$ cells in spleen. CCA also inhibited the age-related decline of splenic IL-2 production. These results suggested that CCA might improve the regression of the lymphadenopathy. Moreover, CCA significantly suppressed the increase of splenic immunoglobulin G secreting cells, and the appearence of serum IgG class-rheumatoid factor and immune complex. In conclusion, it was evaluated that CCA improve the immunological disorders in MRL/l mice by ameliorating the abnormality of the differentiation of T lymphocytes.

Dr. Tsukidate has examined the effect of dihydroheptaprenol (DHP), which enhances a resistance to bacterial infection in mice, with regard to influence on blood neutrophil numbers of experimental animals. Treatment of mice (n=5), guinea pigs (n=4) and rhesus monkeys (n=2) with DHP results in a significant increase in peripheral blood neutrophils. The effective dose of DHP producing the increase of neutrophils was approximately 1.5 mg/head in all species. In rats treated with DHP, hypergranulopoiesis was histologically observed in the bone marrow and spleen, and myeloid-erythroid ratio of myelogram was about 3.4 times higher than that of control rats. DHP was found to increase serum coloney stimulating factor (CSF) in mice after s.c. injection. These results suggest that the mechanism of anti-infectious action of DHP may be, at least in part, its ability to stimulate the generation of neutrophils in hemopoietic tissues via CSF, and also suggest that clinically optimal biological response modifying dose of DHP may be estimated from the optimal dose "per head but not per kg" of experimental animals.

Dr. Shibata has studied on the effect of N-(2-phenylethyl)-3,6,6,-trimethyl-5,6-dihydroimidazo[2,1-b]thiazole-2-carboxamide (TOK-8801) on some immunological inflammations. TOK-8801 inhibited the SRBC-induced DTH reaction by oral administration of 0.1-1.0 mg/kg for 5 days from the sensitization in mice, though it didn't affect the reaction when administered just before the antigen challenge. In the experiment of the MeHSA-induced DTH reaction, TOK-8801 augmented the reaction in low responder (C57BL/6) mice, whereas a little suppression was shown in moderate responder (C3H/He) or high responder (ICR) mice. Despite of lack of inhibitory effect on the carrageenin-induced paw edema in rats, this compound prevented the development of adjuvant- and collagen-induced arthritis which are widely used as the models of rheumatoid arthritis.

Dr. Nishimura investigated autoantibody producing-properties of L-BCDF and effects of an immunomodulating compound, SM-8849, on L-BCDF production and disease process in MRL/lpr mice. L-BCDF obtained from culture supernatant of spleen cells from MRL/lpr mice proved to induce differentiation of unprimed BALB/c cells into anti-DNA antibody-secreting cells, whereas it failed to do as concerns anti-KLH antibody. MRL/lpr mice treated with SM-8849 (25 mg/kg), 5 days a week for 12 weeks, showed reduced L-BCDF production. In addition, SM-8849 was effective in reducing autoantibody titers without suppressing serum IgG levels and anti-KLH antibody titers. These results indicate that, in MRL/lpr mice, L-BCDF is closely related to autoantibody production rather than polyclonal B cell activation. In fact, SM-8849 can reduce autoantibody production and modify the development of immunopathology without affecting polyclonal B cell activation.

Dr. Hishinuma has described that (4R)-3-benzoyl-N-[(1R)-1-penylethyl]-4-thiazolidinecarboxamide (RS-0481) was low toxic, and that its LD_{50} was more than 5g/kg in rodent. RS-0481 showed no cytotoxicity for tumor cells in vitro, but exhibited in vivo antitumor activities in solid tumor system and inhibited metastasis in several tumor models by oral administration. Synergism of RS-0481 with various chemotherapeutic agents, such as FT, MMC, ACNU and CQ, was also observed. Immunological analysis using spleen and lymph node cells obtained from normal and tumor-bearing mice, indicated that RS-0481 had no mitogenic activity but modulated T cell functions. In tumor-bearing mice, RS-0481 augmented tumor specific CTL and T_{DTH} activities. Precursor frequency analysis of IL-2 producing spleen cells according to the limiting dilution method, revealed that RS-0481 restored the number of IL-2 producing cells in tumor-bearing mice.

Dr. Nencioni has compared the synthetic nonapeptide (163-171 peptide fragment of hu IL-1β), previously shown to be devoid of inflammatory effects, to the native protein for its capacity to sitmulate the immmune response in vivo. The nonapeptide could enhance the number of specific antibody-secreting cells in the spleen of mice immunized with both proteic and saccharidic antigens to the same extent as hu rIL-1β. The 163-171 peptide was most active when administered intravenously at 10 pg/kg. However, the same level of immunostimulation was also reached when the nonapeptide was given subcutaneously (10 ug/kg), orally (1 mg/kg) or intraperitoneally (1 mg/kg). Preliminary experiments were then performed in vitro to better understand the mechanism of action of this peptide. After peptide treatment, supernatants of Con A-primed spleen cells contained both IL-2 and IL-4, as assessed by induction of proliferation of the CTLL-2 T cell line and specific blocking by mAb 11.B.11 (anti IL-4) or by mAb PC.61 (anti IL-2 receptor). Thus, it can be suggested that the in vivo adjuvant activity of the 163-171 peptide of hu IL-1β might be the result of helper T lymphocyte activation through the induction of both IL-2 and IL-4 production.

Synthetic Immunomodifiers (II)

MICHAEL A. CHIRIGOS* and TETSUO SHIBA**
*U.S. Army Medical Research Institute of Infectious Diseases, Frederick, Maryland, U.S.A.
**Peptide Institute, Osaka, Japan

In this workshop, 10 presentation were delivered dealing with both new and old synthetic chemicals possessing cellular regulatory function(s) as well as capability of stimulating synthesis and release of specific cytokine(s). Of particular interest was the attempts made to identify not only the specific cell acted on by the immunomodifier (IMM) but also the cytokine(s) induced by the IMM. Such studies would lead to specifically identifying the mechanism(s) of action of the various IMM. Recent reports show that many cytokines administered by the intravenous or subcutaneous route are cleared very rapidly from the peripheral circulatory blood system. It is of value then to seek IMM which induce cytokines leading to higher and longer maintained levels of the induced cytokines. The structural heterogeneity of many of the IMM and the observation that many possess a similar mechanism (e.g., interferon inducers, IL-inducers, etc) would indicate that a specific moiety of the molecular structure is the responsible functional group. The use of crystallography and molecular modeling would be useful in identifying such groups. Use of such technology would lead to the elucidation of their mode of cellular action and increase our knowledge on the interaction of these chemicals with cell surface targets or alterations in cellular enzymatic activity.

In this workshop several of the presentations described the cytokines which were induced, or synergized with, the synthetic IMM. Based on the presentations delivered at this workshop, a brief profile is presented concerning the various compounds. Dr. Kalland (Lund, Sweden) reported on the ability of Linomide (carboxyamide-3-guinoline) to both generate an increase in the number of NK cells as well as augmentation of their activity. Continuous administration of Linomide to C57Bl/6 mice increased a persistent NK activity lasting for two weeks. It appeared that Linomide also increased the number of NK cells. NK cell activity which decreased following lethal irradiation in mice, was found to regenerate much more rapidly following bone marrow transplantation and Linomide treatment. Use of limiting dilution analysis of bone marrow NK cell progenitors showed Linomide increased differentiation of bone marrow cells into mature NK cells. Linomide combined with IL-2 in vitro were synergistic in generating NK cells from immature bone marrow progenitors. Linomide activity was independent of interferon.

Xerosin II, Ribavirin, Bru-Pel (an extract from Brucella abortus), and Ampligen were examined for their ability to stimulate hemopoietic stem cell regeneration, and to enhance survival in irradiated mice. Patchen and Chirigos (Bethesda, MD, USA) reported that prophylactic (treatment 1 day prior to irradiation) IMM administration resulted in some beneficial effects in either increasing endogenous hemopoietic spleen colony-forming units (E-CFU), survival time, or both. Based on E-CFU results, the optimal doses of Xerosin II, Ribavirin, Bru-Pel and Ampligen were 50, 200, 400 and 5 mg/kg. Compared to the 2.8 E-CFU observed in the saline-treated control mice, these agents, respectively, produced 30, 6.0, > 40 and 8.0 E-CFU when they were administered before irradiation (6.5 Gy total body) and 40, 4.8, > 40, and 3.0 E-CFU when administered after irradiation. Significant increases in the percent of mice surviving irradiation were achieved by pretreating mice with Xerosin II (74%), Ribavirin (50%), Bru-Pel (23%) and ampligen (25%) compared to saline controls. Only Xerosin II was found capable of increasing survival (45%) in mice which received treatment following irradiation.

The synthetic acyltripeptide FK-565 and its analogs were shown to activate human blood monocytes by N. Inamura, S. Sone, A. Okubo, J. Yanagawa, A. Nii and T. Ogura of the Tokushima University, Tokushima, Japan. Human peripheral blood monocytes were separated by centrifugal elutriation and incubated with FK565 or its analogs. These monocytes were rendered tumoricidal against the A375 melanoma cell line in a 72hr ^{125}I-IUPR release assay. The tumoricidal activity was dependent on drug concentration and monocyte density. A synergistic tumoricidal activity was achieved by combining FK565 with IFNγ but not with IFN α or β.

The synthetic tripeptides Arg-Lys-Glu (ELS-1) and Arg-Ala-Arg (ELS-2) were reported to have an effect on T cell maturation and function (Kouttab, N., Prada, M., and Brunetti, B. Ellem Ind. Pharmaceuticals, Milan, Italy) reported that these two tripeptides induced the expression of the Thy 1.2 antigen or spleen cells of congenitally athymic (nude) mice. Comparison study of these tripeptides to duodenal peptides, of molecular weight less that 600 d, showed the duodenal peptides failed to induce Th 1.2 antigen. The two tripeptides but not duodenal peptides were capable of enhancing RNA synthesis (activation) and DNA synthesis (proliferation) of peripheral blood mononuclear cells activated with phytohemagglutinin. Inactivated cells did not respond to the tripeptides. Of particular interest was the demonstration that both tripeptides, but not duodenal peptides, could enhance the production by peripheral blood mononuclear cells of B cell growth factor (BCGF and IL-2). ELS-1 and ELS-2 appear to possess the specific capacity of modulating the maturation and function of T lymphocytes.

Y. Kumazawa of Kitasato University, Tokyo, Japan representing his colleagues, focused on defining the structural activity relationship of lipid A by using chemically synthesized subunit analogs of lipid A. The effect of these analogs compared to lipid A were examined for immunopharmacological and toxic activities in several assays, i.e., mitogenicity, macrophage activation, adjuvant activity, mediator induction (tumor necrosis factor, and interferon), pyrogenicity, Shwartzman reaction and lethal toxicity in galactosamine sensitive mice. 4-O-phosphono-D-glucosamine derivatives carrying different amide and 3-O-ester bound acyl groups were investigated. Among the analogs tested, GLA-60, 4-O-phosphono-D-glucasmine carrying N-3-hydroxytetradecanoyl and 3-O-3-tetradecanoyloxytetradecanoyl groups, persistently exhibited the most intensive immunopharmacological activities, indicating the importance of acyl groups and their stereospecificites.

The immunobiological activities of chemically synthesized monosaccharide analogs of lipid A were described by T. Shimizo for his colleagues from the School of Pharmaceutical Sciences, University of Shizuoka, and Fuji Chemical Industries, Takaoka, Japan. The chemically synthesized acylglucosamine-4-phosphate (Acyl-Glc-N-4P), a non-reducing sugar moiety of lipid A, and lipid X, Y are reducing sugar moiety were shown to prolong survival time of mice inoculated with Ehrlich carcinoma. The protection was not as great as natural LPS but was better than control. The compounds exhibited lethal toxicity to mice sensitized to galactosamine, and showed a weak mitogenicity towards splenocytes. The derivatives of Acyl-Glc-N-4P linked 3-deoxy-D-manno-2-octulosonic acid (KDO) exhibited mitogenicity, lethal toxicity, and antitumor activity, but did not cause local Shwartzman reaction. The Acyl-Glc-N-4P linked N-acetylneuraminic acid compounds showed mitogenicity and lethal toxicity, but the activity of Acyl-Glc-N-4P linked N-acetylneuraminic acid appear to be almost the same as N-acetylneuraminic acid free Acyl-Glc-N-4P.

The chemically synthesized lipid A-subunit analogs described by Kumazawa and his colleagues from Kitasato University and Gifu, University Japan, were also investigated for their therapeutic effect on tumor and microbial infections by M. Nakatsuka, representing his colleagues. The lipid A subunit analogs were the 4-O-phosphono-D-glucasamine derivatives carrying N-and 3-O-acylgroups as previously described. Intratumor or intravenous injection of 100μg of GLA-59 or GLA-60 into Meth A-bearing BALB/c mice resulted in marked regression comparable to that produced by 10μg of natural lipid A, administration of both compounds led to markedly decreased numbers of lesions formed on the tail of mice infected with vaccinia virus. Administration of GLA-60 induced a markedly stronger resistance to P. aeruginosa infection when administered 24 hour prior to infection, GLA-59 was shown to be less effective than GLA-60.

A.M. Isetta et al. (Farmitalia Carlo Erba, Milan, Italy) described the effect of a new synthetic immunomodulator FCE 24578. Previous studies showed this compound to act on macrophages, in vitro and in vivo, to exert tumoricidal activity. The compound appears to act as an immune enhancing agent increasing macrophage tumoricidal activity leading to reduced mortality and long term survivors of P388 leukemia inoculated mice as well as bacterial infected mice. Isetta and colleagues focused on the ability of FCE 24578 to induce IL-1 production and secretion. Peripheral monocytes (PM) from mice receiving a single i.p. injection of 10 mg/kg of FCE 24578, were incubated for 24 hours and supernatants tested for the presence of IL-1. Results show that PM collected at different times from treated mice maintained an elevated production of IL-1 for several days, peaking from the 4th to the 7th day. Results of exposing PM to actinomycin D in vitro indicate that activation of macrophages by FCE 24576 to produce IL-1 occurred soon after treatment.

Isoprinosine, another synthetic immunomodulator, was examined by V. Spicak and his colleagues (Faculty Hospital, Bulovka, Prague, Czechoslovakia) as a treatment for asthmatic children. The immunological patterns of asthmatic children, receiving 50 mg/kg of Isoprinosine were evaluated. Asthmatic children showed significant clinical improvement. Phagocytic activity of monocytes and eosinophils was increased and the aggamaglobulinanemia with decreased IgA levels appeared to be alleviated by Isoprinosine treatment. The morbidity and frequency of respiratory infections were decreased significantly following Isoprinosine treatment.

R. Khanna (Dept of Microbiology, J.N. Medical College, Aligarh Muslin University, Aligarh, India) presented their evaluation of vaccination studies in rhesus monkeys with simian malaria using muramyl dipeptide (MDP) as an adjuvant. Using various immunological assays, they found that whole antigen plus MDP was more effective than soluble antigen fractions combined with MDP. The use of MDP as an adjuvant, however, did not provide a stimulation sufficient to produce a vaccine capable of offering total protection.

Lymphokines and Monokines (I)

KEN-ICHI ARAI* and TOSHIO HIRANO**

*DNAX Research Institute, Palo Alto, California, USA

**Division of Cellular Immunology, Institute for Molecular and Cellular Biology, Osaka University, Osaka, Japan

In this workshop, 15 presentations concerning interleukin 1 (IL-1), IL-3 and IL-6 were delivered and discussed.

Various reagents affecting IL-1 response were discussed by several participants. Dr Allison (Syntex Research) demonstrated that glucocorticoids (GC) decreased Il-1β mRNA levels in human peripheral blood cells and monocytic cell line, U937 following LPS induction. GC inhibited IL-1β gene transcription in U937 but not in monocytes. Therefore, GC seemed to have effect on the stability of Il-1β mRNA. GC also inhibited the Il-1- induced Il-6 production in rheumatoid synovial cells. Dr Akahoshi (Kitasato Univ.) showed the GC increased the number of Il-1 receptors without changes in affinity in peripheral blood mononuclear cells as well as fibroblasts. The effect of GC was observed only in B cells but not in T cells, macrophages, LGL or neutrophils. Dr Eugui (Syntex) reported that prostaglandin E2 (PGE2) had no effect on IL-1 production, but inhibited thymocyte response to IL-1. Dr Akahoshi reported that IL-1 upregulated the expression of IL-1 receptors via endogenously produced PGE2 upon stimulation with IL-1 in fibroblasts. Dr Yoshikubo (Otsuka Pharmaceutical Co) demonstrated that IL-2 induced IL-1 production in <u>Staphylococcus aureus</u> Cowan I (SAC)-stimulated B cells. The data indicate that part of IL-2 effects on B cell growth and differentiation may be due to induced IL-1.

IL-1 has been demonstrated to act on a variety of lymphoid and nonlymphoid cells to exert multiple functions, and among these functions, effects of IL-1 on T cells and thymic epithelial cells were discussed. Dr Yamashita (Univ. Occu. Envir. Health) demonstrated that thymocytes obtained from IL-1 treated mice showed an enhanced proliferative response upon the stimulation with hapten-modified self antigens. Furthermore, enhanced cytotoxic T lymphocyte development was also observed. The frequency of $L3T4^+$, Ia^+ and $H\text{-}2^+$ cells was increased, wheras that of $Lyt2^+$ $Thyl^+$ and PNA^+ cells was decreased in Il-1 pretreated thymocytes. Dr Hadden (Univ. South Florida Medical College) reported that IL-1 and IL-2 synergistically induced cell growth of prothymocytes and PAN^+ as well as PNA- thymocytes in the absence of ConA. Dr Galy (Univ. South Florida Medical College) reported that IL-1α,β and IFN-γ were able to induce cell growth of human thymic keratin-positive epithelial cells, whereas IL-2, TNF and thymosin fraction V did not. IL-1β induced morphological change and production of IL-1 in thymic epitherial cells. All the data suggest that IL-1 plays an important role in T cell development in thymus.

The effort to determine the minimal structure responsible for the functions of IL-1 was reported by Dr Kikumoto (Otsuka Pharmaceutical Co.). Utilizing site specific mutagenesis, he demonstrated that Arg ^{4}. Arg ^{98} and Lys ^{93} were essential for the expression of IL-1β activity measured by the growth inhibitory activity against human melanoma A375.S1 cells.

IL-6 has been demonstrated to be a multifunctional cytokine produced by both lymphoid and non-lymphoid cells and regulate immune responses, acute phase reaction and hematopoiesis. Furthermore, unregulated production of IL-6 may be involved in a variety of immunological diseases. Dr Takatsuki (Ajinomoto Co.) reported that human IL-6 acted on murine B cells and enhanced anti-SRBC antibody production <u>in vitro</u> as well as <u>in vivo</u>. The effect of IL-6 was completely neutralized by anti-IL-6 antibody. In the secondary response, the amount of anti-SRBC antibody in serum from mice injected with IL-6 was eleven times higher than than of control mice. Dr Yoshizaki (Osaka Univ.) demonstrated that the germinal centers of hyperplastic lymph nodes of patients with Castleman's disease produce constitutively IL-6. Since several clinical abnormalities, such as hypergammaglobulinemia and elevated levels of acute phase proteins were well correlated with the presence of abnormal lymph nodes and elevated serum levels of IL-6 in these patients, he proposed that continuous production of IL-6 may cause clinical abnormalities in Castleman's disease. Dr Teranishi (Osaka-Minami Natl. Hosp.) reported the presence of large amounts of IL-6 in synovial fluids of affected joints of patients with rheumatoid arthritis. Dr Tanaka (Univ. Occu. Environ. Health) demonstrated that B cells obtained from SLE patients produce B cell stimulatory factor (BFF) capable of inducing growth and differentiation of SAC-activated normal B cells as well as SLE B cells. The BSF preparation was found to contain Il-1α , IL-4 and IL-6. All data suggested that unregulated production of IL-6 and/or the other cytokines affecting B cell growth and differentiation is involved in the pathogenesis of various kinds of autoimmune diseases.

The structures of IL-1, IL-3 and IL-6 receptors and molecules related with IL-3 receptors were discussed. Dr Arai (DNAX) demonstrated that IL-3 receptors consists of two molecules with molecular weight of ~ 70 kd and ~ 120 kd which were cross linked with IL-3 and the cross linking of IL-3 to these molecules was inhibited by monoclonal antibody (F9). F9 antibody was established by Dr Ohta, Nippon Roche which seemed to recognize Il-3 receptor: F9 mimiced biological activities of IL-3 and inhibited IL-3 binding to homologous receptor. Dr Koyasu (The Tokyo Metropolitan Institute) demonstrated that IL-3 induced tyrosine phosphorylation of a 150 kd membrane glycoprotein, indicating that tyrosine kinase is involved in signal transduction mechanism of IL-3-IL-3 receptor system. Dr Resch (Medical School Hannover) demonstrated that IL-1 receptor consists of two chains, one with molecular weight of 41-43 kd and the other with 80 kd which are non-covalently linked to each other. He also demonstrated that 41-43 kd chain was autophosphorylated at tyrosine residue upon the stimulation with IL-1. Dr Yamasaki (Osaka Univ.) reported the cloning of the cDNA encoding human IL-6 receptor utilizing a high efficiency COS7 cell expression system. biotinated recombinant IL-6 and fluorescein conjugated avidin. The IL-6 receptor consists of 468 amino acids, including a signal peptide of ~19 amino acids and a domain of ~ 90 amino acids that is similar to a domain in the immunoglobulin superfamily. The cytoplasmic domain of ~ 82 amino acids lacks a tyrosine-kinase domain. At the moment, the possibility of the presence of a second chains as demonstrated in the cases of IL-1 and IL-2 is not neglected.

Evidence has been accumulating to show that unregulated production of cytokines, such as IL-1 and IL-6 is involved in the pathogenesis of a variety of immunological disorders, such as autoimmune diseases. Therefore, future studies on the regulation of expression of cytokines and their receptors and the mechanisms of signal transduction through the receptors will shed light on the role of these cytokines in the pathogenesis of various diseases. Furthermore, it will provide new diagnostic means and treatment approaches to these diseases.

Lymphokines and Monokines (II)

D. R. WEBB* and I. YAHARA**

*Syntex Research, Palo Alto, California 94303, U.S.A.

**The Tokyo Metropolitan Institute of Medical Science, Tokyo 113, Japan

This was the second workshop convened to discuss the role of cytokines in immune regulation. The variety of topics discussed at this session underscores the vast research effort that continues to focus on the nature and function of cytokines as well as on their potential utility as therapeutic agents.

As one of the chairpersons, Dr. I. Yahara opened the workshop with a few introductory remarks. Due to the availability of various recombinant lymphokines, monokines and other cytokines and to the development of various cloned cell types, we are now able to perform experiments to investigate functions of these agents. Indeed, various functions of cytokines are now demonstrated in vitro. In general, one cytokine affects various cell types (ambiguity of cytokine actions). Conversely, one cell type is affected by various species of cytokines (degeneracy or redundancy of cytokine actions). These properties concerning information transfer from one cell to other cells may be useful to stabilize biological systems which involve cytokines as are in the neuronal network system. At the same time, these results lead one to wonder whether or not all the effects of cytokines observed in vitro are really physiologically significant. If the answer is no, he must further ask what are physiological, in vivo functions of a cytokine in question. Such questions seem to be sound. However, we may suppose that such a question may be useless at present because there is no evidence against the view that a cytokine is doing in vivo all what we observe in vitro. The situation is not altered even for the case that one observed a significant in vitro effect of a cytokine at an unusually high dose. We do not know yet the way how cytokines are released into microenvironments of the in vivo system and how these cytokines are used and depleted. Before solving such a problem, we are free to discuss functions of cytokines based upon in vitro experimental results. In other words, it is important to consider how cytokines act in vivo for correctly interpreting results obtained in vitro.

In the first presentation, Dr. Y. Yamaguchi discussed the role of IL-5 on the growth and function of eosinophils. He noted that IL-5 alone is capable to supporting the development of eosinophils from normal bone marrow cells but not when the cell source is spleen cells from 5-FU-treated mice. This argues that IL-5 affects a cell that has already been stimulated to enter a growth and differentiation pathway possibly by IL-1 or IL-6. IL-5 seems also important in maintaining the growth and functional capabilities of eosinophils. The discussion of this presentation focused on whether when IL-5 induced functional differentiation there was a decrease in eosinophil growth. This is not the case. The possible role of IL-5 in hypereosinophil syndrome was considered a topic for further investigation.

The next presentation continued the theme of the role of cytokines in hematopoesis; in this case the discussant, Dr. J. Talmadge, presented the results of his studies on the restorative capacity of a variety of cytokines to induce myeloid cell recovery following cytoreductive therapy. The injection of G- or GM-CSF, IL-2, IL-1 or IFN-γ all increased CFU-C in all hematopoetic organs in mice treated with cyclophosphamide or irradiation. The key observation was that there was a clear correlation of CFU-C levels and myeloid restoration and survival and thus CFU-C activity may be an early predictor of myeloid reconstitution. As a practical demonstration, Dr. Talmadge presented his results using the B16 melanoma model, using increased amounts of cytotoxic drug and autologous bone marrow transplantation for myelorestoration. IL-1 co-therapy with the bone marrow transplant was more effective than giving bone marrow alone.

The next two presentations by Dr. C. Damais illustrates the fact that many lymphokines have broad regulatory effects. In the first presentation, Dr. Damais showed that the toxin produced by Staphylococcus aureus, responsible for toxic shock syndrome (TSST-1), induces the production of TNF-α as well as IFN-γ and IL-2. The possible synergy of these several factors may very well contribute to the overall pathology of toxic shock. This presentation and the discussion that followed focused attention on a key problem in lymphokine research, that is the difficulty in understanding the natural role of these lymphokines alone or together in vivo in disease. In vitro modeling does not always reflect accurately the in vivo situation. Dr. Damais continued her second presentation by noting that IFN-γ induces chemotaxis of bone marrow cells into the peritoneal cavity. In addition, IFN-γ stimulates an oxidative burst in cells in the peritoneum that is not affected by 5-FU treatment; thus both resident cells as well as migrating cells must participate in oxidative burst induced by IFN-γ. IL-2 appeared to synergize with IFN-γ in this system although by itself IL-2 had no effect. It was speculated that both IFN-γ and IL-2 might synergize during non-specific host residence to infection. The speaker does not yet know whether the IL-2 receptor triggered in this situation is high or low affinity.

Dr. S. Yonehara returned to the topic of tumor necresis factor and described a novel monoclonal antibody termed anti-Fas. This antibody kills target cells in a fashion that could not be discriminated from the killing observed using TNF-α. He also noted that the binding of TNF was not competed out by anti-Fas and the quantity of antigen on the cell surface that reacted with anti-Fas might be different than the amount of TNF receptor on the same cells. The Fas antigen was, however, down-regulated coordinately with the TNF receptor and vise versa in TNF-sensitive cell lines but not in TNF-insensitive ones. Dr. Yonehara and his assocates concluded that Fas may be associated with the TNF receptor on TNF-sensitive cells and only at this case TNF exhibits cytocydal activity through Fas antigen. A number of the participants questioned Dr. Yonehara concerning the nature of the possible information of Fas with the TNF receptor. However, not much additional information is available at this time. Unfortunately, Yonehara and his associates have not been able to demonstrate capping or co-capping the TNF receptor and Fas particularly because the number of the antigen and TNF receptor is not sufficiently large for observation by fluorescence microscopy. They have not yet succeeded in immuneprecipitation with anti-Fas although the antibody detect a protein of 200-kDa on Western blots.

Dr. C. Sautes presented data using cDNAs of both human and mouse FcγRII for transfection experiments in order to show that the cDNAs contain all the information necessary to code for fully functional Fc receptors. These studies reminded one of the chairmen that from a physiological point of view, immunoglobulins are in fact the classical lymphokine.

Dr. S. Murakami refocused the workshop's attention on the problem of newly detected lymphokines by describing a TRF activity present in cell culture fluids of the T-cell hybridoma B151K12. This factor which acts on unstimulated B cells to cause a polyclonal B cell differentiation accompanying autoantibody production appears to bind to N-acetylglucosamine. Using an antibody, J1, that binds to N-acetylglucosamine, Dr. Murakami and his associates demonstrated the presence of a B cell subset that is responsive to the B151-TRF. They hypothesize that the B151-TRF responsive B cells may be crucial to the development of certain autoimmune diseases in mice. In the discussion it was learned that the B151K12 cell line also produces IL-5 which may contribute in some as yet unknown way to the observed phenomenon.

Continuing a discussion of B cell activation and maturation, Dr. T. Hamano presented data that suggests that surface Ia molecules on B cells may be directly involved in the transduction of the maturation signal triggered by IL-5. Precisely how this occurs or what exactly the relationship is between IL-5 and Ia remains unclear.

Dr. I. Kawamura discussed a topic that receives very little attention currently, namely antigen-specific augmentation. He and his associates have found a humoral factor that augments DTH to a specific antigen(s). The factor is apparently quite large (200-400 kDa), is not an immunoglobulin, shows Igh-1-linked restriction but not MHC-restriction and its production requires the interaction of two subsets of T-cells. It is apparently difficult at this time to get a clear sense of the nature of the cell that produces this material. Since the factor is present in the serum of infected mice we should expect to see more thorough going characterization o this material.

The final oral presentation concerned the biochemical and molecular biological properties of a non-specific suppressor factor (SIRS) and was presented by the co-chairman Dr. D. Webb. Dr. Webb also took the opportunity to sum up the session by pointing out that although we now possessed a large number of cytokines with a plethora of biological activities there was still plently to do. In the area of suppressor factors, so far only one factor with suppressor activity has been characterized at the molecular level, TGF-ß. SIRS is a small polpeptide with a molecular weight of 10,000 that acts to block the transition of cells from G2 phase to mitosis apparently by blocking tubulin polymerization. Webb et al., have succeeded in obtaining a 21 residue amino terminal sequence of murine SIRS. This sequence has been used to raise anti-peptide antisera that neutralize SIRS activity; a synthetic oligonucleotide probe has also been constructed from this sequence and used to demonstrate the presence of SIRS messenger RNA in SIRS producing cell only. Southern blot analysis has shown the presence of more than one hybridizing band possibly indicating the presence of more than one gene containing an SIRS-like sequence. Currently both mouse and human cDNA libraries are being analyzed for full length SIRS cDNA sequences.

Future studies in the area of cytokines will undoubtedly focus additional attention on the distribution of receptors for the known cytokines as well as identifying new factors. We still know precious little about the nature of the growth and differentiation signals that induce early stem cells to select either a B cell or T cell differentiation pathway. More work needs to be done to identify the factors involved in suppressor T cell growth and differentiation. Finally, better in vivo models will have to be developed so that we can begin to understand exactly how different cytokines interact in normal and pathophysiological states to exert their biological effects.

Thymic Hormones

H. ISHITSUKA* and G. DORIA**
*Nippon Roche Research Center, Kamakura, Kanagawa, Japan
**Pathology Lab. Enea C.R.E. Casaccia, Rome, Italy

This paper summarizes 8 presentations in the Workshop each dealing with thymic hormones. Four of these were concerned with chemically defined thymic factors, thymosin alpha 1 (peptide consisting of 28 amino acids) and its fragment peptides; and the remaining four were concerned with partially purified lysates of thymus, thymosin Fr. 5, thymomodulin and thymolymphotropin.
Presentations in the Workshop point to the importance of thymic hormones not only in its known, direct role for T-cell maturation and functions, but also in affecting other populations of cells in hemopoiesis indirectly. These effects lead to their practical utility as immunomodulating agents to restore immune functions in various systems with immunomodeficient mice and rats as manifected in these presentations: lymphokine production in nude and aged mice; tumor immunity in mice immunosuppressed by radiation; mitogen responses in immunologically abnormal SHR rats (probably caused by viral infections); opportunistic infections and tumor metastasis in mice pretreated with 5-FU etc. Furthermore, thymomodulin was reported to prevent leukopenia in cancer patients subjected to radiation therapy. In addition to these direct and indirect effects, the effects of thymic hormones on neuroendocrine systems may also contribute in some way to the control of immunoregulation, although no presentation was made on this point in this Workshop.
Thymic hormones have been shown to be practically non-Toxic in the clinical trials performed so far. Thus, thymic hormones will be clinically useful not only for treatment of congenital T-cell defects but also for treatment of secondary immunodeficiencies such as treatment of the aged to improve their immunocompetence and treatment of cancer patients who are receiving myelosuppressive chemo- and radiotherapies.

Brief profiles of the research work presented during this Workshop were as follows:

1. Thymosin

Y. Ohta presented data suggesting that thymosin alpha 1 stimulates the hemopoiesis in immunosuppressed mice indirectly through maturation of T cells capable of producing IL-3. Nu/nu mice were incapable of producing many lymphokines, including IL-2 and IL-3, because of congenital T-cell defects. However, treatment of nu/nu mice with thymosin alpha 1 at a dose of 5 mcg/kg by the i.p. route for 13 times in 6 weeks enabled splenocytes to produce IL-3, but not IL-2, in response to Con A-stimulation *in vitro*. IL-3 activity was determined by the proliferation of IL-3 dependent cell lines and a CFU-S assay. Thymosin alpha 1 itself had no CSF-like activity. She suggested that thymosin alpha 1 enhanced hemopoiesis indirectly through maturation of a particular subtype of helper T-cell precursors, TH_2, recently classified by Mosmann in terms of lymphokine producibility. TH_1 produces IFN-gamma, IL-2, IL-3 and GM-CFS, while TH_2 produces IL-3, GM-CFS and other lymphokines excluding IFN-gamma or IL-2.

Y. Tanaka also argued that thymosin alpha 1 may contribute to hemopoiesis of lymphocytic cell lineage. IL-1 is commonly known to recover cyclophosphamide (CPA)-induced granulocytopenia in mice. However, it did not recover CPA (100 mg/kg, i.p.)-induced lymphopenia or somewhat reduced the number of PBMC at a dose of 2 mcg/mouse, i.p. Although thymosin alpha 1 at doses of 4 and 40 mcg/kg (i.p.) daily for 4 times did not reverse CPA-induced leukocytopenia, its combination with IL-1 recovered granulocytopenia to a greater extent and lymphopenia (reversing the number of PBMC).
In addition, Y. Tanaka discussed the potential application of thymosin alpha 1 as an adjuvant to cancer chemotherapy and radiation therapy. An exposure of non-tumor areas in mice bearing UV2237m fibrosarcoma to X-ray irradiation (1500 rad: upper half body) shortened the survival period ($P<0.02$) as a result of the acceleration of pulmonary metastasis. Thymosin alpha 1 given at a dose of 40 mcg/kg daily for 13 times after X-ray extended the period of survival, possibly through the enhancement of T-cell immunity. In fact, the X-ray destroyed the antitumor T-cell immunity to UV2237m of mice previously immunized with the same tumor cells, and this resulted in the significant growth of the rechallenged tumor. Conversely, thymosin alpha 1 given at 40 mcg/kg daily for 13 times after the X-ray restored the immunity and suppressed the tumor growth completely.

N. Takeichi studied environmental factors to find the cause of immunological abnormalities in spontaneously hypertensive rats (SHR) with congenital T-cell depression. In a conventional environment, T-cell depression (the increase of natural thymocytotoxic autoantibodies and incidence of polyarthritis nodosa) in SHR were evident. This was clearly shown to be associated with viral infection such as mouse hepatitis virus and Sendai virus from facts that antibodies to the viruses were detected in high frequency, and that the experimental infection with the viruses induced the T-cell depression. In SHR, the secretion of thymic hormones was suppressed. Transplantation of thymus (single injection) or administration of a lysate of thymus, thymosin Fr. 5 (2 mg/kg daily for 6 times), reversed the virus induced-T cell abnormalities as well as hypertension.

G. Doria presented evidence that thymosin alpha 1 at a dose of 10 mg/kg improved T-cell abnormalities in aged mice (>12 months old), such as the decreases in function of helper T-cells, in responses to Con A, in productivity of IL-2 and in the number of IL-2 receptor sites (high affinity). N-terminal peptide of thymosin alpha 1 consisting of 14 amino acids (5 mg/kg), but not C-terminal peptide consisting of the remaining 14 amino acids, was shown to have the activity to a similar extent to thymosin alpha 1 (10 mg/kg). However, in young mice (3 months old) thymosin alpha 1 did not influence T cell-functions as determined by IL-2 producibility.

B. Bohn reported that thymosin alpha 1 and its fragment peptides restored immunodeficiencies in mice treated with a cytostatic. Treatment with 5-FU at a dose of 25 mg/kg/day for 10 days made mice susceptible to infection with *Candida albicans* (opportunistic infection). Thymosin alpha 1 and its several fragment peptides (The structures were not mentioned because the patent covering the peptides has not yet been disclosed) given concomitantly with 5-FU counteracted the 5-FU-induced immunosuppression and prevented the Candida infection. Interestingly, some fragment peptides were active even by the oral route. Thymosin alpha 1 and its fragment peptides were also shown to be active in reduction of the incidence of pulmonary tumor metastasis caused by intravenous inoculation of B16 melanoma. Twin-thymosin alpha 1 was also shown to be active or somewhat superior to thymosin alpha 1 in the enhancement of immunocompetencies in newborn mice.

2. Thymomodulin

Thymomodulin is a partial acid lysate of calf thymus, rich in polypeptides which act on the immune systems. It has been used clinically since 1970 in Italy. P. Cazzola discussed the usefulness of thymomodulin as an adjuvant to cancer radiation therapy. He reported that the incidence of leukopenia (WBC <3900/mmc) in cancer patients (breast and genital tract cancers) treated with radiation therapy plus thymomodulin (20 mg/day, i.m. starting 7 days before radiation therapy and for the entire period of radiation therapy, n=30) was much lower than that in patients treated with radiation therapy alone (n=30); 3% (1 case) vs. 46% (14 cases) (P <0.01). This result is impressive, since opportunistic infections as a result of myelosuppression caused by radiation therapy which are often observed is one of the serious problems in radiation therapy.

P. Cazzola explained the above efficacy from his *in vitro* study on the enhancement of cell growth of bone marrow cells by thymomodulin. Although thymomodulin itself had no CSF activity, it was capable of inducing a CSF-like factor in human lymphocyte cultures at concentrations of 10 and 20 mcg/ml. This factor promoted the colony formation in *in vitro* cultures of bone marrow cells from healthy subjects and patients with myelodysplastic syndrome, but not from patients with melanoma and myeloproliferative diseases.

3. Thymolymphotropin

Thymolymphotropin (TLT) is also a partial acid lysate of calf thymus with many components of molecular weight ranging from 1 to 10KD. M. Prada studied the modulation effects of TLT and its purified components on T cell maturation and function. TLT modulated expression of Thy 1.2 antigen on spleen cells of nude mice and of TdT activity in murine bone marrow and thymic cells, promoted mitogen-responses, and enhanced the production of BCGF and IL-2 by human PBL. It was suggested that TLT shows these effects through mechanisms linked to an intracellular increase of cGMP.

Effector Functions of Cytokines in Cancer

E. LOTZOVÁ* and E. TSUBURA**
*University of Texas, M. D. Anderson Cancer Center, Houston, TX, USA
**The Toneyama National Hospital, Osaka, Japan

The area of cytokines has been a topic of substantial therapeutic interest for a number of years, and became a subject of active investigations in both the basic science and clinical arena, in the last few years. The latter activity has been related primarily to the recent advances in the development of cloned molecules with cancer therapeutic potential, like interferons (IFN, primarily α and γ), tumor necrosis factors (α and β) and interleukins (IL 1-6). The research efforts clearly showed that cytokines play an important role in cell-to-cell communication as well as in antitumor response; the latter appears to be executed either directly, or indirectly via potentiation of immune effector mechanisms.

Therapeutically however, neither of these molecules has proved to be a "magic bullet" for the treatment of cancer. One of the reasons for the rather marginal clinical effects of cytokines is undoubtedly the treatment of patients with an advanced disease and a large tumor burden. The other factors which may contribute to the insufficient clinical responses are the suboptimal use of these molecules in a clinical set up and/or their adverse effects, such as cancer-promoting activity. Finally, and most plausibly, no single currently available immunomodulator may be adequate in conquering the cancer. Thus, the trend of the future investigations should focus on the analysis of the mechanisms of cytokine activity, on the understanding how these molecules can synergize with each other, or with other cytoreductive therapies as well as with various effector cell populations, in mediating the most effective anti-cancer responses. Such information may result in optimization of clinical protocols for treatment of cancer in that it might be possible to apply a small dose of multiple cytokines instead of a mega-dose of a single molecule (or combine the cytokines with other therapeutic modalities), and to achieve an optimal clinical effect with minimal toxicity.

The speakers in this workshop as well as those who presented the posters addressed some of these important issues, the synopsis of which is contoured below.

Two presentations dealt with the role of Interleukin-1 (IL-1) in cancer, and described quite a diverse effect of this molecule. Okubo reported that membrane-bound IL-1 is involved in killing of human A375 melanoma cells. He demonstrated that IFN-α, β or γ and/or synthetic des-methyl muramyl dipeptide (MDP) were effective in activating monocytes to mediate lysis of A375 melanoma. The cytotoxicity of IFN-activated monocytes was abrogated by fixation with para-formaldehyde, while fixation of monocytes activated with MDP or LPS, did not affect tumoricidal activity. The latter activity was however, completely inhibited by anti-IL-1α, but not by IL-1β antiserum. Based on these observations, the investigators concluded that the membrane-bound IL-1α may play a role in host defense mechanisms against melanoma.

Data of Tattori and co-workers, on the other hand, showed the role of IL-1 in facilitation of growth of acute myelogenous leukemia (AML) cells. Specifically, culture of AML cells from patients with M-7 stage of leukemia (as classified by French-American-British classification system) with IL-1 resulted in a significant increase in the number of CD25 antigen-positive cells. Also, the leukemic cells expressed IL-1β genes, as detected by northern blot analysis, and the culture supernatant exhibited IL-1 activity. The CD25 antigen expression and proliferation of leukemic cells, as well as the IL-1 activity of the culture supernatants was inhibited by anti-IL-1β antibody. Leukemic cells from another AML patient with M-7 stage neither did respond to IL-1, nor did produce this molecule, suggesting that this phenomenon is not universal. These observations are of concern, since they indicate that the autocrine secretion of IL-1β may play a role in proliferation of some leukemic cells. Consequently, the inhibition of IL-1β activity may be beneficial in treatment of some AML patients.

Interleukin-2 (IL-2) and IL-2 activated killer cells represented the topic of the next few presentations. Suzuki discussed synergistic effect of lentinan and IL-2 in generation of LAK activity in C3H/HeN mice. He demonstrated that the activated effector cells induced by lentinan and IL-2 *in vivo*, as well as their precursors were asialo GM1 positive NK cells. He also reported that two types of killer cells can be generated *in vitro*, NK cells (asialo GM1-positive) and T cells (Thy1-positive). However, since Thy 1 antigen is also present on NK cells, the T cell nature of a subpopulation of *in vitro* generated killer cells was not clearly established. Treatment with lentinan and IL-2 resulted also in induction of LAK activity in tumor-bearing mice and in prominent inhibition of growth of MM46 tumor, as well as in prolongation of survival of C3H/HeN mice. Thus, combination treatment with lentinan and IL-2 may be therapeutically beneficial.

In the next presentation, Koyama et al provided an evidence for the presence of suppressor cells in cultures of peripheral blood lymphocytes of patients with nonresectable carcinoma, after activation with TCGF (cultured supernatant of PHA-stimulated human spleen cells). The suppressor cells, designated lymphokine activated suppressors (LAS), were also detected in peripheral blood of some patients with resectable advanced carcinoma, suggesting that generation of LAS was associated with large tumor burden. Two color flow cytometry analysis demonstrated that LAS expressed $CD8^{+}$, $CD11^{-}$ phenotype. The presence of suppressor cells may be responsible for failure of IL-2 treatment to achieve significant clinical effects in some of the patients with advanced disease.

Hosokawa and Kobayashi presented the data indicating that combined treatment of Lewis lung carcinoma (3LL)-bearing C57BL/6 mice with cyclophosphamide (CY) and recombinant IL-2 resulted in complete cure of the mice, while treatment with CY alone achieved only temporary regression, and IL-2 alone did not show any effect. Even though the combined CY and IL-2 treatment did not result in induction of LAK activity (in contrast to the treatment with IL-2 alone), the ^{111}Indium oxine-labelled, killer cells with LAK activity, were found to accumulate in CY-treated tumors after adoptive transfer more densely, than in tumors of untreated mice. The investigators suggested that the combination of CY and IL-2 treatment may result in improved antitumor effects.

Uchida presented the data on the soluble factor produced by large granular lymphocytes (LGL) of cancer patients. This cytotoxic factor, termed LGL-CF, was found to be cytolytic to autologous and allogeneic fresh human tumor cells, which were resistant to lysis by any of the recombinant cytokines, like TNF-α and β, IFN-α and γ, IL-1, IL-2, or their combination. However, IFN was effective in augmenting lysis by LGL-CF. Treatment of LGL-CF with monoclonal and polyclonal antibodies (separately or in combination) against TNFs, IFNs, and IL-1 did not abolish LGL-CF tumor lytic activity. If further characterized, this factor may have therapeutic potential.

The next few presentations were concerned with the activities of B cell growth factors. Matsuda and his colleagues observed that human B cell stimulatory factor 2(BSF-2) also known as IL-6, promoted the growth of murine plasmocytomas, and more importantly human myeloma cells in vitro. The latter cells were found also to produce BSF-2 and to express BSF-2 receptor. Subsequently, the in vitro growth of myeloma cells was inhibited by anti-BSF-2 antibody. These observations suggest that BSF-2 may be an autocrine growth factor for human myeloma. Consequently, the monoclonal antibodies against BSF-2 or specific inhibitors of this molecule, could be useful in therapy of human myelomas.

The involvement of recombinant IL-6 in generation of cytotoxic T lymphocytes (CTL) was studied by Okada and co-workers. This group reported that IL-6 could function as a killer-helper factor in generation of CTL from human peripheral blood and human thymocytes. IL-6 was not involved in T cell proliferation or in induction of IL-2 production. IL-2 alone was unable to induce CTL generation, however its presence during the early phase of the culture was essential for expression of IL-6 activity in CTL generation. The helper effect of IL-6 was neutralized by anti-IL-6 antibody (but not by anti IL-2 antibody). These observations indicate possible usefulness of IL-6 in generation of antitumor-directed effector mechanisms.

Nishiyama and his colleagues investigated the antitumor effect of recombinant IFN-γ and natural human tumor necrosis factor (TNF)-α and β (lymphotoxin) on 3LL carcinoma in BDF1 mice. Each of the two TNFs demonstrated approximately 20% inhibition of growth of pulmonary metastatic tumors when used alone, and 50-60% inhibition when used in combination with IFN-γ. Additionally, 50% inhibition of tumor growth was observed after administration of both TNF-α and β, suggesting that combination therapy with IFN-γ and TNF-α and β may improve the antitumor effect.

Nakano et al examined the effect of TNF on in vitro generation of murine (C3H/He) cytotoxic T cells against syngeneic tumors, in mixed lymphocyte-tumor cell cultures. The results showed that generation of CTL was augmented in a dose-dependent manner by addition of TNF, and this effect was more pronounced when TNF was added at the initiation of the culture. Also the effect of TNF was augmented when indomethacin was added to the culture. This augmentation of CTL generation by TNF was antigen-specific in that the addition of TNF did not augment nonspecific cytotoxicity. The CTL expressed L3T4$^-$ and Lyt2$^+$ phenotype. Thus, TNF may exert antitumor activity through immune effector mechanisms.

Maeda and his co-workers investigated the synergistic effect of hyperthermia and TNF α and β on in vitro proliferation of human colon cancer cell line (RPMI 4788) and on the growth of Meth A sarcoma cells in vivo. The synergistic effects of hyperthermia and TNF-α or β was observed in both systems when the temperature was elevated above 42°C. These studies showed that TNFs in combination with hyperthermia were synergistic in mediating an antitumor effect.

Another group of investigators (Miyake et al) examined the synergistic effect of TNF α and β in inhibition of clonogenic growth of human colon cancer cell line, RPMI-4788. The results of these studies showed that the tumor-inhibitory effect of TNF-α was stronger than that of TNF-β, and the combination of both of these biologicals was more effective than each of these molecules alone.

Similarly to the above study, Shiiki, et al investigated the combination of cytotoxic effects of TNFs (α and β) and IFNs (α and γ) on various human cancer cell lines. Results of these investigations demonstrated that TNFs and IFNs either acted synergistically or at least their combination resulted in increased cytotoxicity. Furthermore, when TNFs were combined with IFNs, the spectrum of killer effects was extended to cancer cells, which were insensitive to TNFs or IFNs alone.

The study of Klein et al showed that TNF administered to rats by continuous intravenous infusion for three hours peaked later and stayed elevated in the serum longer than when given as a single bolus administration. TNF infusion resulted in increased blastogenic responsiveness and augmented IL-1 production by splenocytes.

Iwagaki and colleagues studied the mechanism by which IFN-β and γ transmits its message from the cell surface into the inner part of the cell. Since calcium controls variety of cellular processes, these investigators examined the changes associated with the transmembrane processing of the IFN signal, using Ca^{2+} indicator and membrane potential-sensitive dye. Results showed that the membrane was depolarized shortly after exposure to IFN-γ, but not to IFN-β. These studies indicate that IFN-γ-induced Ca^{2+} signal was caused by the membrane-potential-dependent Ca^{2+} channel.

Yamamoto et al investigated the relationship between in vivo therapeutic effect of OK-432 against murine Meth A fibrosarcoma and the levels of serum-borne tumor-cytotoxic factor (CF). Cytotoxic factor became detectable in the sera of mice after two intravenous OK-432 injections. Negligible activity of this factor was detected in the sera after administration of OK-432 by different than intravenous routes. Similarly, regression or even the complete rejection of Meth-A fibrosarcoma was observed after two intravenous injections of OK-432. This suggests that serum cytotoxic factor, may be responsible for tumor rejection in this model.

Yamaue and co-workers examined the possible synergistic effect of IL-2 and OK-432 on in vitro generated killer cells from spleens of BALB/c mice. They found that after simultaneous stimulation with IL-2 and OK-432 the LAK activity was inhibited in comparison to that induced by IL-2 alone. After depletion of macrophages, however the synergistic effect of these two immunomodulators in generation of LAK activity was noted. This indicated that OK-432 may have adverse effect on induction of LAK activity, and suggest that the mechanism of interaction of various biologicals should be carefully analysed before combination treatments are applied clinically.

The report of Nagamuta et al was concerned with the ability of OK-432 to induce cytotoxic factors. The overnight stimulation of blood monocytes of normal donors or patients with hepatoma with OK-432 resulted in production of soluble factors with lytic activity against L929 cell line. Such lytic activity was completely neutralized with a monoclonal antibody against human TNF-α. Similar anti-L929 lytic activity was detected in sera of healthy donors; in contrast, sera from patients with hepatoma contained factors that enhanced growth of the target cells. However, this L929 growth-enhancing activity in the sera of patients was reduced 6 to 9 hours after intravenous administration of OK-432, indicating the potential of this biological in reversion of tumor-promoting activity in sera of patients with hepatoma.

In conclusion, the presentations in this workshop clearly showed that the combination of several currently available biologicals (or combination of biologicals with other treatment modalities) may synergize in mediating the most effective antitumor activity. It is hoped that these observations will be instrumental in future development of new therapeutic modalities for treatment of cancer.

Clinical Applications of Cytokines

M. S. MITCHELL* and N. OHSAWA**
*University of Southern California, Los Angeles, U.S.A.
**University of Tokyo, Tokyo, Japan

In this workshop, 15 abstracts were submitted for poster presentation and 8 papers from them were presented orally and discussed fruitfully by a large and active audience

This workshop handled a wide variety of topics related to various aspects of the clinical applications of cytokines. Cytokines discussed were; interferon α (IFN), interferon γ (IFN), interleukin 1 (IL-1), interleukin 2 (IL-2), tumor necrosis factor (TNF), colony stimulating factor (CSF) and so on, and applications were; for malignancy, hepatitis, bone marrow transplantation and autoimmune diseases.

Among the various contributions, two topics were especially interested by many attendants. The first topic was the favorable effect of IL-1 on thrombocytopenia induced by irradiation presented by Dr Nakai and the second topic was the clinical effect of allogeneic LAK cell treatment by Dr Shimizu et al. and Dr Kimoto et al.

Based on the abstracts and presentations, brief comments on the topic with regard to each cytokine are given in the following sections.

IFNα:

The favourable effect of human recombinant IFNα in the treatment of patients with hairy cell leukemia was reported by Dr Stonicki (Krakow, Poland). Daily doses of 10^6 x 5 units of IFNα for 3 months and 2 times per week for subsequent 3 months (i.m.) resulted in 9 cases of complete and 2 cases of partial remission out of 14 cases with minimal side effects. Dr Fuchimoto (Okayama, Japan) reported the useful combination therapy of h-IFNα and h-TNF with or without anticancer drugs to patients with recurrent or progressive solid tumors. Their results were impressive but evaluated that they needed the comparison of the efficacy of the combination therapy with the individual cytokine therapy.

IFNγ:

Antimetastatic effect of IFNγ was analyzed by Dr Murata (Sapporo, Japan) using a mouse-mouse system. Mouse recombinent IFNγ in appropriate multiple treatment modalities resulted in the reduction of lung metastasis in mice. This simulation experiment suggested the application of h-IFNγ for the possible anti-metastatic effect in man. Besides the antitumor effect, beneficial effect of h-IFNγ for the treatment of patients with rheumatoid arthritis was tested by a double blind study with placebo by Dr Veys (Ghent, Belgium). Subcutaneous administration of h-IFNγ (100 µg) for 6 months yielded superior effects in various parameters with minimal side effects. The results were encouraging.

TNF :

As far as the antitumor effect of TNF in man is concerned, there have been many equivocal reports. Dr Terata (Ohtsu, Japan) is concerned with the problems of TNF in clinical use, especially its side effects. Their experience revealed that the adverse reactions were frequently observed and dose limiting factor of TNF was hypotension. Dr Taguchi (Osaka, Japan) tested combination therapy of TNF with various anticancer agents using murine and human tumors transplanted in mice. Their results showed augmentation of anticancer effects of various cytotoxic agents by TNF, suggesting the possible usefulness of the combination therapy in humans.

IL-1 :

Possible clinical usefulness of IL-1 in cancer therapy using recombinant human IL-1 and animal models was studied by Dr Nakai (Tokushima, Japan). Although their results told us the considerable antitumor effects of IL-1 in animal tumors in vivo., the most impressive data were the enhancement by IL-1 of granulopoietic and thrombopoietic recovery in mice treated with 5-FU or X-ray irradiation. The mechanism of accelerated recovery from leucopenia was due to the release of CSF by IL-1 but the mechanism of thrombopoietic recovery was not known. Since there is no efficient therapeutic procedure for thrombocytopenia, the IL-1 effect is extremely important.

Biological Response Modifiers (BRM):

Various BRMs are believed to exert their anticancer effects through the activation of macrophages or lymphocytes with subsequent release of cytokines, especially IL-1 and TNF. Using the model of colon cancer metastasis in rat, Dr Jeannin (Dijon, France) studied the anticancer effects of endotoxins, OK 432 and lentinan with regard to their potency of releasing IL-1 and TFN. His analysis showed that there was no correlation between the therapeutic effect of endotoxins, lentinan or OK432 and their ability to activate macrophages in vitro., especially to induce the production of TNF and IL-1.

IL-2 :

Adoptive immunotherapy of malignant diseases with IL-2 and LAK cells have recently been an important topic in cancer therapy. Usually autologous LAK cells are used for the treatment. In this workshop, there were two reports of adoptive immunotherapy with allogeneic LAK cells. Dr Shimizu (Osaka, Japan) dealt with brain tumors and Dr Kimoto (Osaka, Japan) studied cases with breast and laryngeal carcinomas. They obtained the appreciable anticancer effects with minimal side effects. No immunological side effect such as anaphylaxis or graft versus host reaction were experienced. Clinical studies on antiviral effect of IL-2 were reported by Dr. Onji (Ehime, Japan). Immunological parameters have been changed following the administration of recombinant IL-2 in patients with chronic type B hepatitis. These effects may favor the elimination of virus in infected hepatocytes.

Colony Stimulating Factor (CSF):

Clinical effect of CSF from human urine (M-CSF) in bone marrow transplantation was tested by Dr Masaoka (Osaka, Japan) in a phase II study. Steady and rapid recovery of leucocytes and granulocytes was observed, indicating that M-CSF seems to be a promising agent for bone marrow transplantation. However, the use of CSF or other cytokines in bone marrow translantation needs caution. Dr Imamura (Sapporo, Japan) reported that IL-2 or G-CSF increased alloreactive MLRs in murine bone marrow chimeras.

Miscellaneous :

Dr Orgawa (Izumo, Japan) reported that MNSF (monoclonal nonspecific suppressor factor, a murine T-T hybridoma-derived lymphokine) has a preventive effect of autoimmune hemolytic anemia in NZB mice, suggesting a possible clinical implication. Dr Yachi (Sapporo, Japan) reported a new pancreas cancer-associated antigen MUSE11, which seems to be useful for detection of pancreas cancer.

Summary MDP and Derivatives

H. FROST* and S. KOTANI**

*CIBA-GEIGY Limited, CH-4002 Basel, Switzerland
**Osaka College of Medical Technology, Osaka, Japan

INTRODUCTION

The 3 main areas muramyldipeptides are developed for in preclinical and clinical research were briefly reviewed by H. Frost with the historical note on the host country Japan where major initial discoveries on MDP were made approximately 15 years ago by S. Kotani simultaneously with the groups of Drs. Lederer and Chedid in France. The progress since has focused the activities of MDPs

1. on new adjuvants in novel vaccines
2. on the stimulation of non-specific immunity against infections
3. on macrophage activation for the induction of tumoricidal activities in malignancies.

Several MDPs are already in clinical development, particularly the lipophilic MDP derivatives muramyltripeptide-phosphatidyl-ethanolamine (MTP-PE) and the $\underline{N}^{\alpha}$-($\underline{N}$-acetylmuramyl-L-alanyl-D-isoglutamine)-$\underline{N}^{\varepsilon}$-stearoyl-L-lysine [MDP-Lys(L18)] which found broad coverage during the workshop.

MDPs AS ADJUVANTS IN VACCINES

A. Allison gave an overview on the threonine analogue of MDP (MDP-Thr) which is formulated in a stable emulsion of squalene with Pluronic Polymer L121. MDP-Thr is suitable in this formulation as adjuvant in influenza and hepatitis B virus vaccines. Using inactivated oncoviruses and surface antigens of herpes virus protective immunity in animals has been obtained. MDP-Thr had a low toxicity in preclinical studies and is being predicted as a safe adjuvant for clinical use.

The poster by H. Iinuma et al on the induction of cytotoxic lymphocyte activity by influenza MDP-virosome showed the induction of antibody and cell mediated immunity against influenza using subunit vaccine by a combination of 6-O-(2-tetradeoylhexadecanoyl)-MDP (B30-MDP) and cholesterol.

The augmentation of tumor specific immunity against either syngeneic X5563 tumor cells in C3H/He mice or BCL1 leukemia in Balb/c mice was reported by H. Nakajima et al and J. Shima et al both using a new haptenic MDP-derivative (L4-MDP) cross reactive with Mycobacterium bovis BCG. Mice primed with BCG contained L4 MDP-reactive helper cells enhancing the induction of tumor specific immunity to L4-MDP-coupled syngeneic X5563 tumor cells or MDP modified

BCL1 cells. The combination of specific immunity to BCG and to the tumor cells are thus augmenting tumor rejection.

MDPs FOR STIMULATION OF NON-SPECIFIC IMMUNITY AGAINST INFECTION

A novel approach for anti-viral activity was presented by V. Strnadová et al using the anti-influenza drug amantadine coupled to a desmuramyl dipeptid. This complex induced similar changes in the chemiluminescence of blood cells as MDP.

Leukocytosis and recovery from induced leukopenia was demonstrated for MDP-Lys(L18) by R. Nakajima et al for murine experimental systems. The data by F. Yamaguchi et al could attribute this activity of MDP-Lys(L18) to the induction of colony stimulating factors induced in macrophages. Future will show if correction of leukopenia and induction of leukocytosis by MDPs will be clinically important. A pharmacokinetic study with MDP-Lys(L18) in healthy adult male volunteers was shown by H. Naruse et al. With the use of a sensitive EIA maximal drug concentrations could be detected 1 to 2 hours after s.c. injections of up to 200 μg daily. The preclinical toxicity of MDP-Lys(L18) was demonstrated by Y. Ono et al showing large species differences, i.e. arthritis, liver injury and thrombus formation in some species but not in others.

MACROPHAGE ACTIVATION BY MDPs FOR THE INDUCTION OF TUMORICIAL ACTIVITIES

Species differences for macrophage activation were shown by S. Nagao et al. Peritoneal exsudate cells could be activated by MDP in rats and guinea pigs but not in mice. S. Nagao et al demonstrated a synergistic macrophage mediated anti-tumor effect of MDP-Lys(L18) with murine recombinant interferon γ on Lewis lung adenocarcinoma (3LL).

Several other presentations focused on the generation of cytotoxic mediators from macrophages. These and other reports on general mechanisms are summarized in the following chapter.

IMMUNOPHARMACOLOGICAL MECHANISMS OF MDPs

The binding of MDPs to cellular structures can be investigated using a radioactive iodine containing aryl-azide MDP derivatives as reported by J.F. Petit et al. While this compound bound to the surface of activated murine B cells binding could only be discovered intracellularly in macrophages. The binding of MDP to surface receptors of macrophages remains controversial. However, M. Akasaki et al presented data on the binding of sites of MDP-Lys(L18) to be located on the murine macrophage membrane. As binding was not inhibited by MDP, binding of MDP-Lys(L18) via the stearoyl residue was suggested.

The *in vitro* and *in vivo* enhancement of monokine induction by lipophilic muramyl peptides using monoclonal anti-MDP antibodies was demonstrated by G.J. Riveau et al. Binding of MDP to Fc receptors and endocytosis may be one of the explanations for this interesting phenomenon.

The induction of interleukin 2 receptor expression on B cells but not on T cells was presented by T. Saito-Taki et al.

A bacterial peptidoglycan-specific T cell line specific for the peptidoglycan subunit of bacterial cell wall, disaccharide tetrapeptide (GM-53) consisting partly of MDP, could be generated by T. Koga et al and used for transferring *in vivo* DTH against GM-53 indicating that previous specific host response to bacterial peptidoglycans could participate in immunological mechanisms of MDPs.

Y. Noso *et al* reported pretreatment of mice with several hydrophilic or lipophilic MDP derivatives leading to increased TNF levels induced by LPS as compared to LPS alone. The same group had also evidence that MDP primed for the induction of TNF in nude mice by LPS or bacterial vaccines suggesting that T cells are not required for TNF production stimulated by MDPs.

H. Usami *et al* had similar *in vivo* data on MDP as a priming agent for LPS-induced TNF production by macrophages.

SUMMARY

In summary presentations and discussions at the workshop reflected the rapid progress on MDP and derivatives. Molecular mechanisms by which MDPs interact with cellular components of the immune system were presented. Further progress has been achieved on using MDP derivatives in clinical situations, as modern adjuvants in vaccines, or as macrophage activators against tumors or as stimulators of non-specific resistence against infections.

Allergy and Antiallergies

A. L. DE WECK* and T. MIYAMOTO**

*Institut fur Klinische Immunologie, Inselspital Bern, Switzerland
**Dep. of Med. & Physical Therapy, Univ. of Tokyo, School of Med., Tokyo, Japan

In this workshop, 7 oral presentations and 7 posters were presented. Each dealt with allergy or antiallergic drugs. This is rapidly advancing field and the workshop was interesting.

Each presentation dealt with different subject. So some of them will be summarized briefly.

N. Uchibayashi (Osaka, Japan) discussed their production of the recombinant soluble Fc_{ε} RII as a secretory molecule instead of a proteolytic product of membrane receptor. He discussed that the product of the chimeric gene as well as the soluble receptor from B cells bind to IgE and competitively inhibit IgE binding to eosinophils, suggesting that soluble Fc_{ε} RII plays a role in the prevention of the effector phase of allergy.

T. Okada (Aichi, Japan) presented a time-lapse cinematography showing the degranulation of mast cells and their recovery. The inhibitory effect of antiallergic drugs was also shown. Anti-allergic drugs such as tranilast, glycyrrhizin, repirinast and amoxanox inhibited histamine release and degranulation of mast cells.

A. L. de Weck (Bern, Switzerland) presented a new instrument consisting in an inverted fluorescence microscope with a vidicon camera which is useful to investigate the effect of lymphokines or immunopharmacological agents in a small number of cells.

K. Kurosawa (Maebashi, Japan) stated that the protein kinase C may play a crucial role during mediator release from rat mast cells, as staurosporine, a novel protein kinase C inhibitor, inhibited histamine release from stimulated rat mast cells.

K. Hirai (Tokyo, Japan) discussed that human basophil histamine release are regulated by GM-CSF and IL-3, and that basophils have functional receptors for both factors based upon this experiment.

N. Inagaki (Gifu, Japan) mentioned that glucocorticoids display anti-allergic activity through a mechanism different from that of anti-inflammatory activity based upon their experiments.

T. Noma (Tokyo, Japan) reported that induction of IL2 responsiveness of the peripheral blood lymphocytes to stimulation with nominal antigen may reflect immune response to the allergen in patients with allergy. Ketotifen seems to be capable of blocking the response in pathogenic processes of allergic disease.

4 of 7 posters presented the immunopharmacological action of newly developed anti-allergic agents such as KW-4679 (a product of Kyowa Hakko Kogyo, Japan), OKY-046 (a product of Kissei Pharmaceutical Co., Japan), IPD-1151T (a product of Taiho Pharmaceutical Co., Japan), Neurotropin (a product of Nippon Zoki Pharmaceutical Co., Japan). Some of them have inhibitory action to PAF, histamine, leukotriene, substance P, or thromboxane A2 synthesis.

Also some of them show the inhibitory effects upon chemical mediator release from inflammatory cells. They are under clinical assessment, aiming to effective drugs in allergic diseases.

Other papers suggested that PAF and leukotrienes may be able to modify inflammatory and immunological events in liver tissue (Y. Sakagami, Osaka, Japan).

All presentations related somewhat to clinical application of substances and active discussions were carried out to make the session quite fruitful.

Pharmacology of Immunocytes

JEAN-FRANCOIS PETIT* and TAKESHI OGURA**
*Biochimie-Biophysique, Universite Paris-SUD, Paris, France
**Internal Medicine, Tokushima, Japan

Three topics were raised in this workshop: 1) effector mechanisms involved in cancer immunotherapy, 2) pharmacology and biochemistry of immunocytes, 3) relations between the central nervous system and the immune system.

1) Effector Mechanisms Involved in Cancer Immunotherapy.

This topic was the predominant topic of the session.

A) A first series of papers dealt with various aspects of the action of OK432, a streptococcal preparation, which has been widely used in adjuvant immunotherapy for patients with cancer.

Dr. Hoshino's (Fukui, Japan) interest was an overview of the immunopharmacological effects of OK432 *in vitro* and *in vivo*. *In vitro*, he was able to show that OK432, when cultured with effector cells from cancer patients, increases the cell-mediated cytotoxicities against allogeneic and freshly prepared autologous tumor cells. He also observed increases of productions of cytokines: IFNα and γ, IL1, IL2, TNF, NK cytotoxic factor (CF), MCF and GCF, a granulocyte derived factor which he has recently identified.

In vivo, he examined various immunological parameters of the patients treated by intradermal OK432 injections after surgical resection of stage I-cancers. The results were that both cytotoxicities of NK, ATK (autologous tumor killer) and LAK cells and the capacity to produce TNF, IL1, IL2 IFNα and γ, NKCF, MCF and GCF were augmented siginificantly. He observed also that the doses and frequency of OK432 administration necessary to produce an adequate augmentation of the immunological parameters were related to the baseline values at the onset of the treatment, low baselines-needing more intense treatment.

To study a possibility of increasing ADCC against a human salivary adenocarcinoma (HSG), Dr. Sato (Tokushima, Japan) raised an mouse IgG2a monoclonal antibody (5B/10) reacting to a nonsialylated carbohydrate epitope. Treatment of peripheral blood leukocytes with OK432 *in vitro* did not enhanced ADCC. However, treatment with both the monoclonal antibody and OK432 significantly increased the ADCC activity and the survival period of the mice inoculated intraperitoneally with the tumor. A new approach to examine the ability of OK432 to modulate target cell susceptibility to effector cells was presented by Dr. Uchida (Kyoto, Japan). He found an increased sensitivity of tumor cells binding OK432 to autologous LGL, small T lymphocytes and monocyte/marcophages as well as to novel soluble cytotoxic factors produced by LGL and macrophages.

In experimental studies with animals, two papers stressed the action of OK432 on NK cells. Dr. Murakami (Okayama, Japan) noticed that a single portal injection of OK432 significantly enhanced the NK activity of hepatic lymphocytes in Wistar rats: the peak of action was at day 1 and returned to normal level at day 4. Similar effect was observed 4 days after single injection of a protein bound glucan, PSK. By contrast, r-IL2 was necessary to be injeceted repeatedly for increase of NK activity.

Dr. Yamaue (Wakayama, Japan), by resensitizing mice spleen cells in vitro with OK 432, observed an increase of NK activity in Thy 1^-, asialo GM^+ cells associating with productions of IL-2 and IFN-γ activities. He injected locally these activated NK cells into mice bearing intraperitoneal SP2 myeloma cells and those bearing subcutaneous C26 colon adenocarcinoma, resulting in remarkable tumor inhibition in both cases.

Regarding effect of OK432 on chemotactic activity for PMN's, Dr. Inoue (Kyoto, Japan) measured PMN's migration through filter membrane applied to the turned peritoneum of rats. With proper use of OK432 and/or normal human serum with inhibitors to complement or arachidonic metabolism, he could show that the both complement and arachidonic cascade played a role in the chemotactic activity of OK432.

These results indicate variety of anticancer effector mechanisms activated by OK432.

B) Two papers were devoted to new drugs or association of drugs.

Dr. Riccardi (Perugia, Italy) presented biological activities of PCF39 (N-alpha-5-(hypoxanthin-9-yl)pentyloxycarbonyl-L-arginine), which has already known to protect mice from tumor and bacterial challenges. In this session, it was shown that addition of PCF39 and PMN to an inoculum of human tumor cells in nude mice led to rejection of the tumor graft. Pretreatment with the agent in immunocompetent mice could also cure infection of Aspergillus fum.

Dr. Kato (Kyoto, Japan) showed that oral administration of K18a, conjugated product of human IgG and melphalan, combined with an i.p. injection of PSK, could increase the survival period of mouse bearing ascites Meth A tumor. In vitro cytotoxic activity was found to be augmented by the peritoneal cells from tumor-bearing mice injected with K18 and in those of normal mice treated in vitro with K18, suggesting that this compound, besides the known direct cytotoxic effect of melphalan, could have an immunotherapeutic efficacy.

C) Two papers dealt with the effects of chemotherapeutic drugs on immunological parameters.

Dr. Iwaguchi (Tokyo, Japan) devised a procedure to monitor the modulation of suppressor cells. He analysed the histograms of lymphocyte mobility in a cell electrophoretic apparatus (Parmoguant L) and established that suppressor T cells induced by con A had a lower mobility than normal T cells. His device allowed him to monitor the disappearance of con A induced suppressor cells by in vivo treatment with 5-FU.

Dr. Vecchi (Milan, Italy) analysed the effects of administration of doxorubicin, cyclophosphamide and 5-FU in vitro on generations of LAK, CTL and NK activities from splenocytes. Although the effect was variable according to combination of anticancer drug with target cytotoxic activity, Doxorubicin was found to be rather inactive to affect cytotoxic activity, and allospecific cytotoxic activity seemed more sensitive to anticancer drug.

These two papers may offer a new fundamental consideration in designing regimen of chemoimmunotherapy.

2) Parmacology and Biochemistry of Immunocytes

Dr. Resch (Hannover, FRG) analysed the pathways involved in the induction of IL2 receptor (IL2-R) and IL2 secretion in human periheral blood lymphocytes. Anti-CD3 or anti-TCR-CD3 monoclonal antibodies induce IL2 production, IL2-R expression and lymphocyte proliferation. Stimulation by TPA and ionomycin leads to the same pattern. By contrast, stimulation by dioctanoylglycerol (di-C8) and ionomycin, which should give similar results, only induced IL2-R; addition of polyinsaturated fatty acids restored IL2 production and proliferation. Dr. Resch noticed that whereas di-C8 + inomycin activated phospholipase A2 with a peak at 30 min, the peaks of phospholipase A2 and of lysophosphotidacyltransferase activity were at 4 h upon stimulation with monoclonal antibodies or ionomycin + TPA. It thus seems that long term activation of phospholipid metabolizing enzymes is necessary signals for IL2 production and lymphocyte proliferation.

Dr. Florentin studied the in vivo effects of α/β IFN on the chemoluminescence (CL) of mouse peritoneal macrophages. Contradictory results led the authors to take into account the age of the mice. Usually, IFN α/β decreases the chemoluminescence induced by TPA except in mice of around 7 weeks of age: the increase of CL induced by IFN α/β at this age was related to the presence of a population of adherent asialo $GM1^+$, LGL^- like cells without NK activity.

In another paper, she presented two new tuftsin derivatives: formylated tuftsin (f-tuftsin) and formyl-methionyl-tuftsin (f-Met-tuftsin). In binding experiments, f-tuftsin competed slightly with tuftsin and f-Met-tuftsin not at all: these new derivatives may thus have acquired affinity for the receptor for formylated peptides. The most interesting finding is that the formylated peptides, although having almost the same properties as tuftsin do not have depressive effects on lymphocytes: this might be due to their lesser induction of PGE2 production by macrophages.

3) Relations between The Central Nervous System and The Immune Systems

Four papers dealt with the very quickly developing field of

of the connections between nervous and immune systems.

Dr. Hadden looked for endocrine factors involved in a link between pituitary and thymus. He obtained an extract of bovine pituitary and showed that the agent prolifereted human thymic epithelial cells (HUTE) in vitro like fibroblast and epidermal growth factors and produced IL-1 like substance. Preliminary characterization indicates that the factor involved is a polypeptide (MW >10 kD precipitates with ammonium sulphate). Further studies using antibody have shown a relationship with Fibroblast Growth Factor. Chromatographic studies to isolate the factor are currently in progress.

Dr. Li presented an impressive set of data on the action of metenkephalin on various aspects of the activity of the immune system. Almost many others, Met-Enk enhances in vitro the blastogenesis of mouse splenocytes stimulated by suboptimal concentrations of Con A and PHA whereas it inhibits blastogenesis induced by LPS. In vitro and in vivo it increases IL-1 production induced by LPS from peritoneal macrophages.

Dr. Renoux used parkinsonian inducing drug, 1-methyl-4-phenyl-1,2,3,6-tetrahydropyridine (MPTP), to stress his previous findings on the role of the neocortex on T cell balance. MPTP, which depresses dopamine striatal levels, also affects the T cell balance. Imuthiol (diethyldithiocarbamate) restored the dopamine striatal levels and T cell dependent responses. Thus, by the elegant use of MPTP, Dr. Renoux brings new arguments in favor of a dopaminemediated role of the neocortex on T cell functions.

Dr.Gontova presented results on acetylcholine inhibition of immune responses which could be blocked by indomethacin and ware thus in part mediated by prostaglandins produced by macrophages.

In conclusion, results presented at this workshop stressed the complexity in the cellular and molecular network involved in cancer immunotherapy by immunomodulator and related cytokines: this complexity is now analysed more and more carefully in vivo and in vitro in man and in experimental animals and it should lead to an improved use of these agents.

The possibility of modulating suppressor cells by chemotherapeutic agents is an interesting trend as well as the fact that experiments are in progress in animal models to select drugs which will not h nder later use of immunotherapy.

The complexity of the action of defined agents at the cellular level is well known and was stressed by some presentations. As a final conclusion, complexity is not limited to the immune system and its network of cells and mediators: this system is in constant interplay through receptors and mediators with the neural and endocrine system: convincing data were presented which tell us that the in vivo functioning of the immune system must be approached in the broad context of integrated physiology.

Immunotoxicology

ENRICO MIHICH[1] and KEIJI UDAKA[2]

[1] *Grace Cancer Drug Center, Roswell Park Memorial Institute, 666 Elm Street, Buffalo, New York 14263, USA*

[2] *Nippon Roche Research Center, 200 Kajiwara, Kamakura, Kanagawa, Japan*

Immunotoxicology is acquiring increasing importance not only as a consequence of recent advances in immunological approaches to therapeutics, which involve the clinical evaluation of new biological response modifiers (BRMs) and biological agents, but also as a result of increased knowledge about the existence and action of noxious reagents in the environment, inclusive of allergens and agents causing pseudoallergic reactions. In parallel with the expanding needs for immunotoxicological evaluations in preclinical and clinical investigations, there is the need to develop new approaches and new models which when integrated with appropriate classical toxicological approaches would provide relevant information useful in the advancement of new treatments to the clinical level or in the management of immunological syndromes.

In a broad sence, the field of immunotoxicology can be grossly divided into the three areas mentioned below.

1) Immunotoxicity of drugs, chemicals and biologicals which most often lead to suppression of immune effectors development and/or function; in this context, effectors of host defenses are to be considered in a global functional sense, beyond the limiting classical definition of "immune effectors". Autoimmune reactions may occur consequent to such phenomena as a disregulation of the host response, a haptenic function provided by the causative agent or antigen availability or increased expression resulting from the cellular action of the causative agent. Thus, the selective toxicity of certain agents, while potentially exploitable for therapy, may also cause imbalances inducing toxicities based on immunological mechanisms.

2) Tissue toxicities of BRMs as currently viewed seemingly may be unrelated to their effects on host-defenses however they may actually become reconciled with these effects once the mechanisms of toxicity are more completely understood. Two recent examples are those of the increased vascular endothelium permeability caused by Interleukin 2, which leads to the development of edema in humans, and the vascular endothelial proliferation and synovial changes induced in animals by certain macrophage activators of the MDP type.

3) Hypersensitivity reactions to drugs have been known for a long time as related mainly to antibiotics. Recently these reactions have acquired a broader scope of importance as they can be induced by a number of cytokines, peptides, adjuvants, antibodies and chemicals in the environment. The immunotoxicology of peptides will require increasing attention in the future as the number of

peptide agents developed for medicinal purposes is rapidly expanding; indeed major efforts are being made to mimic or inhibit cytokines or other regulators which can now be identified, produced and tested thanks to the availability of modern molecular technologies. Pseudoallergic drug reactions should also be given proper attention in immunotoxicology given the increasing evidence of their importance in parallel with that of strictly defined allergic reactions.

In this Workshop only some aspepcts of the broad area of Immunotoxicology could be considered, particularly those concerned with the toxicity of drugs and chemicals on host defense mechanisms. Seven presentations were delivered. These presentations dealt with either methodologies for evaluating drug immunotoxicity and hypersensitivity or immunotoxicity or selectie toxicity of specific immunomodulating agents such as aminocarb, dieldrin and cadmium.

Methodologies for evaluating drug immunotoxicity in the process of drug assessment were described by Mr. Horii (Kamakura, JAPAN). Immune function tests on anti-SRBC antibody production, allograft tumor rejection, responses to CSF and resistance to Psudomonas infection were conducted in rats and mice given 5-FU [5-fluorouracil] or its derivative cytostatics (Tegafur [1-(2-tetrahydrofuryl)-5-fluorouracil], UFT [Tegafur+uracil], 5'DFUR [5'-deoxy-5-fluorouridine]). These immune function tests proved to be effective on short-term administration (one-week) since immunotoxic effects were mostly transient or reversible and parameters were normalized on longer administration (4-week). Comparative data confirmed that all drugs tested were immunosuppressive to various degrees, and changes in T-cell and bone marrow functions accompanied by morphological changes of the thymus were noted at lower doses for some drugs. In combination with the conventional standard toxicity tests for drug evaluation, in which hematological and various other parameters, i.e. weight and histopathological changes of immunoresponsible organs, have been used to evaluate immunotoxicity to a limited extent, these functional tests were noted to serve as a reliable method in determining the immunotoxic potential of drugs.

Methodologies for evaluating immunologically-mediated drug hypersensitivity, both allergenicity and immunogenicity, were introduced by Mr. Inoue (Kamakura, JAPAN). Test drugs, penicillin G and 4-aminoantipyrine, were subjected to the following tests: active systemic anaphylaxis test, skin test and lymphocyte transformation test. Among the species employed in each test, guinea pigs were found to be most suitable for the evaluation. Guinea pigs were the only animals that reacted with positive allergenicity and negative immunogenicity for penicillin G. The active systemic anaphylaxis test proved to be the most sensitive immunological test, and for carrier proteins of immunogen, heterogeneous proteins were more effective in detecting hypersensitivity than homogeneous proteins. Establishment of animal models for drug hypersensitivity is still an area requiring concentration.

Aminocarb [p-dimethylamino-m-tolyl N-methylcarbamate], a carbamate insecticide, was presented as a potential immunomodulatory factor by Dr. Bernier (Quebec, CANADA). Aminocarb induces transient and reversible immunosuppression of humoral response by gavage and dermic exposure of inbred C57BL/6 mice. These tests were conducted on single administration on account of spontaneous degradation of the compound if it were placed in the environment. Oral aminocarb is not immunosuppressive and causes no major effects on antiviral resistance in mice. The target for immunomodulatory aminocarb interaction is not clear; however, data suggesting interference with the B-cell at the activation sequence, but not the antigen processing, were noted.

Immunosuppression by dieldrin [1,2,3,4,10,10-hexachloro-6,7-epoxy-1,4,4a,4,6,7,8,8a-octo-hydro-endo-exo-1,4,5,8-dimethanonaphtalene], an organochlorine pesticide, was discussed by Dr. Fournier (Quebec, CANADA). Dieldrin is known to cause transient but significant immunosuppression of humoral and cellular responses and affect antibacterial and antiviral resistance in mice. The dieldrin level in the tissue and changes in tissue glutathione content in mice exposed to dieldrin correlated, and a significant decrease in total glutathione concentration was observed in parallel to the transient immunosuppressive effects. The mechanism by which dieldrin exerts immunosuppressive effects is still unresolved. Available data, however, indicate that the action is not directly related to any cytotoxicity on immunocompetent cells but rather to disruption of some cooperative system involving the macrophage.

Two presentations were made on the capacity of cadmium to induce autoimmune or immunosuppressive responses. The capability of cadmium to induce antinuclear antibodies in vitro and in vivo was examined by Dr. Ohsawa (Kanagawa, JAPAN). Antinuclear antibodies were detected in the sera of ICR and other mice exposed to subcutaneous cadmium (cadmium chloride), whereas only apparent induction was noted after administration of mercury or lead. Cadmium also successfully induced antinuclear antibodies in an in vitro test employing spleen cell cultures. It was concluded that antinuclear antibody induction in mice treated with cadmium can serve as an effective model for chemically-induced autoimmune response.

The capacity of cadmium to affect human lymphocyte responses in vitro and the mechanism by which cadmium inhibits human lymphocyte proliferation were discussed by Dr. Alesse (ITALY). Cadmium (cadmium chloride) was found to inhibit PHA- or PMA- induced lymphocyte proliferation. Biochemical evaluation indicated that after PHA stimulation, IP3 was rapidly eliminated and IP1 produced in the presence of cadmium. Additional data show that PKC activity is decreased consequent to the addition of cadmium, and it is speculated that cadmium inhibits lymphocyte proliferation through inhibition of some steps in signal transduction. It was additionally noted that zinc was the only element that could restore this suppression.

Macrophage exocytosis of processed antigen was discussed by Dr. Krzystyniak (Quebec, CANADA) as a potential site of zenobiotic-induced immunosuppression of humoral responses. Immunomodulating (aminocarb, dimethyldithiocarbamate, dieldrin, cadmium) and lysosomotropic (ammonium chloride, chloroquine) agents were tested for effects on macrophage antigen processing in vivo and in vitro, respectively, with a single protein antigen, avidin. It was reported that only suppression of the macrophage antigen processing could be attributed to the effect on macrophages caused by the immunomodulating agents studied. Rim damage of the macrophage did not decrease phagocytosis. An increase in macrophage antigen processing could not be supported by drug-related immunopotentiation.

Novel Aspects and Approaches in Immunomanipulation

A. C. ALLISON* and T. TADA**

*Institute of Biological Sciences, Syntex Research, Palo Alto, California, U.S.A. and
**Department of Immunology, Faculty of Medicine, University of Tokyo, Japan

The presentations in this workshop concerned previously unrecognized activities of known drugs, cytokines and other factors and novel applications of existing therapies. No radically new approaches to immunomanipulation emerged.

S. Sozzani and colleagues (Milan) reported that while high doses of Cyclosporin A (CsA) (150 mg/kg/day) inhibited the formation of antibodies against sheep red blood cells in mice, lower doses (50 mg/kg/day) increased the number of antibody-forming cells about threefold. The same dose of CsA was found to decrease the generation of T-cells suppressing the formation of antibodies against type III pneumococcal polysaccharide. The authors suggest that moderate doses of CsA can inhibit the generation of T-cells suppressing antibody formation.

N. Tanaka and colleagues (Okayama) reported that CsA can increase the rate of regeneration of mouse liver following partial hepatectomy. This operation was found to induce spontaneous IL-2 production by spleen cells, and administration of recombinant IL-2 significantly inhibited liver regeneration. CsA was thought to increase regeneration by inhibiting IL-2 production. Neither CsA nor IL-2 in the doses used had any direct effect on cultured regenerating liver cells, suggesting that IL-2 activates effector cells exerting a cytostatic or cytotoxic effect on regenerating hepatocytes. These observations have interesting implications for the pathogenesis of virus-related and autoimmune hepatitis, in which regeneration of hepatocytes as part of the repair process may be impaired by IL-2 production and perhaps LAK cell activation.

Infusion of activated LAK cells into subcutaneously implanted gliomas, followed by daily intraperitoneal administration of IL-2, was reported by T. Yamaki and colleagues (Sapporo) to have marked anti-tumor activity. The regressing tumor contained many T-cells, which was attributed to the induction of strong immunity of the host against the tumor. Infusion of activated LAK cells and IL-2 into brain tumors could induce local anti-tumor effects with minimal systemic side effects. However, potential local side effects, notably edema, might limit the use of this strategy.

Activation of blood by extracorporeal circulation through polystyrene fibers to which lipopolysaccharide (LPS) was immobilized, as a strategy for inducing anti-tumor effects while reducing side effects, was proposed by K. Numa et al. (Shiga). Using this procedure in rabbits bearing transplanted tumors, 80% survivors were obtained, as compared with no survivors in controls. The proportion of survivors was further increased by hemoperfusion with BCG as a priming agent. Hemoperfusion with de-acylated LPS on fibers was ineffective. The mechanism by which immobilized LPS activates blood to produce anti-tumor effects remains unknown. Especially with allogeneic tumors, as in rabbits, several possible mechanisms might be operating.

The complexity of factors controlling cytotoxic mechanisms was illustrated by a study of T. Yamasaki and colleagues (Kyoto) of the effects of dimethylsulfoxide (DMSO) and interferon-γ (IFN-γ) on the susceptibility of mouse lymphoma cells (YAC-1) to lysis by NK cells and specific cytotoxic T-cells (CTL). DMSO and IFN-γ augmented expression of H-2 glycoproteins on YAC-1 cells, which increased their sensitivity to CTL but decreased their sensitivity to NK cells. DMSO treatment did not affect the binding of NK cells to target cells, so protection against lysis is due to an event following binding. In a variant of YAC-1 lacking β_2-microglobulin, DMSO exposure did not of course induce H-2 expression or decrease sensitivity to NK cells.

Variants of the mouse AKR lymphoma with high malignancy (HM) and low malignancy (LM) were reported by O. Klein et al. (Tel Aviv) to differ in susceptibility to growth inhibition effects of macrophages activated in different ways. LM cells were sensitive to macrophages activated by Aerobacter levan (poly-fructose) or levamisole whereas carrageenan increased the growth of LM-cells while depressing the growth of the HM variant. The authors point out that during tumor progression phenotypic changes occur, including allerations in sensitivity to immune responses.

For these and other reasons responses to immunotherapy vary and are not always favorable. G. Mathe and colleagues (Paris) reported that the effects of chemotherapy with an oxalato-platinum complex on a transplantable murine mammary tumor were not significantly improved by hormonotherapy with an LHRH analog and/or immunotherapy with zinc gluconate and bestatin.

Allograft-induced antibody responses are an important cause of transplant failure and chronic graft-versus-host reactions. A. Gorski and colleagues (Warsaw) used human mixed lymphocyte reactions MHC (MLR) as a model for studying effects of monoclonal antibodies against class II antigens and IL-2 receptor. Antibodies against class II inhibited MLR-induced Ig synthesis, the effect of anti-DP being less than that of anti-DR and anti-DQ. Such differences were not observed when PWM was used as stimulant. Antibody against the IL-2 receptor also inhibited MLR-induced Ig synthesis although with different kinetics. The authors suggest that such monoclonal antibodies may be useful to treat diseases with hyperactivation of B-cells.

The capacity of neurotropin to restore IL-2 production and proliferative responses of spleen cells in aging (NZB/NZW) F1 mice was reported by M. Naiki et al. (Hyogo). Neurotropin is a substance extracted from inflammatory skin of rabbits inoculated with vaccinia virus. An extract of the plant Eleutherococcus senticosus was reported by B. Bohn et al. (Heidelberg) to increase the number of T-cells and NK cells in humans. These remarkable effects were attributed to pleiotropic effects in the neuroendocrine-immunological network.

T.Y. Ha and colleagues (Chonju, Korea) reported the presence in human seminal plasma of high- and low-molecular weight factors suppressing delayed hypersensitivity to intravaginally administered antigens. Other investigators have suggested that the former are prostaglandins and other eicosanoids. Convenient routine tests for immunomodulators are useful, and K. Nouza et al. (Prague) described a package of investigations suitable for study in normal mice and mice with selectively suppressed immune functions.

Immune Manipulation in Infectious Diseases

A. G. JOHNSON* and K. NOMOTO**

*Department of Medical Microbiology/Immunology, University of Minnesota, Duluth, MN
**Medical Institute of Bioregulation, Kyushu University,
Fukuoka 812, Japan

Workshop number 19 focussed on the most relevant issue of immunopharmacology, that of intelligent interference with the establishment of infectious agents and their diverse pathogenic processes. Of the thirteen posters displayed, nine were presented orally.

The session started with three presentations on the immunomodulating capabilities of muramyl di-peptides and their derivatives. Dr. C. Ishihara, from the Institute of Immunological Science, Hokkaido University in Sapporo, Japan presented evidence for the efficacy of MDP-Lys (L18) against Herpes, type 1 infection in young (5 week old) cyclophosphamide treated, immunodepressed Balb mice. In this model, injection of 50 μg of this MDP derivative on days -3 and -1 before i.v. infection with $10^{2.4}$ pfu of HSV, type 1, protected mice against the impairment of host resistance by this immunosuppressive drug. Unfortunately, treatment after the initiation of infection did not deter the virus; however, heightened resistance was evidenced for as long as 7 days after MDP-Lys (L18).

This group also presented the results of attempts to enhance host resistance against Sendai virus infection by a multiplicity of biological response modifiers. MDP-Lys (L18), a deacetylated chitin preparation, poly L arginine, murine gamma interferon, human granulocyte colony stimulating factor and interleukin 1 beta, all exhibited various degrees of elevation of host resistance when given intranasally to 5 week old Balb/c mice. Again the compounds were prophylactic, being given 3 or 1 day before infection. Challenge was with $10^{1.7}$ $TCID_{50}$ of Sendai virus.

Dr. Monique Parant of the Institut Biomedical des Cordeliers, Paris, France continued the emphasis on MDP derivatives. Using 12 derivatives of MDP, she demonstrated a positive correlation between the ability of the derivative to synergize with lipopolysaccharide from Gram negative bacilli to induce high levels of tumor necrosis factor and their ability to protect against infectious challenge.

Discussion then centered on 3 presentations concerning the ability to protect against bacterial and viral infections of PSK, a protein bound polysaccharide isolated from the Basidiomycetes, Coriolus vesicolor Quiel. Drs. Y. Minamishima and M. Okada, from the Department of Microbiology and 1st Department of Surgery, Miyazaki Medical School, Miyazaki, Japan, presented data showing this biological response modifier (as well as a Streptococal preparation OK 432) protected mice against murine cytomegalovirus, both acute and cyclophosphamide induced exacerbation of latent infection. A positive correlation was evident between the ability of these two preparations to increase NK cell activity and induce resistance.

This was followed by Drs. H. Saito and H. Tomioka from the Department of Microbiology and Immunology, Shimane Medical University, Izumo, Japan, who reported the capacity of PSK to protect mice against Listeria monocytogenes. This was true regardless of the timing of the injection from 10 to 4 days before infection. This time exposure was shortened, however, for Pseudomonas aeruginosa infected mice. Resistance against this organism was highest when PSK was given 4 days before infection. Acceleration of wound healing and elimination of organisms were noted when an ointment containing Solbase and PSK was applied to experimentally burned surfaces of mice. Intraperitoneal administration of PSK also was found to enhance oxygen metabolism in peritoneal macrophages 4-7 days following injection.

In further studies with PSK, T. Kawana and M. Hashido from the Department of Obstetrics and Gynecology at Tokyo University Branch Hospital, Tokyo, Japan, treated 30 patients with recurrent genital herpes with a daily dose of 3-5 grams per os. In most patients, PSK reduced the duration of illness and frequency of reoccurrence.

Oxalysine, an antibiotic metabolite isolated from a new species of Streptomyces roseoviridofuscus found in North China, was the subject of an investigation by Drs. X. Y. Li, L. M. Tong, J. F. Lin, C. Y. Cao, J. F. Wang and P. P. Zhu from the Shanghai Institute of Materia Medica in Shanghai, China. They reported this simple compound inhibited the growth of several animal transplanted tumors and protected the liver from injuries following acute or chronic carbon tetrachloride poisoning. In addition, clinical trials revealed improvement in liver function and blood flow in patients with chronic viral hepatitis. In C57Bl mice, oxalysine at 100 mg/kg ip. or po. for 5 days elevated splenic PFC and serum hemolysin, IgG and $C^{1}3$ levels. At 50-100 mg/kg ip. for 3 days, splenic lymphocyte transformation and delayed hypersensitivity were elevated.

Dr. P. R. J. Gangadharam and R. Taylor from the Mycobacteriology Research Laboratories at the National Jewish Center for Immunology and Respiratory Medicine in Denver, CO reported on the effect of anti-lymphocyte serum, anti-thy 1.2, anti-L3T4 and anti-Lyt-2 monoclonal antibodies on Mycobacterium avium complex (MAC) infection in Beige mice. The latter have been shown to be very susceptible to infection with these organisms. These organisms cause a serious disseminated disease in normal and immunodeficient individuals as well as in AIDS patients. Anti-thymocyte serum did not affect significantly the in vivo growth of MAC. It also did not influence the mitogenic response of T cells or Thy-1 responding cells, or the release of H_2O_2 from macrophages. However, it caused a decrease in L3T4 and LyT-2 responding T cells. Specific monoclonal antibodies also failed to alter in vivo growth of MAC or affect splenomegaly. On the other hand, anti-thy 1.2 monoclonal antibody reduced all T cell populations while anti-L3T4 and anti-LyT-2 antibodies caused a transient reduction in the suppressor and helper cells respectively.

The session concluded with a portrayal of Ia antigens in the rat intestinal epithelium by Drs. H. Nagura, S. Nakamura and Y. Sumi from the Institute for Disease Mechanism and Control at Nagoya University School of Medicine in Nagoya, Japan. Germfree and nude rats were studied to determine whether microbial antigen free environments and/or T cells were required for Ia expression. The Ia antigen was found using an immunoperoxidase technique in conventional adult rats to be restricted to the absorptive epithelial cells on the villus and those covering the Peyer's patches. The distribution was similar in nude rats. Germfree adults rats however were negative in this respect, but could be induced to express Ia antigens on microbial contamination. Ia antigens were absent from the epithelial cells of the neonatal gut until 4 weeks of age. The authors concluded that T cells were not obligatory for Ia expression and that antigenic stimulation may be required.

Novel Vaccines

A. OYA* and F. AUDIBERT**
*National Institute of Health, Tokyo, Japan and
**College of Medicine, University of South Florida, Tampa, USA

In this workshop,7 papers were presented dealing with a new type of vaccine development. Those presentations may be divided into 3 categories: 1) Introduction of new idea to develop vaccine to prevent disease, 2) Development of a vaccine as a strategy to control a newly described disease, and 3) Application of unique technology to develop a vaccine. Dr.Rong's paper presenting vaccine against insecticide poisoning and Dr.Sasaki's paper analysing action of BCG as a vaccine against tumors may be categorized in the first group. Dr.Yamanishi's paper presenting a vaccine development for prevention of an infection with a newly discovered HFRS virus (hemorrhagic fever with renal syndrome virus) is the second type of presentation. The other 4 presentations may be grouped in the third category dealing with the introduction of newly developped biotechnology in the vaccine production. Those 3 categories represent a current progress of vaccine development in the world, and presented papers provided many valuable hints or suggestions to the audience.

Dr.K.Rong,Institute of Pharmacology and Toxicology,Beijing reported his trial to develop vaccines against chemicals to prevent poisoning with those. Application of insecticides for agricultural purpose is common in China and poisoning of farmers with those chemicals become a problem in agriculture in China. The purpose of his study is to develop vaccines to prevent poisoning. More than 50 artificial antigens were prepared and development of vaccines against organophosphate and tricothecene compounds was attempted. The method he used is to combine chemicals with carriers to make effective immunogens. Anti-VX vaccine was successfully developed and immunization of rabbits with this vaccine induced partially protective antibody. Passively immunized mice with this antibody survived after 1 LD VX challenge. He concluded that the vaccination against chemicals is feasible only when a target chemical is of high toxicity and fully immunogenic inducing high titer of antibody which reacts specifically to the chemical.

Dr.J.Sasaki,Department of Bacteriology,Hirosaki University,Hirosaki,Japan showed close similarity of some surface antigens from BCG to some tumor associated antigens. This study is based on the current application of BCG as one of BRM treatment for cancer patients. Water extraction method was devised to isolate surface antigens from tumor cells and BCG. Antigenical analysis between them were performed by indirect immunofluorescent technique, SDS-PAGE and Western blotting methods. It was found that all the animal tumor cells used shared the common antigens with BCG. Two bands of tumor associated antigens (TAA) were detected by SDS-PAGE, which were lacking in normal liver cells from guinea pigs. Major band of TAA corresponded with the surface isolate from BCG. Two bands of TAA and one band of surface isolate from BCG were sensitive to pronase. Further studies are in progress on the clinical application of BCG surface antigen as a tumor marker and a vaccine against tumors.

Dr.K.Yamanishi et al of Research Institute for Microbial Diseases, Osaka University, Japan attempted to develop a vaccine against hemorrhagic fever with renal syndrome, etiological agent of which was recently isolated as hantavirus. Some antigenic variability among strains was found to exist in hantavirus. Therefore, a vaccine to be developed should cover infection with a variety of hantavirus strains. B-1 strain was serially passaged in newborn mouse brain. Inactivated vaccine by formalin was prepared from the infected mouse brain employing purification procedure by ultracentrifugation. Potency of vaccine bound to aluminum hydroxide gel was assayed in BALB/C mice. After two immunization, antibodies were detected by immunofluorescence and hemagglutination-inhibition tests. When immunized mice were challenged with B-1 virus and heterologous strain, virus titers in lungs and spleens of immunized mice were significantly less than those of control mice.

Dr.Y.Kino et al of Chemo-sero-therapeutic Research Institute,Kumamoto and Department of Virology, School of Medicine,Kyushu University,Japan presented their studies on herpes simplex virus vaccine employing recombinant DNA technology. They used one of the structural protein gB-1 to produce component vaccine. Glycoprotein gB-1 gene was cloned and gB-1 related protein was successfully expressed in yeast (ygB-1). Immunogenecity of ygB-1 was examined in mice and guinea pigs. Mice immunized with alum-precipitated ygB-1 developed neutralizing antibody, ELIZA antibody and delayed type hypersensitivity reaction. They were protected from intraperitoneal and corneal challenge with herpes simplex virus type 1. Latent infection in the trigeminal ganglia was restricted. Guinea pigs immunized with alum-precipitated ygB-1 showed neutralizing antibody to both type 1 and 2 herpes simplex virus, delayed type hypersensitivity reaction and lymphoproliferative reaction. Those guinea pigs were resistant to primary infection and subsequent recurrent infection after intravaginal challenge with type 2 herpes simplex virus.

Dr.K.Okuma et al of Chemo-sero-therapeutic Research Institute,Kumamoto and National Institute of Health, Japan reported the construction of virosome employing a derivative of muramyl dipeptide aiming at development of effective component vaccine for influenza. A virosome was constructed with influenza virus hemagglutinin, neuraminidase which were inserted on the surface of liposome consisted of 6-O-(2-tetradecyl-hexadecanolyl)-N-acetyl-muramyl-L-alanyl-D-isoglutamine (B30-MDP) and cholestrol. MDP-virosome with approximately100 nm in diameter was injected to mice to examine immunogenicity. Cell-associated immunity was induced in the immunized mice as well as high titer antibody. In the challenge experiment with influenza virus, significant increase of survival rates was observed. Discussion was made on the applicability of MDP to humans.

Dr.H.Fujita et al of Research Foundation for Microbial Diseases of Osaka University, Metropolitan Institute of Medical Science, Tokyo and Institute of Tropical Medicine, Nagasaki University introduced their attempt to develop Japanese encephalitis (JE) component vaccine employing gene technology since the currently available purified mouse brain vaccine is expensive though they are sufficiently safe and effective. JE virus envelope protein gene was expressed in yeast cells. Yeast derived protein (yE) was shown to lack some epitopes which strongly related to neutralization of JE virus so that multiple injections of yE protein were required to induce detectable amount of neutralizing antibody in mice. Mammalian cell drived envelope protein (mE) showed weak immunogenicity though it contained epitopes for production of neutralizing antibody. They are seeking more effective approach to develop JE vaccine after careful examination of envelope gene sequence of various strain of JE virus.

Dr.A.Kojima et al of National Institute of Health, Japan and Nippon Zeon Co.,Ltd.,Kawasaki presented paper on their attempt to develop safe and effective live recombinant vaccine by using low-neurovirulent vaccinia virus LC16m0 (m0) or LC16m8 (m8) strains as vectors. The hepatitis B surface antigen gene has been inserted into the genome of the highly attenuated m0 or m8 strain. These vaccinia recombinants (recVV) expressed hepatitis virus surface antigen particles consisting of 24K protein and 28K glycoprotein. Rabbits inoculated intradermally with recVV produced high titers of antibody to hepatitis virus surface antigen for at least 16 months. Revaccination with recVV worked as a booster in antibody production. RecVV preserved almost the same pathogenicity as their attenuated parent strains. rabbits inoculated intracerebrally with recVV showed similar lesions in the meninges to those caused by m0 or m8 strains. No detectable or only trace amount of virus was recovered from the brains of rabbits. They concluded their live recombinat vaccine may be used as safe and effective hepatitis B vaccine.

Immunosuppressive Agents (I) Deoxyspergualin and Other Interesting Agents

H. AMEMIYA and J. E. TALMADGE

Department of Surgical Research, National Cardio-vascular Center Research Institute, Osaka, Japan and Department of Immunology, Smith Kline & French Laboratories, King of Prussia, PZ, USA

A total of 15 abstracts: seven on 15-deoxyspergualin and/or FK-506 and one each on histamine, ferritin, promethazine, etretinate, triptolide, the combination of Metipranolol plus Tergurid, glucocorticoid and viral peptides, were accepted for the poster presentation in the Section "Immunosuppressive Agents (1)". Of these 15 abstracts, four on 15-deoxyspergualin and one on histamine, ferritin, promethazine and etretinate were selected for oral presentation. Regrettably, the two abstracts on promethazine and etretinate, were cancelled.

15-deoxyspergualin originates from a substance isolated by Hamao Umezawa (1981) from the culture fluid of Bacillus lacterosporus (Takeuchi et al., 1987). This substance has antitumor activity and its structure consists of a spermidinic and a guanidinic group. Thus the substance was designated as spergualin (Umezawa et al., 1981). It was found to exert a strong antitumor effect on intraperitoneally and subcutaneously allografted mouse leukemic cell lines, Ehrlich tumor cell and sarcoma 180 (Takeuchi et al., 1987). Subsequently, many derivatives of spergualin were synthesized and their antitumor effects studied. 15-deoxyspergualin (DSG) was confirmed to be effective in a wider dose range than spergualin (Iwasawa et al., 1982), and in April 1987, DSG entered the Phase I clinical study as an anti-cancer drug.

In addition to its antineoplastic activity, spergualin was found to suppress in vitro lymphocyte blastogenesis against Con A and lipopolysaccharide, in vivo production of antibody against SRBC, delayed type hypersensitivity and rat skin graft rejection (Umezawa et al., 1985). DSG has been further shown to suppress graft versus host reaction in mice (Nemoto et al., 1985), to prolong graft survival after allogeneic heart transplantation in the rat (Suzuki et al., 1987), to prolong allogeneic renal transplantation in the dog (Amemiya et al., 1988), and, to "cure" rejection arising after allogeneic heart transplantation in rat (Suzuki et al., in press). However, the mechanism of action for this immunosuppression has not been clarified. Nemoto et al. (1987) reported that the production of IL-1 and IL-2 was stimulated rather than suppressed in spleen cells from DSG treated rats. This suggests that DSG has a different immunosuppressive mechanism compared to that of cyclosporine (CsA) which is used clinically for organ transplantation to slow or prevent rejection.

Takahara et al. (WS 21-1) pointed out in their presentation "The immunopharmacological outlines of FK 506, 15-deoxyspergualin, mizoribine and cyclosporine" that induced gastrointestinal disorders are one side effect of DSG, and proposed it would be better to use the agent as a pulse (intermittent) therapy during rejection, but not for long-term administration or as a prophylactic regime. Adverse reactions of DSG occurred most strongly in dogs but are relatively infrequent in rats and monkeys. All these adverse reactions appear to be related to gastrointestinal disorders. DSG is now under Phase 1 clinical study, and adverse reactions in humans will be reported in near future. However, it appears that the incidence of adverse reaction to DSG between species vary considerably in incidence and severity. At least in humans, the possible side effect may be mild, and it seems most reasonable to use this agent for pulse therapy to treat acute rejection as proposed by Fukuda et al. Note that this is a conclusion common to all the reports on DSG published in the present congress. The immunosuppressive mechanism of FK 506 is similar to that of CsA (i.e., reduced IL-2 production) while DSG appears to have a different mechanism. Briefly, using deoxymethylspergualin (MeDSG), which is not hydrolyzed, instead of DSG in the cultures (normal human peripheral blood mononuclear cells), Takahara et al. observed the immunosuppressive effect of MeDSG on a MLR and mitogen-induced blastogenesis, at doses >100 nm. They reported that MeDSG suppressed allostimulation and that the suppression of the MLR was not seen in the early stage of culture, but the immune response was suppressed in the late stage of culture, i.e., from the time when the Tc cell induction was established. In this experiment, a dose of MeDSG as high as 100 μg/ml was required to obtain the suppression in 5-day cultured MLR system. In relation to this point, K. Nemoto (Nippon Kayaku Co., Tokyo, Japan) stated that by prolonging the culture period to 7 days, a MLR-suppressing effect similar to that observed in Takahara's experiment could be obtained at 1.0 μg MeDSG/ml. Together, these results suggest that DSG exerts a strong suppressive effect on a MLR during the late stage of MLR culture. This is in contrast to cyclosporine or FK-565, which reduce IL-2 production and receptor expression early in MLR co-cultures.

Additional studies by H. Fujii et al. (WS 21-11) on antibody production showed that DSG suppress not only the primary antibody but also secondary antibody production, i.e., both IgG and IgM antibody production in response to T cell dependent and independent antigens (SRBC, DNP-LPS and DNP-Ficoll). This was contrasted to cyclosporine activity which did not inhibit antibody response to DNP-LPS. They also reported that deoxyspergualin prolonged the survival of skin allografts in rats but increased MLR and IL-2 production. This was also contrasted to cyclosporine which depressed both the MLR from allografted rats as well as IL-2 production.

Because MeDSG, an analog of DSG, is less susceptible to hydrolysis, it is stable enough for in vitro experiments, as compared to DSG. Using this analog, Takada et al. (WS 21-9) found that MeDSG acted on the MLR of both human and mouse lymphocytes in the late stage of culture and suppressed the MLR at doses higher than 0.1 μg/ml. Further studies on the mechanism of action of DSG (MeDSG) by K. Nishimura et al. in their presentation "Mode of action of 15-deoxyspergualin (DSG): Effects on induction and effector function of cytotoxic T lymphocytes (CTL)" (WS 21-2), revealed that DSG suppressed the induction of alloreactive secondary CTL in vivo and in vitro. However, DSG could not suppress the effector function of CTL once they were induced. Furthermore, the suppressive action of DSG on CTL induction was mimicked by exogenous IFN-γ, and DSG suppressed the differentiation of bone marrow cells in response to colony-stimulating factor. From these results, they suggested that DSG might suppress the generation of effector CTL (late G_1) from CTL-precursors (early G_1) by inhibiting the production of INF-γ by T_H cells.

In the presentation "In vivo mechanism of action DSG in rat heart transplantation" (WS 21-3), Suzuki et al. reported a mean survival time of 30 days for rat heart allografts and a 10% survival for longer than 100 days in animals treated with DSG for 15 days from the day of transplantation, while allografts of non-treated animals survived only for 9.0 ± 2.6 days. In 50% of animals treated with DSG for 14 days from the confirmation of the onset of rejection evidenced by elevation of Pi/Pcr ratio on NMR spectrogram, the allografts survived for longer than 100 days. Furthermore, the administration of spleen cells from these long-term tolerant rats to syngeneic rats transferred the immunotolerance to these third party rats. They concluded that DSG might selectively attack a lymphocyte clone which expanded during graft rejection and induced tolerance, which was maintained by suppressor cells probably specific to the donor antigen.

As mentioned before, there have been a variety of reports on the effectiveness of DSG as an immunosuppressive agent. Nemoto et al. also reported (WS 21-10) that DSG was very effective for the treatment of immunologically-mediated lethal aplastic anemia in rat, and that an i.p. dose of 1 mg/kg was as effective as oral dose of 30 mg/kg. Y. Fukuda et al. (WS 21-4) stated that DSG effectively prolonged the survival time of rat liver allograft. They also observed that IL-2 production was suppressed by this substance. However, in a canine renal allograft model it induced sever side effects, but if administered as a pulse therapy during the rejection episode it had significant activity with acceptable toxicity.

Among the non-spergualin presentations, the one by Khan et al. (WS 21-5) reported data on a series of congeners of histamine which have unique biologic activity for lymphocyte function in vitro. These analogs suppress MLRs and LPS induced B cell proliferation, but not IL-2 dependent T cell proliferation. They were also shown to suppress in vivo immune responses including antibody responses to specific antigens and CTL induction by P-815. However, none of the analogs affected a DTH response. These ligands were suggested to be specific for lymphocytes since they did not interact with H1 or H2 receptors on myocardium or aorta and did not block the activity of Imidazal on these tissue receptors. These investigators, however, have not yet examined the activity of these unique analogs on H3 receptors.

Harada et al. (WS 21-6) reported on the effect of ferritin and its suppressive activities for DTH and Arthus-type responses to footpad challenges for specific soluble or particulate antigens. Ferritin appears to decrease DTH, but not antibody response and acts at the effector cell phase since it does not impact on the ability to do a cellular transfer experiment. In the DTH reaction it effects either the induction or expression of activity depending upon the time of injection. In addition, ferritin inhibits peritoneal exudate macrophage migration and partially inhibits antigen presentation as well as depresses a MLR at levels >200 μg/ml.

H. Raskova et al. ("Combined behavioral and immunomodulatory effects of Metipranolol and Tergurid") discussed the immunomodulatory and therapeutic properties of a beta blocker (Metipranolol) and the dopaminergic ergoline derivative with antidopaminergic potency (Tergurid) for calves and mice. These agents reduced transportation induced stress, respiratory infections (shipping fever) and reduced DTH in calves and mice. Both ligands had sedative effects on behavior and Tergurid enhanced a DTH response while Metipranolol had no effect on DTH. Regardless, therapeutic effect was significant for both agents with decreased incidence of respiratory infections and a lower incidence of mortality to shipping stress in calves.

Studies by Mitani et al. (WS 21-15) discussed the immunosuppressive properties of retrovirus and their peptides. They reported that purified HIV-1 and FeLV enhanced PBL IgG synthesis although they depressed IgG production in response to mitogens. This depression is also observed for the U937 production of Factor B such that Sendi and NDV enhance production as did FeLV; however, they suppressed PMA induced Factor B production. In other studies by M. Lukie (WS 21-14) glucocorticoids were shown to induce a factor which inhibited mitogen induced T cell proliferation. This factor is a high molecular weight protein produced by macrophages or endothelial cells. It was suggested to reduce IL-2 production and receptor expression but not proliferation in response to exogenous IL-2. Further, it appeared that the glucocorticoid immunoregulatory factor produced by macrophages and endothelial cells may act as an inhibitor of IL-1 activity. Triptolide, an active principle from Tripterygium hypoglacum (L. Pu et al., WS 21-12) was reported to reduce T and B cell proliferation induced by Con A and LPS. Similarly, IL-2 production was suppressed by this substance.

In summary, a number of potentially useful immunosuppressive strategies were discussed. Most notably, these included the use of DSG, FK 506, and the discussion based on preliminary data of the use of classic ligands as immunomodulatory agents. These included histamine with the suggestion that a lymphocytic specific pharmacophore could be designed as well as agents active at beta or dopamine receptors for use against shipping fever in cattle. These strategies point toward the utility of studying classic receptors as immunomodulators as well as the difficulties associated with all immunosuppressive strategies including the toxicity of many immunosuppressive agents such as DSG and the limitations of the various in vivo and in vitro biologic assays currently available.

REFERENCES

Amemiya, H. et al. (1988). Transplant. Proc. 20, suppl. 1:229.
Iwasawa, H. et al. (1982). J. Antibiot. (Tokyo), 35:1665.
Nemoto, K. et al. (1985). J. Antibiot. (Tokyo), 38:283.
Nemoto, K. et al. (1987). J. Antibiot. (Tokyo), 40:1062.
Suzuki, S. et al. (1987). Transplantation 44:483.
Suzuki, S. et al. (in press). Transplantation.
Takeuchi T. et al. (1987). J. Antibiot. (Tokyo), 34:1619.
Umezawa, H. et al. (1981). J. Antibiot. (Tokyo), 24:1622.
Umezawa, H. et al. (1985). J. Antibiot. (Tokyo), 38:283.

Immunosuppressive Agents (II)

P. C. HIESTAND* and T. OCHIAI**

*Preclinical Research, Sandoz Pharmaceuticals Ltd., CH-4000 Basel, Switzerland
**Department of Surgery II, School of Medicine, Chiba University, 1–8–1 Inohana, Chiba 280, Japan

This workshop was divided into two parts. The first dealt with the macrolide FK 506 and its immunosuppressive effects *in vitro* and *in vivo*, while various non-related topics, dealing with modulation of immune responses, were presented and discussed during the second part of this session.

The introduction of Sandimmune® (Cyclosporine A) as a non-cytostatic, non-cytotoxic immune suppressive agent has had a tremendous impact on transplantation. Extended clinical trials also suggest that specific immune suppressive agents, like cyclosporine, may be very effective in many autoimmune diseases. Therefore it is not surprising that many investigators from industry and university are trying to find new drugs to manipulate immune responses.

One of the few new compounds is the macrolide lactone FK 506, which has been isolated from Streptomyces tsukubaensis (Tanaka 1987). FK 506 was found during a search for new structures from microbiological origin which inhibit specifically the production and release of lymphokines from activated lymphocytes. FK 506 was shown to have antimicrobial properties against Aspergillus fumigatus and Fusarium oxosporum (Kino 1987). It also inhibited the proliferative response of lymphocytes in a mixed lymphocyte culture *in vitro*, the formation of antibody producing cells, a localized graft-versus-host reaction, and a delayed type hypersensitivity reaction in mice (Kino 1987). In *in vitro* studies, FK 506 proved to be 100 times more potent than cyclosporin A. *In vivo*, however, FK 506 is only about 3 to 20 times as active as cyclosporin A. In later studies the immunopharmacology of FK 506 has been investigated in depth in rat skin allograft (Inamura 1988), heterotopic heart transplantation in rats (Ochiai 1987a, 1987b, Lim 1987, Murase 1987), renal allograft in dogs (Ochiai 1987c, 1988, Todo 1988), orthotopic liver allograft in dogs (Todo 1987a, 1987b), Pancreas transplantation in dog (Kenmochi 1988) and xenotransplantation of mouse skin and heart into rats (Ochiai 1987d). Low doses (0.04-0.4 mg/kg/day) of FK 506 in rodents given by either i.m. or s.c. route regularly led to continued graft acceptance. Combination of suboptimal doses of both FK 506 and cyclosporin A were shown to behave synergistically (Murase 1987). In dogs, however, somewhat higher doses (1.0 mg/kg/day) were needed to prevent kidney or liver allograft rejection.

Development of a new immunosuppressive agent calls for a drug with a wide therapeutic window. Hence; a thorough toxicological evaluation must be undertaken with any new entity in more than one species over a long period of time. This is especially true for drugs intended for use in autoimmune disorders, where lifelong treatment is often necessary for a non-life threatening condition.

Unfortunately only limited information is available on the side effects of FK 506. Virtually no toxicity was observed in rats over a wide range (0.02-1.28 mg/kg/day) by s.c. route (Todo 1988). There was less impairment of kidney function by FK 506 than with cyclosporin A. Oral administration of FK 506 to dogs, however, at doses of greater then 0.5 mg/kg/day caused weight loss and manifold evidence of toxicity (Todo 1987a). Lower doses of FK 506 (0.5 mg/kg/day) administered in combination with cyclosporin A to dogs with a kidney allograft were void of toxicity, and showed also the best survival rates (Todo 1987a). It seems therefore that only a thorough toxicological investigation of FK 506 can provide the necessary information about a safe dose range.

Additional information on the effectiveness of FK 506 was provided in this session and is summarized below.

Dr. S. Sakuma (Osaka, Japan) presented a comparison on the effects of FK 506 and cyclosporin A on IL-2 production and expression of its mRNA. An IL-1 dependent T cell lymphoma which produces IL-2 was stimulated with IL-1 and mitogen in the absence or presence of drug. The IL-2 secreted was assayed measuring the proliferation of an IL-2 dependent cell line. Messenger RNA transcription was assayed using a filter hybridization assay and the following cDNA probes: IL-2, IL-2R, c-myc and actin. Both, FK 506 and cyclosporin A selectively inhibited the production of IL-2 by the T cell lymphoma without interfering with the proliferation of the cell line. Both drugs inhibited the expression of mRNA for IL-2 but not for IL-2R, c-myc or actin. The concentration used for FK 506 to suppress IL-2 production was 100 times less than the one for cyclosporin A. He concluded that FK 506 mediates its immunosuppressive effects by a similar mechanism than cyclosporin A.

In a study to determine the effects of FK 506 on B cell activation, Dr. N. Suzuki (Shimane, Japan) compared the effects of FK 506 to those of cyclosporin A using various means of B cell activation. He also tried to delineate differential mechanisms by which the two drugs inhibit B cell proliferation and/or differentiation in response to mitogens. He found that both drugs inhibit T cell dependent B cell activation in a similar fashion, while T cell-independent B cell activation is relatively refractory to the effects of both drugs. FK 506 seems to interfere with T_H cell - B cell interaction and T_H cell - monocyte interaction. B cells activated by poke-weed mitogen, but not by Staphylococcus aureus Cowan I, are sensitive to FK 506 as soon as they differentiate into Ig-secreting cells in response to helper factors. Again, the effects of FK 506 exceeds that of cyclosporin A by 100 fold. He concluded that FK 506 mainly interferes with interaction of T cells and other cells which are essential for B cell activation.

Dr. K. Nakajima (Chiba, Japan) reported data on long-term cardiac allograft survival following short term treatment by FK 506. The study was undertaken to investigate the mechanisms leading to induction and maintenance of long-term allograft acceptance by FK 506. The primary effect of FK 506 is on responder lymphocytes reacting to donor antigens in the induction phase. Cell and serum transfer experiments suggest that donor-specific suppresser cells and humoral factors were induced by treatment with FK 506 in the presence of the allograft. These cells and factors may play a role in the maintenance of long term graft survival.

Dr. K. Yamamoto (Tokyo, Japan) presented data on the effectiveness of FK 506 in an autoimmune disease model. He used the MRL/lpr mice which develop lupus like symptoms, anti-DNA antibodies, rheumatoid factors and a lymphoproliferative disease. Most animals die of renal failure attributable to deposition of immune complexes in kidney glomeruli. FK 506 at doses of 0.2, 0.8 and 2 mg/kg/day was used to treat eight week old female MRL/lpr mice. The high and the intermediate dose of FK 506 prolonged survival of these mice while increased proteinurea was only suppressed by the high dose. The lymphoproliferative disease was affected only by the high dose of FK 506. It has to be determined if FK 506 has beneficial effects in this autoimmune disease model when treatment starts at a later stage of the disease. Nevertheless these results show that FK 506 may have the potential to interfere with autoimmune disease processes.

The second part of the workshop was devoted to topics unrelated to FK 506.

Dr. H. Yagi (Osaka, Japan) investigated the effects of BCG injections on the course of diabetes type I in NOD mice. He found that a single injection of BCG prevents the development of diabetes in NOD mice and transfer of spleen cells from BCG-treated animals into prevents the appearance of disease in recipient NOD mice. He concluded that some sort of suppressor cell is generated by BCG treatment. Flow cytofluorometry revealed that Mac-1+ and Mac-2+ cells increased upon BCG treatment. Spleen cells of BCG vaccinated mice responded only poorly to mitogens such as Con A, PHA, PWM, LPS and alloantigens. Removal of plastic adherent cells from BCG-treated NOD mice restored the response to mitogens. Addition of FACS-sorted Mac-1+ cells from BCG-treated mice suppressed the Con A response of macrophage-depleted spleen cells. These data suggest that suppresser macrophage are generated by BCG-treatment and that these cells may play a role in the autoimmune pathogenesis leading to diabetes in NOD mice.

Dr. P. R. J. Gangadharam (Denver, USA) presented results showing that infection by Mycobacterium avium complex (MAC) of low virulence in S/W mice caused an increase in PGE_2 release and reduction in both gamma-interferon and IL-2 release by T lymphocytes. The studies were extended to assess the ability of high (101) and low virulent (1403) strains of MAC to induce the release of superoxide anions ($O_2^{\cdot}$) and PGE_2 from S/W mice and compared with beige mice, which have been shown to be the most susceptible mouse strain to MAC infection. Both low and high virulent strains caused a gradual increase in PGE_2 release with the progression of MAC infection. There was no difference between the two MAC strains or the two strains of mice with respect of PGE_2 release after MAC infection. The results suggest that the increased susceptibility of the beige mouse to MAC infection is not due to unusually high production of PGE_2. The low virulent MAC strain induced more $O_2^{\cdot}$ release than the highly virulent strain in both strains of mice.

The presentation by D. S. Cammisuli (Basel, Switzerland) aimed to clarify the controversy as to whether cyclosporin A interferes with antigen presentation or not. It has been reported that Sandimmun (SIM, cyclosporin A) inhibits antigen presentation to T cells. However, these studies may be biased by the fact that drug carried over by the pretreated antigen presenting cells (APCs) directly inhibits antigen induced T cell activation, in spite of normal antigen presentation. To avoid this problem he used $CD4^+$, class II restricted antigen specific T cells, able both to proliferate in response to, and to kill antigen pulsed EBV transformed B cells (EBV-B) acting as APCs. SIM did not inhibit the latter activity. He reported that EBV-B, pulsed with antigen either in presence or absence of SIM, were equally susceptible to killing by class II restricted T cells, whereas EBV-B, pulsed with antigen in the presence of SIM, partially inhibited T cell proliferation. This inhibitory activity was abrogated if the pulsed APCs were fixed with glutaraldehyde before coculture with the antigen specific T cells. This finding suggests that the inhibition seen at the T cell proliferation level is due to a carry-over of SIM by the unfixed APCs. The results show that SIM does not affect uptake, processing and presentation of soluble antigens by EBV-B cells.

The presentation by Dr. K. Sugimura (Sapporo, Japan) dealt with a new monokine isolated from the human macrophage cell line U937. The factor (LBIF, lymphocyte blastogenesis inhibitory factor), which blocks proliferation of lectin-stimulated lymphocytes by arresting them in G_1, was purified to homogeneity using HPLC. LBIF is a glycosylated single chain acidic protein with an pI of 4.28-4.56. Its molecular size of about 57,000 was estimated by SDS-gel electrophoresis. In addition to its inhibitory effects on lymphocytes, LBIF inhibits the proliferation of a human melanoma cell line (A375). No effect was seen on 14 other tumor cell lines. LBIF has no cytotoxic potential. From its chemical and biological properties it was concluded that LBIF is distinct from other cytokines such as IL-1, TNF (alpha and beta), TGF (beta-1 and beta-2), leukoregulin or oncostatin M.

REFERENCES

Inamura, N., Nakahara, K., Ochiai, T., *et al.* (1988). *Transplantation 45*, 206-209.

Kenmochi, T., Asano, T., Enomoto, K., *et al.* (1988). *Transplant. Proc. 20*, 223-225.

Kino, T., Hatanaka, H., Hashimoto, M., *et al.* (1987). *J. of Antibiotics 40*, 1249-1255.

Lim, S.M.L., Thiru, S. and White, D.J.G. (1987). *Trandplant. Proc. 19*, 68-70.

Murase, N., Todo, S., Lee, P.-H., *et al.* (1987). *Transplant. Proc. 19*, 71-75.

Ochiai, T., Nakajima, K., Nagata, M., *et al.* (1987a). *Transplant. Proc. 19*, 1284-1286.

Ochiai, T., Nakajima, K., Nagata, M., *et al.* (1987b). *Transplantation 44*, 734-738.

Ochiai, T., Nagata, M., Nakajima, K., *et al.* (1987c). *Transplantation 44*, 729-733.

Ochiai, T., Nagata, M., Nakajima, K., *et al.* (1987d). *Transplant. Proc. 19*, 84-86.

Ochiai, T., Sakamoto, K., Nagata, M., *et al.* (1988). *Transplant. Proc. 20*, 209-214.

Tanaka, H., Kuroda, A., Marusawa, H., *et al.* (1987). *J. Am. Chem. Soc. 109*, 5031-5033.

Todo, S., Demetris, A.J., Ueda, Y., *et al.* (1987a). *Transplant. Proc. 19*, 57-61.

Todo, S., Podesta, L., ChapChap, P., *et al.* (1987b). *Transplant. Proc. 19*, 64-67.

Todo, S., Murase, N., Ueda, Y., *et al.* (1988). *Transplant. Proc. 20*, 215-219.

Endotoxins

T. W. KLEIN* and M. NAKANO**
*College of Medicine, University of South Florida Tampa, Florida, USA
**Jichi Medical School, Tochigi-Ken, Japan

The workshop on bacterial endotoxins consisted of ten oral presentations by scientists from Japan, France, Germany, and the United States. Data were presented on the influence of endotoxins on B lymphocyte maturation and function, interleukin 1 production, and biological responses ranging from shock to analgesic action. It was clear to those attending the workshop that, with the chemical synthesis of lipopolysaccharide now accomplished, critical studies are being designed to establish the molecular basis of endotoxin effects and to explore the possible application of endotoxin combination therapy with other drugs as biological response modifiers. Synthetic lipid A derivatives, which are nontoxic but biologically active, are being constructed and tested as possible therapeutic agents in cancer and infectious diseases.

The session began with a presentation by Kawji, wherein endotoxin injection was used as a stimulus to study B lymphocyte ontogeny in rats. Data were presented suggesting that i.v. injection of Enterobacteriacae LPS was useful in inducing the differentiation of the B lineage in the bone marrow of recepient animals. Data presented by Hosokawa et al. also dealt with the effect of LPS on B lymphocytes. Using a mouse adoptive cell transfer system, these scientists were able to show that LPS administered with a T independent antigen suppressed the induction of B cell memory. No such effect by LPS was seen in the memory response to a T dependent antigen. Other results indicated that the induction of B lymphocyte memory for a T independent antigen is quite sensitive to endotoxin treatment. Another report on the modulation of the biology of B lymphocytes was presented by Vacheron et al. They reported on studies with the glycoprotein extract from Klebsiella pneumoniae 01K2 referred to as RU-41740. The data presented suggested that the chemical extraction of RU-41740 with cetyl trimetylammonium bromide resulted in the formation of a glycoprotein fraction. This P1 fraction was shown to be mitogenic for B lymphocytes in C3H/HeJ mice, insensitive to polymyxin B treatment, and able to induce the production of IL-1 and TNF in macrophages from these animals.

The influence of endotoxin on the induction of interleukin 1 was the subject of three workshop papers. Loppnow et al. presented two papers dealing with the LPS structural requirements for IL-1 induction as well as the cellular requirements for this effect. They examined IL-1 production and release from human mononuclear cells when stimulated in culture with a variety of LPS preparations, including naturally occurring LPS, sythetic lipid A, and synthetic lipid A analogues. The results presented suggested that intact lipid A is the major active ingredient for IL-1 induction, in that the removal of either acyl or phosphate groups reduced the IL-1 inducing potency. Il-1 inducing potency by the various endotoxins and lipid A preparations also varied with the type of mononuclear phagocyte population studied. Terada et al. in another paper explored using molecular biology techniques the chemical basis of LPS nonresponsiveness in cells from C3H/HeJ mice. Peritoneal macrophages from C3H/He mice can produce IL-1 in response to either LPS or the calcium ionophores. However, the macrophages from C3H/HeJ mice cannot produce IL-1 following these stimuli. The defect in IL-1 production was traced by Northern blot analysis to an absence of IL-1 beta mRNA production in the C3H/HeJ macrophage. A calmodulin inhibitor (W7) when added to cultures of C3H/He macrophages suppressed the calcium ionophore induced IL-1 beta mRNA expression. An inhibitor of the protein kinase C pathway (H7) had no effect in this regard. The authors concluded, by extrapolation to the C3H/HeJ system, their results suggested that the unresponsiveness may be related to calmodulin dependent events rather than protein kinase C events.

A variety of studies were also presented examining the biological consequences of endotoxin injection either alone or in conjunction with other biological response modifiers. Schade et al. reported on the attenuation of toxicity in endotoxin shock by a vasoactive drug currently used for circulatory disorders. This drug, Pentoxyfylline (Trental^{R}) when injected i.p. into mice 24 hr before or up to 2 hr after LPS injection significantly shifted the LPS LD_{50} dose. Drug treatment also significantly inhibited the LPS induced leukopenia. Takada et al. reported on an anaphylactoid reaction induced in mice by injection of Bacteroides LPS in muramyl dipeptide-primed animals. LPS from a variety of oral bacteria other than Bacteroides lacked the ability to induce the anaphylactoid reaction. Also, not all mouse strains were susceptible to the LPS induced reaction, including BALB/c and DBA/2. However, the LPS nonresponsive strain, C3H/HeJ, did respond to LPS injection with the development of the anaphylactoid reaction. The interesting phenomenon of the analgesic action of LPS was studied and presented by Kawamura et al. Doses of LPS ranging from 30 to 1,000 ug/kg, injected intravenously into mice were shown to have an analgesic effect when evaluated by the tail pressure method. Not all mouse strains displayed the analgesic effect and low responders were BALB/c and C57BL6. C3H/HeJ mice also did not present an analgesic response to LPS treatment. Chronically stressed mice presenting with a decreased pain threshold, responded to the analgesic effect of LPS. Further studies are continuing on this interesting LPS-associated biological phenomenon. The workshop session concluded with a paper by Matsumura et al. dealing with an immunotherapy model employing interferon gamma and LPS. These two biological response modifiers previously had been demonstrated to exert a synergestic effect on the activation of macrophages in culture. In the present report the *in vitro* studies were extended to an *in vivo* infection model. Several mouse strains including the beige mutant mouse were infected with virulent *Salmonella* organisms. All mouse strains tested, including the mutant mouse strain, were protected by pretreatment with combinations of interferon gamma and LPS. The protective doses observed in drug combination studies suggested synergistic drug effects occurring *in vivo*.

New insights were gained from the workshop presentations concerning the molecular and cellular basis of the biological effects of endotoxins. However, many challenges in this field remain. The development of synthetic lipid A and lipid A analogues should aid future studies designed to understand the molecular basis of endotoxin effects. Also, the possibility that some of these substances may be relatively nontoxic justifies continued attempts to incorporate these potent substances into immunotherapy protocols.

Drug Delivery Systems Including Liposomes as Carriers

CARL R. ALVING* and YOSHIYUKI HASHIMOTO**

*Department of Membrane Biochemistry, Walter Reed Army Institute of Research, Washington, DC 20307–5100 USA

**Department of Hygienic Chemistry, Pharmaceutical Institute, Tohoku University, Aobayama Sendai 980 Japan

In this workshop a broad range of topics on drug derivery systems involving liposomes and other carriers was presented and discussed among 14 posters and 8 oral presentations. The workshop reflected many of the diagnostic, therapeutic, and toxicology issues that are currently active in this field. The diseases addressed included cancer (numerous types) and infectious diseases (Plasmodium falciparum malaria and Mycobacterium avium infection). The chemical and physical approaches discussed included liposomes as drug carriers, and targeting of liposomes, antibodies and other macromolecules as carriers of drugs or prodrugs. Localized drug delivery to an experimentally heated skin tumor using thermosensitive liposomes containing cisplatin is one example of a specialized biophysical approach presented by K. Iga, et al (Osaka, Japan). The range of strategies discussed in the workshop included: diagnostic tumor scintigraphy; selective targeting of drugs to tumors or to infections; reduction of drug toxicity either through direct blocking of toxicity (a "prodrug" approach) or through selective targeting of drugs to tumor cells or infected cells; and utilization of liposomes as carriers of vaccines.

Although liposomes are currently in Phase II human clinical trials as carriers of an immunomodulator (muramyl tripeptidephosphatidylethanolamine, MTP-PE) there was no discussion of that approach in this workshop. However another amplification technique is to use liposomes as carriers of vaccines. A successful example of this is to utilize liposomes as carriers of synthetic antignes and adjuvants for production of humoral immunity against Plasmodium falciparum. C.R. Alving (Washington, DC, USA) presented the most recent data (Richards et al.) from the Walter Reed malaria vaccine program in which liposomes containing a recombinant protein antigen from the P. falciparum circumsporozoite protein was encapsulated within liposomes. Lipid A was included in the liposomes as an adjuvant, and the pyrogenicity of the lipid A was blocked by incorporation of lipid A into liposomes. The resulting formulation, when absorbed with aluminum hydroxide adjuvant, caused much higher antibody titers in monkeys than the titers obtained without liposomes and lipid A.

Lipid A is an example of a potent adjuvant that has numerous physiological effects such as pyrogenicity and neutropenia. Both of these side-effects are exerted through secretion of mediators, and both can be eliminated by incorporation of lipid A into liposomes. However, liposomes themselves were reported by Alving (Wassef et al.) to cause cardiovascular effects in pigs resulting from activation of complement. Complement activation led to massive secretion of thromboxane, and the complement activation itself was caused by naturally-occurring autoantibodies to liposomal cholesterol in pig serum. The cardiovascular effects were not seen when liposomal lipids lacking cholesterol were used. The adverse systemic effects of thromboxane were eliminated by pretreating the pigs with indomethacin before administering the liposomes.

Several presentations were given describing drug targeting using liposomes or other macromolecules as carriers. Y. Hashimoto, et al. (Sendai, Japan) described the preparation of "chemoimmunoliposomes" (CIL) in which a murine monoclonal antibody to human bladder cancer cells was conjugated to sonicated small unilamellar liposomes. The liposomes were then loaded with adriamycin and were found to have marked cytotoxicity in vitro against human bladder cells expressing the antigen. The cytotoxicity was proportional to antigen expression, and nonspecific antibodies provided 40-fold less effectiveness. Cytotoxicity was much greater than that caused by free adriamycin. A CIL preparation loaded with actinomycin D was also much less effective.

Liposomes administered by aerosol inhalation were used in a human clinical trial by Le Pape et al. (Tours, France) as a unique method for delivering a bacterial immunomodulator (Nocardia Soluble Peptidoglycan Derivative, NSPD) into the blood circulation. The theoretical rationale underlying the study was based on preliminary observations that NSPD selectively bound to a model of activated macrophages. Since such macrophages would be expected to be in the vicinity of micrometastases of tumors, the NSPD should seek out and provide diagnostic recognition of such areas. In their study, a total of 34 patients with possible residual tumors (lung, melanoma, breast) were injected with lipsosomes containing 99m-Tc-labelled NSPD. Very small areas of residual tumor (as small as 0.5 cm as determined by histological examination) were successfully detected by this technique of scintigraphy.

In another clinical trial, Kitamura et al. (Kyoto, Japan) utilized a monoclonal antibody (MAB) conjugated to neocarzinostatin to treat a total of 41 patients with colorectal cancer. The antibody was a murine MAB (A7) obtained by immunization with human colon cancer. The MAB induced relatively minor adverse effects (fever, leukocytosis) and the antibody was found in resected tumor tissue. Three of eight patients with postoperative liver metastasis had evidence of tumor reduction, but no benefit was observed in lung or peritoneal metastasis.

In other antibody-drug studies M. Page et al. (Quebec, Canada) and K. Shibuya et al. (Tokyo, Japan) conjugated cytoxic drugs to antibodies. The former group found enhanced in vitro activity of chlorambucil- and daunomycin-antibody conjugates against sarcoma cells. The latter group used an IgM antibody (ST433) that recognizes Lewis Y blood group. The antibody was conjugated to peplomycin and was used to treat nude mice transplanted with human gastric cancer. The antibody was proposed to have potential benefit for immunodiagnosis and therapeutics. N. Umemoto et al. (Tokyo, Japan) demonstrated in vitro cytotoxicity of methotrexate conjugated to an antibody via a short oligopeptide spacer arm. The methotrexate was a prodrug that could be released by lysosomal digestion after internalization of the conjugate. T. Iwahashi et al. (Tokyo, Japan) conjugated cytorhodin-S to a monoclonal antibody directed against carcinoembryonic antigen (CEA). The conjugate was used to inhibit the growth of a cell line secreting CEA.

Drugs were also conjugated to macromolecules other than antibodies. Daunomycin conjugated to transferrin was successfully targeted to transferrin receptors on malignant cells by Lemieux et al. (Quebec, Canada).

Liposomes have been proposed as an excellent method for delivering drugs to macrophages. Liposomes are delivered to macrophages in the absence of special targeting procedures. Therefore liposomes can be used as drug carriers to treat infectious diseases involving macrophages. Mycobacterial infections have been cited as one possible situation in which liposomes might be effectively employed. Pattisapu et al. (Denver, USA) used liposome-encapsulated or free amikacin to treat

Mycobacterium avium complex (MAC) that resided in macrophages from immunocompromised beige mice. In the treatment of MAC in beige mice, use of liposome-encapsulated amikacin was much more effective than use of free amikacin.

In summary, it is evident that in the field of drug carriers, including liposomes, antibodies, and macromolecules, intense activity is proceeding in development of treatments involving cytotoxic drugs and antimicrobial agents, and in development of novel carriers of antigens, adjuvants, and vaccines.

Immunomodulatory Effects of Traditional Medicines

CHAO WEIKANG and SEIJI MORISAWA*

Department of Biochemistry, Shanghai College of Traditional Chinese Medicine, Shanghai, China

**Department of Biochemistry, Osaka City University Medical School, Osaka 545, Japan*

This workshop dealt with the immunomodulatory effects of traditional medicines and their active components on immune competent cells (ICC), especially on macrophages and T cells; on release and activity of various immune effective factors such as interleukin 2 (IL-2), SRF and MIF, and on the relationship between neuroendocrine and immune systems such as hypothalamic-pituitary-gonadal thymic (HPGT) axis in physiological aging. The above effects were observed both in clinic and in experimental animal models in vitro and in vivo.

According to the presentations at this workshop, the immunomodulatory effects of traditional medicines on immune system are to be summarized into two aspects: immunopotentiation and immunosuppression.

IMMUNOPOTENTIATION EFFECTS OF SOME TRADITIONAL MEDICINES

Juzen-taiho-to (TJ-48) which consists of ten kinds of herbs, has several immunostimulating activities. Some immunomodulatory effect of TJ-48 on experimental tumors in animal models were presented. H. Ito reported that TJ-48 suppressed the growth of Ehrlich ascites carcinoma. The number of lung metastatic foci were reduced by the intravenous injection of peritoneal macrophages activated with TJ-48. It was shown that TJ-48 (2g/kg, po) was significantly effective to prolong the life span in tumor-bearing host, mouse leukemic cell (EL-4) in C57BL/6 mice, as well as to augment the reduced activity of macrophage chemotaxis. By histological observation, macrophages were accumulated in situ of tumor inoculation where massive areas were necrotic in the experimental group (S. Yanagisawa et al.). With the same animal model, PFC value and tumor-size were apparently decreased especially when the mice were injected ip with cyclophosphamide. But after administration of TJ-48, PFC values were increased to the normal level (H. Koshimo et al.).

In order to study further the immunopharmacological effects of TJ-48, H. Yamado et al. fractionated the crude polysaccharide fraction (F-5) of TJ-48, and found that only major acidic fraction (F-5-2) had potent mitogenic activity and highest anti-complementary activity. F-5-2 was indicated to be a mixture of some pectin-like acidic polysaccharides, which consists of carbohydrate blocks termed as hairy region and polygalacturonan region (PG). The latter is essential for the expression of the mitogenic activity.

N. Takemoto et al. also reported that TJ-48 and its active fraction(F-5-2) had the mitogenic activity in splenocyte. F-5-2 seems to induce the proliferation of mature B cells.

Y. Ohnishi et al. analyzed the effects of TJ-48 on the recovery of hemopoietic systems from radiation injury in C57BL/6 female mice. In the assay of bone marrow cells for CFU-s. d14, the mice injected with TJ-48-treated bone marrow cells showed better general condition heavier spleen weight, and larger and more numerous colonies in the spleen than the control mice. The results showed that TJ-48 might enhance the function of stem cells to recover from injury due to radiation.

Sho-Saiko-to (TJ-9) is effective against various acute or chronic febrile and inflammatory diseases. J. Matsuda further discussed the immunoregulatory mechanism of TJ-9 from the effects of the culture supernatant of monocytes incubated with TJ-9 on lymphocyte functions employing T-cell colony formation, which shows the function of helper T-lymphocytes, as an indicator. The peripheral blood monocytes, drawn from HIV antibody-positive homosexual men (HS) and hemophilics (HP) were incubated with various concentrations of TJ-9 medium and its components, to obtain the supernatant [CM(+)]. It was found that in HS and HP the colony formation was enhanced by addition of CM (+). CM(-) of HS and HP depressed the colony formation in healthy adults, but the depressed colony formation was recovered by addition of CM (+). The above results suggest that TJ-9 is a biological response modifier which induces IL-1 from monocytes.

S. Kakumu studied the effect of TJ-9 on interferon production of human peripheral blood mononulcear cells (PBMC). When PBMC from 7 healthy subjects were cultured with TJ-9, low but definite amounts of immune interferon (IFN ranging from 12.1±5. 6U/ml to 35.4±11.3 U/ml were detected. When TJ-9 was added to the cultures together with Con A, maximum amounts of IFN(363±85U/ml were produced. This value was significantly higher (P .0.01) than that with Con A alone (232±59U/ml). These findings indicate that TJ-9 has immunomodulatory activities and may explain the therapeutic effect of TJ-9 on certain types of chronic liver disease.

Xu-Hui Liu et al. investigate the putative effects of Kang-Fu Xin (KFX), a traditional Chinese medicine, on macrophages and NK cell activity. Phagocytosis-induced chemiluminescence of mouse peritoneal macrophages after ip injection of KFX was strongly enhanced. The stimulatory effect was maximal on day 1 but still detectable on day 15. Peritoneal macrophages, purified by adherence, were also found to be cytostatic for tumor cells one to eight days after KFX ip injection. Measurement of NK activity of peritoneal cells against YAC-1 targets showed an increased cytotoxic ptential in mice. It is, therefore, suggested that the therapeutic effect of KFX may be due at least in part, to its stimulatory effect on non-specific cellular defense mechanisms.

H. Mori et al. examined the immunological mechanisms regarding the antitumor activity of 4 kinds of Chinese herbs including A. capillaris (CH1, S. doederleinii (CH2), A. macrocephala (CH3) and S. subprostrata (CH4). The results indicated that CH1 showed the antitumor activity through mainly a direct cytotoxicity, while the others display the activity through the enhancement of T cell-mediated tumor immunity, particularly tumor specific DTH.

In recent years, the relationship between neuroendocrine and immune systems have been heavily emphasized. Chao Weikang et al. reported the effect of Essence-Restoring Decoction (ERD), an aging retarding prescription which is mainly composed of tonifying kidney medicines, on HPGT axis in senile animals. The results showed that with age, thymus gland was atrophyed, the ultrastructures of thymus changed, the concentrations of thymic cytoplasmic protein and nuclear RNA, DNA decreased, the quantities of thymic nuclear estradiol E_2 and dihydrotestosterone (DHT) receptors increased significantly while that of thymic cytoplasmic E_2 and DHT receptors decreased, the activity of serum thymic factors declined and the quantities of hypothalmic E^2 and DHT receptors reduced. ERD, however, was capable of improving the above mentioned changes of HPGT axis in senile animals to varying degrees, suggesting that ERD might retard the functional degeneration of thymic endocrine by means of weakening the effect of E_2 and DHT on thymus and of improving the feedback regulation of hypothalamus to E_2 and DHT, which in turn enhances thymus-dependent immunity.

IMMUNOSUPPRESSIVE EFFECT OF SOME TRADITIONAL MEDICINES

T. Nishiyori et al. reported the inhibitory effect of Saiboku-to (SBT), a Chinese blended medicine which had long been used for treatment and prevention of allergic diseases such as bronchial asthma and bronchitis, on type IV hypersensitivity reaction. It was indicated that SBT might inhibit the antigen-induced release of lymphokines including SRF, MIF or MCF from lymphocytes. The erythema caused by an id injection of lymphokine in guinea pig was also inhibited by SBT. The above results suggested that SBT displays the inhibitory activity on type IV hypersensitivity reaction through the suppression of effector phase.

T. Kabuki et al. Observed the effect of SBT on induction of Dermatophagoides Farinae (DF)-induced IL-2 responsiveness in lymphocytes of asthamatic children. It was suggested that SBT is capable of suppressing DF-induced IL-2 responsiveness in lymphocytes from asthmatic children.

Y. Ono et al. reported the immunodepressive effects of Unsei-in, another Chinese blended medicine which is effective against aphthous stomatitis and ulcus vulvae acutum of Behcet's syndrome, on type IV allergic reactions and humoral antibody production. It was found that Unsei-in might inhibit the induction phases rather than the effector phases of type IV allergic reactions. The medicine also inhibited the GvH reaction and the formation of IgG-PFC and IgM-PFC in spleens. The therapeutic effect of Unsei-in Behcet's syndrome may be due to the inhibitory effect on the early phases of cellular immune response.

Y. Mizoguchi et al. discussed the protective effects of GOMISIN A, a lignan component from Shizandra chinensis, in an experimental massive heptatic cell necrosis model. The result showed that GOMISIN A not only inhibited the activation of liver adherent cells and suppressed the release of the cytotoxic factor, but also directly affected the hepatocytes and protected them from the cytotoxic factor.

The above presentations show that traditional medicines have potent immunomodulatory effect on various links of immune system both in clinic and in experimental animal models. Some medicinal herbs are immunopotentiators, others are immunosuppressants. It was also reported that some traditional medicines had biphasic effects.

Most of the contributors carried out their studies on immunopharmacological effects of traditional medicines with compound prescription, which is in accordance with the theories and clinical practices of traditional Chinese medicine. Upon the basis of studying compound prescription, it is necessary to fractionate the active component, which is advantageous to understand deeply the mechanism of the compound prescription and to find new effective immunoregulators.

It had been well known that there are at least two regulatory ways in immune system. One is the self-regulations among various cells of immune system, the other is the external regulations of nervous and endocrine systems to immune system. Most subjects fo the presentations dealt with the former, but a few studies begin to investigate the pharmacological effects of traditional medicines on neuroendocrine-thymic net.

The immunomodulatory effects of traditional medicines on immune deficient models such as tumor, radiation injury, allergic reaction and aging in vivo and in vitro present fascinating and promising prospects worthy of further investigations.

Author Index

Subject Index

The page numbers refer to the first page of the article in which the index term appears.